APPROXIMATE EQUIVALENTS FOR METRIC, APOTHECARY, AND HOUSEHOLD WEIGHTS AND VOLUMES

APPROXIMATE EQUIVALENTS FOR WEIGHT

Metric	Apothecary
1 kg (1000 g)	2.2 lb
1 g (1000 mg)	15 gr
60 mg	1 gr

APPROXIMATE EQUIVALENTS FOR VOLUME

Metric	Apothecary	Household
4000 mL	1 gal (4 qt)	
1 L (1000 mL)	1 qt (2 pt)	
500 mL	1 pt (16 fl oz)	
240 mL	8 oz	1 cup
30 mL	1 oz (8 dr)	2 tbsp
15 mL	½ oz (4 dr)	1 tbsp (3 tsp)
5 mL	1 dr (60 M)	1 tsp (60 gtt)
1 mL	15 M	15 gtt
	1 M	1 gtt

CELSIUS AND FAHRENHEIT TEMPERATURE EQUIVALENTS

Conversion Chart		
Celsius	to	Fahrenheit
35.0		95.0
35.5		95.9
36.0		96.8
36.5		97.7
37.0		98.6
37.5		99.5
38.0		100.4
38.5		101.3
39.0		102.2
39.5		103.1
40.0		104.0
40.5		104.9
41.0		105.8
41.5		106.7
42.0		107.6

To convert from Fahrenheit to Celsius:
$$°C = (°F - 32) \div 1.8$$

To convert from Celsius to Fahrenheit:
$$°F = °C \times 1.8 + 32$$

°C = temperature in degrees Celsius
°F = temperature in degrees Fahrenheit

Clinical Calculations Made Easy

SIXTH EDITION

Solving Problems Using Dimensional Analysis

K

KCL. *See* potassium chloride (KCL)
kilogram (kg), 32, 32b, 32f, 39

L

labor, premature, case study of, 229
lactulose, dosage calculation for, 85, 102
    one-factor, 180
    using drug label, 102
leukemia, case study of, 231
lidocaine, dosage calculation for, two-factor, 190
lincocin (lincomycin), dosage calculation for, one-factor, 184
lipids, dosage calculation for, 206
liquid medication
    cup administration, 81f, 82
    syringe administration, 81f, 82
liter (L)
    conversions, 32, 32f, 32t, 38t
    dimensional analysis conversion, 48
lithium, dosage calculation for, one-factor, 188
lot number, of a drug, 75
lung cancer, small cell, case study of, 221
lyme disease, case study of, 255–256

M

macrotubing, 125, 125t
magnesium sulfate, dosage calculation for
    one-factor, 183
    using drug label, 104
manufacturer, of a drug, 75
measurement systems, 31–33
    apothecaries', 33–36
    household, 33, 34b, 34f
    metric, 31–32
    for temperature, 36, 37f
    for time, 36–37
medication administration, six rights of, 5, 64–67
medication administration record (MAR), 67–68
    defined, 67
    electronic, 67
    military time for, 37
medication cups, 34f, 38t, 82f
medication errors, prevention of, 64
medication label, *see* drug label medication orders, interpretation of
medication problems
    one-factor, 68–74
        defined, 69
        problem solving using, 69–74, 77–80, 82
        random method, 69
        sequential method, 68–69
    three-factor, 149–159
        defined, 149, 155
        problem solving using, 149–169
    two-factor, 112
        defined, 112
        involving drop factors, 129
        involving intermittent infusion, 129–133
        involving IV therapy, 121–125
        involving reconstitution, 116–125
        involving weight, 112–116
        problem solving using, 133–142
medication route, *see also* administration routes
    in medication administration, 65
meperidine, dosage calculation for, 91
    two-factor, 140
    using drug label, 82
meter, 31
methylphenidate hydrochloride, dosage calculation for, using drug label, 80
methylphenidate (Ritalin), dosage calculation for, using drug label, 98
metric measurement system, 31–32
    abbreviations, 32b, 39
    defined, 31
    other system equivalents for, 38t, 39, 43
    volume in, 31, 32b, 32f, 38t
    weight in, 31, 32b, 32f, 38t
mezlin (mezlocillin), dosage calculation for
    IV therapy, 135
    two-factor, 120, 194, 197

microgram (meg), 31, 32b, 32f
micronase (glyburide), dosage calculation for one-factor, 187
    using drug label, 101
microtubing, 125
military time, 36–37, 37f, 40, 45
milligram (mg), 31, 32b, 32f, 38t
milliliter (mL)
    conversions, 32, 32f, 32b, 38t
    dimensional analysis conversion, 49
    minim (M), 33b, 33f, 38t
mirapex (pramipexole), dosage calculation for, one-factor, 186
morphine sulfate, dosage calculation for
    one-factor, 176, 178
    three-factor, 165
    two-factor, 115, 142, 190
    using drug label, 87–88
multiplication
    of decimals, 3, 13, 19, 21
    of fractions, 3, 9–11, 18, 21
mycostatin, dosage calculation for, 205

N

naloxone, dosage calculation for
    one-factor, 179
    using drug label, 105
neupogen, dosage calculation for, three-factor, 160
nipride, dosage calculation for, 207
    three-factor, 158–159, 161, 200–201
nitroglycerin, dosage calculation for, two-factor, 190
normal saline, dosage calculation for, 204
    IV therapy, 126, 129
    two-factor, 198
NS. *See* normal saline
    numbers
        Arabic, 5
        Roman, 5, 6t
    numerator
        in dimensional analysis, 47
        in fractions, 9

O

one-factor medication problems, 68–74
    defined, 68
    problem solving using, 69–74, 77–80, 82–105
    random method, 68
    sequential method, 68
oral (PO) medications, 81–86
orders, medication, interpretation of, 64–66
orinase, dosage calculation for, using drug label, 96
otitis media, case study of, 239–240
ounce (oz)
    conversions, 33b, 34f, 38t
    dimensional analysis conversion, 48–49
output, monitoring of, 35, 35f

P

pain management, case study of, 225–226
parenteral medications, 86–92
    routes for, 86
    syringes for, 86–88
patient, in medication administration, 64
persantine, dosage calculation for, using drug label, 97
phenergan, dosage calculation for, two-factor, 115
phenobarbital, dosage calculation for, 85
    one-factor, 188
pint (pt), 33b, 33f, 38t
pipracil, dosage calculation for, 207
pneumonia, case study of, 225
potassium chloride (KCL), dosage calculation for, 206
    two-factor, 190
pound (lb), 33b, 33f, 38t
prednisolone, dosage calculation for, three-factor, 181
prednisone, dosage calculation for
    one-factor, 176, 181
    three-factor, 204
preeclampsia, case study of, 228
premature labor, case study of, 229
procholorperazine, 83

Q

quantity
  given
    in dimensional analysis, 48, 71
    in three-factor problem solving, 160
    in two-factor problem solving, 117
  wanted, in dimensional analysis, 48
quart (qt), 33b, 33f, 38t

R

random method of dimensional analysis
  defined, 68, 73
  problem solving using, 73
reconstitution
  defined, 121
  medication problems involving, 116, 121–126
  yield of, 121
renal failure, end-stage, case study of, 244
respiratory syncytial virus (RSV), case study of, 230–231
rights, of medication administration, 5, 67–68
Roman numeral system, 5, 6t
  converting between Arabic and, 3, 6–9, 18, 21
  defined, 5
rounding, of decimals, 13
route, in medication administration, *see* administration routes

S

saline, dosage calculation for, 204
  IV therapy, 126, 129
  two-factor, 198
seizures, case study of, 24
sepsis, case study of, 232–233
sequential method of dimensional analysis
  defined, 68
  problem solving using, 69–70
sickle cell anemia, case study of, 222–223
small cell lung cancer, case study of, 221
solu-Medrol, dosage calculation for
  one-factor, 179
  three-factor, l69
  two-factor, 118–119
  using drug label, 105
spontaneous abortion, case study of, 235–236
standard time, 36–37, 37f, 40, 45
staphcillin, dosage calculation for, 206
symbols, 5, 6t
syringes
  insulin, 86, 86f
  for insulin administration, 86, 86f
  3-mL, 86, 86f
  for oral medication administration, 82, 82f
  for parenteral medications, 86, 86f
  tuberculin, 86, 87f

T

tablespoon (tbsp or T), 34b, 34f, 38t
tablets, administration of, 80, 81f
tagamet (cimetidine)
  dosage calculation for
    three-factor, 149–152, 160
    two-factor, 116, 194
    using drug label, 82, 103
drug label, components of, 76
teaspoon (tsp or t), 34b, 34f, 38t
tegretol (carbamazepine), dosage calculation for, using drug label, 84
temperature, 36, 36f
  Celsius, 36, 36f
  conversions, 36b, 36f, 40, 43
  Fahrenheit, 36, 36f
thorazine (chlorpromazine), dosage calculation for,
  defined, 155
  problem solving using, 149–169
  three-factor medication problems, 149–159
  two-factor, 194

3-mL syringe, 86, 86f
Tigan (trimethobenzamide)
  dosage calculation for, 96
    drug label, components of, 77
    one-factor, 179, 185
    using drug label, 77–79, 81, 86, 103
time, 36–37
  considerations in IV therapy, 112
  conversions, 37f, 40, 45
  in medication administration, 65
  military, 36–37, 37f
  standard, 36–37, 37f
titration
  purpose of, 149
  three-factor problem solving for, 149–150
Tolinase, dosage calculation for, using drug label, 79
trade name, of a drug
  defined, 75
  identification of, 65, 76–81
transplantation, bone marrow, case study of, 224
transurethral resection of prostate (TURP), case study of, 241
trimethobenzamide HCL, 78, 81
tuberculin syringe, 86, 86f
tylenol (acetaminophen), dosage calculation for, 72
  one-factor, 176, 182
  two-factor, 133
  using drug label, 102

U

unasyn (ampicillin), dosage calculation for, 205
  IV therapy, 131, 132
  three-factor, 169
  two-factor, 121, 133
unit path, in dimensional analysis, 47, 68

V

vancomycin, dosage calculation for, 205
  three-factor, 202
  two-factor, 134, 192
vantin, dosage calculation for, one-factor, 185
venoglobulin, dosage calculation for, three-factor, 201
verapamil, dosage calculation for, two-factor, 133
vincasar (vincristine sulfate), dosage calculation for, two-factor, 194
vitamin Bi2, dosage calculation for, using drug label, 80
volume
  in apothecaries' measurement system, 33, 33b, 33f
  conversion table, 38t
  in metric measurement system, 31, 32b, 32f

W

wanted quantity, in dimensional analysis, 47, 68
warfarin, administration of, 87
weight
  in apothecaries' measurement system, 33, 33b, 34f
  conversions, 38t, 113
  medication problems involving, 112–115
  in metric measurement system, 31, 32b, 32f
wellbutrin (bupropion hydrochloride), dosage calculation for, two-factor, 197

X

Xanax, dosage calculation for, one-factor, 187

Y

yield, of reconstitution, 116

Z

zantac, dosage calculation for, 85
  IV therapy, 132
  two-factor, 133, 197
zaroxolyn, dosage calculation for, 98
zinacef (cefuroxime), dosage calculation for, two-factor, 198
zofran (ondansetron hydrochloride), dosage calculation for, two-factor, 196
zovirax (acyclovir), dosage calculation for, two-factor, 197

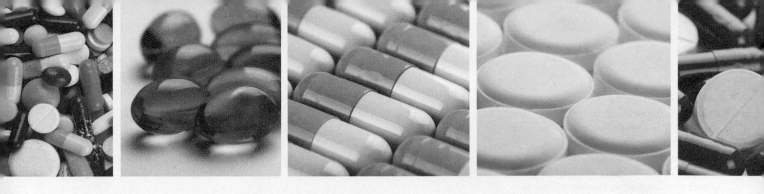

Clinical Calculations Made Easy

SIXTH EDITION

Solving Problems Using Dimensional Analysis

Gloria P. Craig, EdD, MSN, RN
Professor
South Dakota State University
College of Nursing
Brookings, South Dakota

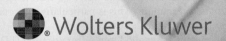

. Wolters Kluwer

Philadelphia • Baltimore • New York • London
Buenos Aires • Hong Kong • Sydney • Tokyo

Publisher: Julie Stegman
Executive Editor: Sherry Dickinson
Product Development Editor: Helen Kogut
Marketing Manager: Dean Karampelas
Editorial Assistant: Dan Reilly
Production Project Manager: Joan Sinclair
Design Coordinator: Holly McLaughlin
Illustration Coordinator: Jennifer Clements
Manufacturing Coordinator: Karin Duffield
Prepress Vendor: Aptara, Inc.

Sixth edition

9 8 7 6 5 4 3 2 1

Printed in China

Library of Congress Cataloging-in-Publication Data

Craig, Gloria P., 1949- , author.
   Clinical calculations made easy : solving problems using dimensional analysis / Gloria P. Craig. – Sixth edition.
      p. ; cm.
   Includes index.
   ISBN 978-1-4963-0282-3
   I. Title.
   [DNLM: 1. Drug Dosage Calculations–Nurses' Instruction. 2. Drug Dosage Calculations–Problems and Exercises. 3. Pharmaceutical Preparations–administration & dosage–Nurses' Instruction. 4. Pharmaceutical Preparations–administration & dosage–Problems and Exercises. 5. Mathematics–Nurses' Instruction. 6. Mathematics–Problems and Exercises. 7. Problem Solving–Nurses' Instruction. 8. Problem Solving–Problems and Exercises. QV 18.2]
   RS57
   615′.1401513–dc23

2015011066

LWW.com

This sixth edition of my text is dedicated to my children, Lori (and her husband, Michael) and Randy (and his wife Samantha), and to my granddaughters, Zoë, Ava, and Lily.

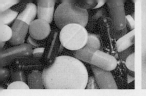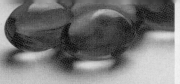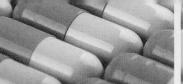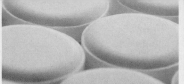

Reviewers

Michele Bach, MS
Professor of Mathematics
Kansas City Community College
Kansas City, Kansas

Rita Bergevin, RN-BC, MA, CWCN
Clinical Associate Professor
Decker School of Nursing
Binghamton University
Binghamton, New York

Emma Bissell, BSN, RN
Practical Nursing Faculty
University of Arkansas Community College at Hope
Hope, Arkansas

Karen Bloomfield, MS, RN, PMHCNS-BC
Assistant Professor of Nursing
Piedmont Virginia Community College
Charlottesville, Virginia

Patricia F. Garofalo, MS, RN
Director of Faculty Support for Simulation and
Adjunct Faculty
Adelphi University, College of Nursing and Public
Health Garden City, New York

Marybeth A. Gillis, MSN, RN
Associate Professor
Elmira College
Elmira, New York

Terry A. Kania, MSN, RN
Assistant Professor of Nursing
Nursing Student Retention Specialist
Joliet Junior College
Joliet, Illinois

Jorie L. Kulczak, MSN, RN
Associate Professor
Joliet Junior College
Joliet, Illinois

Shevellanie Lott, MSN, RN
Chairperson, Assistant Professor
Hampton University School of Nursing
Virginia Beach, Virginia

Jody Myhre-Oechsle, MS, BS, CPhT
Pharmacy Technician Program Director
Chippewa Valley Technical College
Eau Claire, Wisconsin

Valerie M. O'Dell, DNP, RN, CNE
Associate Professor of Nursing
Youngstown State University
Youngstown, Ohio

Marilyn Parker, MSN, RN
Nursing Resident Faculty
Mohave Community College
Lake Havasu, Arizona

Jason Raether, MS, RN
Instructor
South Dakota State University
Brookings, South Dakota

Sheri Wright, MEd, BN, RN
Interim Chair, SPHERE (Simulation)
Centre for Health and Wellness
Lethbridge College
Lethbridge, Alberta, Canada

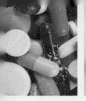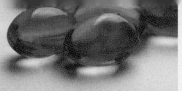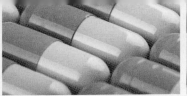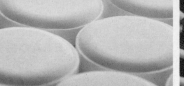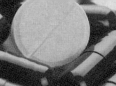

Preface

Many people experience stumbling blocks calculating math problems because of a lack of mathematical ability or associated "math anxiety." Even people with strong math skills often set up medication problems incorrectly, putting the patient at an increased risk for incorrect dosages and the ensuing consequences. However, dosage calculation need not be difficult if you use a problem-solving method that is easy to understand and to implement.

As a student, I experienced anxiety related to poor mathematical abilities and consequently had difficulty with medication calculations. However, a friend introduced me to a problem-solving method that was easy to visualize. By using this method, I was able to easily understand medication problems and thereby avoid the stumbling blocks that I had experienced with other methods of dosage calculations. Later, as a practicing nurse and nursing instructor, I realized that many of my colleagues and students shared my experience with "math anxiety," so I began sharing this problem-solving method with them.

During my baccalaureate nursing education, this problem-solving method became my teaching plan. During my master's education, it became my research. During my doctoral education, it became my dissertation. Now, I would like to share this method with anyone who ever believed that they were mathematically "challenged" or trembled at the thought of solving a medication problem.

The method, called dimensional analysis (also known as factor-label method or conversion-factor method), is a systematic, straightforward approach to setting up and solving problems that require conversions. It is a way of thinking about problems that can be used when two quantities are directly proportional to each other, but one needs to be converted using a conversion factor in order for the problem to be solved.

Dimensional Analysis as a Teaching Tool

Dimensional analysis empowers the learner to solve a variety of medication problems using just one problem-solving method. Research has shown that students experience less frustration and create fewer *medication errors* if one problem-solving method is used to solve *all* medication problems. As a method of reducing errors and improving calculation *abilities,* dimensional analysis has many possibilities. Whether it is used in practice or education, it is a strong approach when the goals are improving medication dosage-calculation skills, reducing medication errors, and improving patient safety. Ultimately, this improved methodology has the potential to reduce the medication errors that occur within the discipline of nursing.

Dimensional analysis helps the learner see and understand the significance of the whole process, since it focuses on how to learn, rather than what to learn. It provides a framework for understanding the principles of the problem-solving method and supports the critical thinking process. It helps the learner to organize and evaluate data, and to avoid errors in setting up problems. Dimensional analysis thus supports the conceptual mastery and higher-level thinking skills that have become the core of curricula at all levels of nursing education.

Organization of the Text

This text uses the simple-to-complex approach in teaching students clinical calculations and is, therefore, divided into four sections.

Section 1: Clinical Calculations

Chapter 1 provides an arithmetic pretest to help gauge the amount of time a student will need to spend reviewing the basic arithmetic skills presented in this chapter.

Chapter 2 reviews systems of measurement, common equivalents, calculating patient intake and output, and converting standard time and military time.

Chapter 3 introduces the student to dimensional analysis and uses common equivalents to help the student practice problem solving with this new method.

Chapter 4 builds on the previous chapter by introducing one-factor conversions.

Chapter 5 continues the growth process by presenting two-factor conversions.

Chapter 6 completes the student's understanding of clinical calculations by introducing three-factor conversions.

Section 2: Practice Problems

Section 2 allows the student the opportunity to refine the skills presented in Section 1 by providing additional one-, two-, and three-factor practice problems followed by comprehensive questions to ensure accurate understanding of clinical calculations.

Section 3: Case Studies

Section 3 helps the student relate dosage calculations to real clinical situations. Fifty case studies that are related to different fields of nursing are included in this section.

Section 4: Comprehensive Post-Tests

Section 4 contains two post-tests of 20 questions each, allowing the instructor to assess the student's mastery of solving clinical calculations using dimensional analysis. The answers to these questions are available to instructors on thePoint®.

Special Features

Each chapter in *Section 1* contains *numerous* **Examples** with detailed explanations. **Thinking it Through** provides additional explanations to help students more fully understand complex topics. *In-chapter* **Exercises** occur after the presentation and explanation of each new concept, providing an opportunity for the student to gain ability and confidence in the material before proceeding to the next concept. Additional **Practice Problems** are provided at the end of the chapter so that students can practice the skills and assess areas where more review may be necessary. An **Answer Key**

for all Exercises and Practice Problems is also located at the end of each chapter. Additionally, a **Post-Test**, designed so that students can tear it out of the book and hand it in to their instructor, appears at the end of each chapter. Answers for all Post-Tests are available to instructors on thePoint®.

In addition:

- **Actual drug labels** are liberally used throughout the text to provide the student with clinically realistic examples.

- A special feature, **Preventing Medication Errors,** helps identify key concepts necessary for avoiding clinical calculation errors.

- A special icon identifying **pediatric medication problems** allows students and teachers to quickly find all pediatric problems in the text.

New to This Edition

The sixth edition provides many opportunities for students to practice their skills. Additional practice problems have been added to Chapters 4, 5, and 6 to further strengthen the student's dosage calculations skills. New information related to vaccines has been added to Chapter 4 along with tables for administering vaccines to adults and children. In addition, there are practice problems related to the tables to help students understand how to use these types of tables effectively.

Additional problems have also been added to the chapter Post-Tests. This edition also includes two Comprehensive Post-Tests at the end of the book. As in past editions, all answers to Post-Test questions are available for instructors on thePoint®.

Resources on thePoint®

There is a wealth of related content available to Students and Instructors on thePoint® website that accompanies this book: http://thepoint.lww.com/Craig6e.

Student Resources

Calculations in Action, an exciting new tool for students to use, includes animated problems that are solved step-by-step with a voice-over explaining each step.

In addition, students will find the following helpful resources to enhance their learning experience:

- Learning Objectives
- Spanish/English Audio Glossary
- Drug Monographs
- Dosage Calculations Quizzes

Instructor Resources

Upon adoption, instructors will receive access to all Student Resources *plus*:

- PowerPoint Presentations
- Answer Key for Pre-Tests in the book

- Answer Key for Post-Tests in the book
- Instructor's Manual
- Strategies for Effective Teaching

By using this text and all of its resources, it is my hope that this sixth edition will help students find that clinical calculation can indeed be made easy using dimensional analysis.

Gloria P. Craig

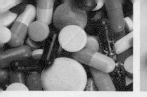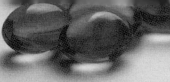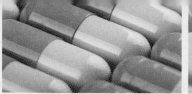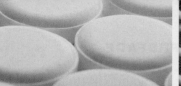

Acknowledgments

There are many people who have assisted me with my professional growth and development, including:

Pauline Callahan, who believed that I would be a great nurse and nursing instructor when I could not believe in myself.

Jackie Kehm, who introduced me to dimensional analysis and helped me pass the medication module that I was sure would be my stumbling block.

Dr. Sandra L. Sellers, for her expertise and guidance throughout the process of writing my thesis and dissertation and her encouragement to write a textbook.

Margaret Cooper, for her friendship and editing support throughout the writing of this textbook.

My students, colleagues, and reviewers, for helping me develop my abilities to explain and teach the problem-solving method of dimensional analysis.

The numerous pharmaceutical companies listed throughout this book that supplied medication labels and gave permission for the labels to be included in this textbook.

Selected drug images are included with permission and copyrighted by First Databank, Inc. This copyrighted material is not for distribution and is intended to supplement, not substitute for, the expertise and judgment of healthcare professionals. The information is not intended to cover all possible uses, directions, precautions, drug interactions or adverse effects, nor should it be construed to indicate that use of a particular drug is safe, appropriate or effective for you or anyone else. A healthcare professional should be consulted before taking any drug, changing any diet, or commencing or discontinuing any course of treatment.

To the faculty at South Dakota State University, College of Nursing, for allowing dimensional analysis to be integrated into the curriculum as the problem-solving method for medication calculation.

To the Lippincott editorial and production teams, for all of their hard work: **Sherry Dickinson,** Executive Editor; **Helen Kogut,** Product Development Editor; and **Holly McLaughlin,** Design Coordinator.

To these people and many more, I would like to express my sincere appreciation for their mentoring, guidance, support, and encouragement that have helped to turn a dream into a reality.

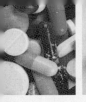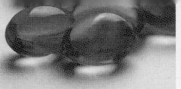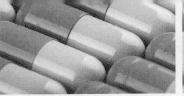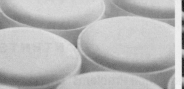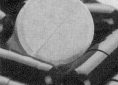

Contents

SECTION 1

Clinical Calculations 1

ARITHMETIC PRE-TEST 3

CHAPTER 1
Arithmetic Review 5

Arabic Numbers and Roman Numerals 5
EXERCISE 1.1 Arabic Numbers and Roman Numerals 6
Fractions 9
Multiplying Fractions 9
EXERCISE 1.2 Multiplying Fractions 10
Dividing Fractions 10
EXERCISE 1.3 Dividing Fractions 11
Decimals 12
Rounding Decimals 13
EXERCISE 1.4 Rounding Decimals 13
Multiplying Decimals 13
EXERCISE 1.5 Multiplying Decimals 14
Dividing Decimals 14
EXERCISE 1.6 Dividing Decimals 15
Converting Fractions to Decimals 16
EXERCISE 1.7 Converting Fractions to Decimals 16
Practice Problems 18
Post-Test 21
Answer Key 23

CHAPTER 2
Systems of Measurement
and Common Equivalents 31

Systems of Measurement 31
The Metric System 31
The Apothecaries' System 33
The Household System 33

Intake and Output 35

Temperature 36

Time 36

Common Equivalents 37
Practice Problems 39
Post-Test 43
Answer Key 45

CHAPTER 3
Solving Problems Using
Dimensional Analysis 47

Terms Used in Dimensional Analysis 47

The Five Steps of Dimensional Analysis 48
EXERCISE 3.1 Dimensional Analysis 51
Practice Problems 55
Post-Test 57
Answer Key 59

CHAPTER 4
One-Factor Medication Problems 64

Interpretation of Medication Orders 64
Right Patient 64
Right Drug 65
Right Dosage 65
Right Route 65
Right Time 65
Right Documentation 66
EXERCISE 4.1 Interpretation of Medication Orders 66
Medication Administration Record 67
EXERCISE 4.2 Medication Administration Record 67

One-Factor Medication Problems 68

Principles of Rounding 72

EXERCISE 4.3 One-Factor Medication Problems 74

Components of a Drug Label 75

Identifying the Components 75

EXERCISE 4.4 Identifying the Components of Drug
Labels 76

Solving Problems With Components of Drug Labels 77

EXERCISE 4.5 Problems With Components of
Drug Labels 79

Administering Medication by Different Routes 81

Enteral Medications 81

EXERCISE 4.6 Administering Enteral Medications 85

Parenteral Medications 86

EXERCISE 4.7 Administering Parenteral Medications 90

Vaccines 92

EXERCISE 4.8 Administering Vaccines 95

Practice Problems 96

Post-Test 101

Answer Key 107

CHAPTER 5
Two-Factor Medication Problems 112

Medication Problems Involving Weight 112

EXERCISE 5.1 Pediatric Medication Problems
Involving Weight 114

Medication Problems Involving Reconstitution 116

EXERCISE 5.2 Medication Problems Involving
Reconstitution 120

**Medication Problems Involving Intravenous
Pumps 121**

EXERCISE 5.3 Medication Problems Involving
Intravenous Pumps 124

Medication Problems Involving Drop Factors 125

EXERCISE 5.4 Medication Problems Involving
Drop Factors 129

**Medication Problems Involving Intermittent
Infusion 129**

EXERCISE 5.5 Medication Problems Involving
Intermittent Infusion 131

Practice Problems 133

Post-Test 139

Answer Key 145

CHAPTER 6
**Three-Factor Medication
Problems 149**

EXERCISE 6.1 Medication Problems Involving Dosage,
Weight, and Time 155

Practice Problems 160

Post-Test 165

Answer Key 171

SECTION 2
Practice Problems 175

One-Factor Practice Problems 175

Two-Factor Practice Problems 189

Three-Factor Practice Problems 199

Comprehensive Practice Problems 205

Answer Key 209

SECTION 3
Case Studies 219

Case Study 1 **Congestive Heart Failure 219**

Case Study 2 **COPD/Emphysema 220**

Case Study 3 **Small-Cell Lung Cancer 221**

Case Study 4 **Acquired Immunodeficiency
Syndrome (AIDS) 222**

Case Study 5 **Sickle Cell Anemia 222**

Case Study 6 **Deep Vein Thrombosis 223**

Case Study 7 **Bone Marrow Transplant 224**

Case Study 8 **Pneumonia 225**

Case Study 9 **Pain 225**

Case Study 10 **Cirrhosis 226**

Case Study 11 **Hyperemesis Gravidarum 227**

Case Study 12 **Preeclampsia 228**

CONTENTS

Case Study 13 Premature Labor 229

Case Study 14 Cystic Fibrosis 229

Case Study 15 Respiratory Syncytial Virus (RSV) 230

Case Study 16 Leukemia 231

Case Study 17 Sepsis 232

Case Study 18 Bronchopulmonary Dysplasia 233

Case Study 19 Cerebral Palsy 234

Case Study 20 Hyperbilirubinemia 234

Case Study 21 Spontaneous Abortion 235

Case Study 22 Bipolar Disorder 236

Case Study 23 Anorexia Nervosa 237

Case Study 24 Clinical Depression 238

Case Study 25 Alzheimer's Disease 238

Case Study 26 Otitis Media 239

Case Study 27 Seizures 240

Case Study 28 Fever of Unknown Origin 241

Case Study 29 TURP with CBI 241

Case Study 30 Hypercholesterolemia 242

Case Study 31 Hypertension 243

Case Study 32 Diabetic Ketoacidosis 244

Case Study 33 End-Stage Renal Failure 244

Case Study 34 Fluid Volume Deficit 245

Case Study 35 Increased Intracranial Pressure 246

Case Study 36 Breast Cancer 247

Case Study 37 Severe Abdominal Pain 248

Case Study 38 Acute Asthma Attack 248

Case Study 39 Right Total Hip Replacement 249

Case Study 40 Colon Resection 250

Case Study 41 Left Total Knee Replacement 251

Case Study 42 Chest Pain 251

Case Study 43 Pneumococcal Meningitis 252

Case Study 44 Diabetic Ketoacidosis 253

Case Study 45 C-Section Delivery 254

Case Study 46 Iron Deficiency Anemia 254

Case Study 47 Lyme Disease 255

Case Study 48 Infectious Mononucleosis 256

Case Study 49 H1N1 Influenza (Swine Flu) 257

Case Study 50 Bronchiolitis 258

SECTION 4
Comprehensive Post-Tests 275

Comprehensive Post-Test 1 277

Comprehensive Post-Test 2 280

APPENDIX
Educational Theory of Dimensional Analysis 283

Index 285

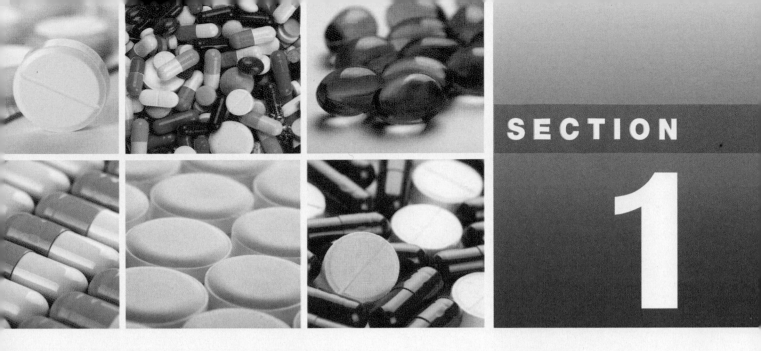

Clinical Calculations

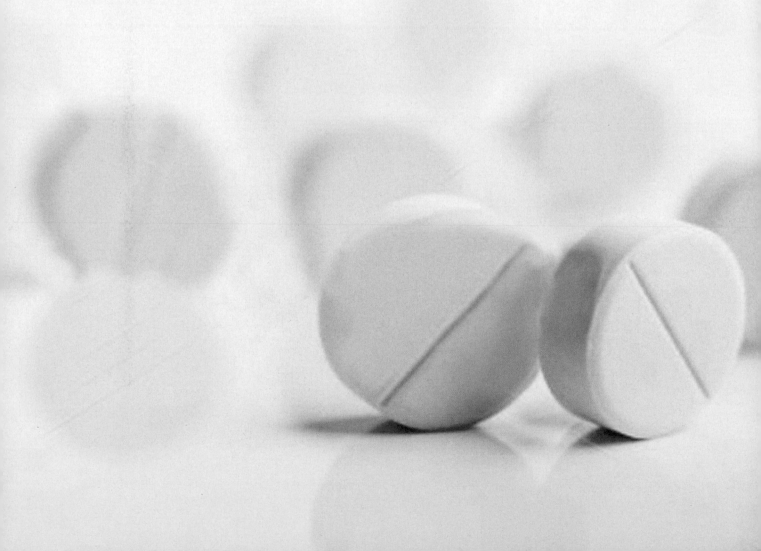

Chapter 1 Pre-Test

Arithmetic Review

Name _____ Date _____

Converting Between Arabic Numbers and Roman Numerals

1. 7   = _____

2. XI   = _____

3. 17   = _____

4. XVI = _____

Multiplying and Dividing Fractions

5. $\dfrac{2}{8} \times \dfrac{2}{2}$ =

6. $\dfrac{2}{5} \div \dfrac{1}{10}$ =

7. $\dfrac{2}{6} \times \dfrac{1}{2}$ =

8. $\dfrac{1}{3} \div \dfrac{3}{9}$ =

9. $\dfrac{3}{4} \times \dfrac{2}{3}$ =

10. $\dfrac{2}{4} \div \dfrac{1}{2}$ =

Converting Fractions to Decimals

11. $\dfrac{4}{8} =$

12. $\dfrac{2}{6} =$

13. $\dfrac{5}{9} =$

14. $\dfrac{1}{4} =$

Multiplying and Dividing Decimals

15. $2.75 \times 1.25 =$

16. $0.25 \div 0.4 =$

17. $4.50 \times 0.75 =$

18. $10.50 \div 4.5 =$

19. $1.2 \times 2 =$

20. $1.5 \div 0.75 =$

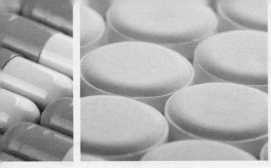
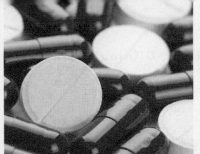

Objectives

After completing this chapter, you will successfully be able to:

1. Express Arabic numbers as Roman numerals.

2. Express Roman numerals as Arabic numbers.

3. Identify the numerator and denominator in a fraction.

4. Multiply and divide fractions.

5. Multiply and divide decimals.

6. Convert fractions to decimals.

Every nurse must know and practice the six rights of medication administration, including the:

1. Right drug
2. Right dose
3. Right route
4. Right time
5. Right patient
6. Right documentation

Although the right drug, route, time, patient, and documentation may be readily identified, the right dose requires **arithmetic skills** that may be difficult for you. This chapter reviews the basic arithmetic skills (multiplication and division) **necessary for calculating** medication dosage problems using the problem-solving method of dimensional analysis. Calculating the **right dose** of medication to be administered to a patient is one of the first steps toward preventing **medication errors**.

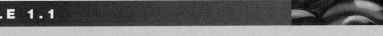

ARABIC NUMBERS AND ROMAN NUMERALS

Most medication dosages are ordered by the physician or the nurse practitioner in the metric and household systems for weights and measures using the Arabic number system with symbols called **digits** (ie, 1, 2, 3, 4, 5). Occasionally, orders are received in the apothecaries' system of weights and measures using the Roman numeral system with numbers represented by **symbols** (ie, I, V, X). The Roman numeral system uses seven basic symbols, and various combinations of these symbols represent all numbers in the Arabic number system.

Table 1.1 includes the seven basic Roman numerals and the corresponding Arabic numbers.

The combination of Roman numeral symbols is based on three specific principles:

1. Symbols are used to construct a number, but no symbol may be used more than three times. The exception is the symbol for five (V), which is used only once because there is a symbol for 10 (X) and a combination of symbols for 15 (XV).

EXAMPLE 1.1

III = (1 + 1 + 1) = 3
XXX = (10 + 10 + 10) = 30

PREVENTING MEDICATION ERRORS

Correctly identifying Roman numerals will assist in preventing **medication errors**. Some medication orders may include a Roman numeral.

Example: Administer X gr of aspirin, which is correctly interpreted as administer 10 gr of aspirin.

However, according to the Institute for Safe Medication Practices (ISMP), abbreviations increase the risk of medication errors. Additionally, while some health care providers may still use roman numerals and the apothecaries' system, the ISMP recommends using the metric system.

2. When symbols of lesser value follow symbols of greater value, they are *added* to construct a number.

EXAMPLE 1.2

VIII = (5 + 3) = 8
XVII = (10 + 5 + 1 + 1) = 17

3. When symbols of greater value follow symbols of lesser value, those of lesser value are *subtracted* from those of higher value to construct a number.

EXAMPLE 1.3

IV = (5 − 1) = 4
IX = (10 − 1) = 9

TABLE 1.1   Seven Basic Roman Numerals

Roman Numerals	Arabic Numbers
I	1
V	5
X	10
L	50
C	100
D	500
M	1000

Exercise 1.1   Arabic Numbers and Roman Numerals

(See page 23 for answers)

Express the following Arabic numbers as Roman numerals.

1. 1 = _____

2. 2 = _____

3. 3 = _____

4. 4 = _____

5. 5 = _____

6. 6 = _____

7. 7 = _____

8. 8 = _____

9. 9 = _____

10. 10 = _____

11. 11 = _____

12. 12 = _____

13. 13 = _____

14. 14 = _____

15. 15 = _____

16. 16 = _____

17. 17 = _____

18. 18 = _____

19. 19 = _____

20. 20 = _____

Although medication orders rarely involve Roman numerals higher than 20, for additional practice, express the following Arabic numbers as Roman numerals.

21. 43 = _____

22. 24 = _____

23. 55 = _____

24. 32 = _____

25. 102 = _____

26. 150 = _____

27. 75 = _____

28. 92 = _____

29. 64 = _____

30. 69 = _____

Express the following Roman numerals as Arabic numbers.

31. II   = _____

32. IV   = _____

33. VI   = _____

34. X   = _____

35. VIII = _____

36. XIX = _____

37. XX   = _____

38. XVIII = _____

39. I   = _____

40. XV   = _____

41. III   = _____

(Exercise continues on page 8)

42. V   = _____
43. IX   = _____
44. VII   = _____
45. XI   = _____
46. XIV   = _____
47. XVI   = _____
48. XII   = _____
49. XVII = _____
50. XIII = _____

To increase your abilities to use either system, convert the following Arabic numbers or Roman numerals.

51. 19   = _____
52. XII   = _____
53. 7   = _____
54. IX   = _____
55. IV   = _____
56. 11   = _____
57. VIII = _____
58. 16   = _____
59. XX   = _____
60. 5   = _____
61. I   = _____
62. 18   = _____
63. VI   = _____
64. 2   = _____
65. III   = _____
66. 10   = _____
67. XIII = _____
68. 14   = _____
69. XV   = _____
70. 17   = _____

FRACTIONS

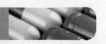

Medication dosages with fractions are occasionally ordered by the physician or used by the pharmaceutical manufacturer on the drug label. A **fraction** is a number that represents part of a whole number and contains three parts:

1. **Numerator**—the number on the top portion of the fraction that represents the number of parts of the whole fraction.
2. **Dividing line**—the line separating the top portion of the fraction from the bottom portion of the fraction.
3. **Denominator**—the number on the bottom portion of the fraction that represents the number of parts into which the whole is divided.

$$\frac{3}{4} = \frac{numerator}{denominator}$$

To solve medication dosage calculation problems using dimensional analysis, you must be able to identify the numerator and denominator portion of the problem. You also must be able to multiply and divide numbers, fractions, and decimals.

Multiplying Fractions

The three steps for multiplying fractions are:

1. Multiply the numerators.
2. Multiply the denominators.
3. Reduce the product to the lowest possible fraction.

EXAMPLE 1.4

$$\frac{2}{4} \times \frac{1}{8} = \frac{2}{32} = \frac{1}{16}$$

or

$$\frac{2\,(numerator)}{4\,(denominator)} \times \frac{1\,(numerator)}{8\,(denominator)} = \frac{2\,(numerator)}{32\,(denominator)}$$

$$= \frac{1}{16}\ (\text{reduced to lowest possible fraction})$$

EXAMPLE 1.5

$$\frac{1}{2} \times \frac{2}{4} = \frac{2}{8} = \frac{1}{4}$$

or

$$\frac{1\,(numerator)}{2\,(denominator)} \times \frac{2\,(numerator)}{4\,(denominator)} = \frac{2\,(numerator)}{8\,(denominator)}$$

$$= \frac{1}{4}\ (\text{reduced to lowest possible fraction})$$

PREVENTING MEDICATION ERRORS

Understanding fractions will assist in preventing **medication errors**. A medication order may include a fraction.

Example: Administer 1/150 gr of nitroglycerin.

Exercise 1.2   Multiplying Fractions
(See pages 23–24 for answers)

To increase your abilities when working with fractions, multiply the following fractions and reduce to the lowest fractional term.

1. $\dfrac{3}{4} \times \dfrac{5}{8} =$

2. $\dfrac{1}{3} \times \dfrac{4}{9} =$

3. $\dfrac{2}{3} \times \dfrac{4}{5} =$

4. $\dfrac{3}{4} \times \dfrac{1}{2} =$

5. $\dfrac{1}{8} \times \dfrac{4}{5} =$

6. $\dfrac{2}{3} \times \dfrac{5}{8} =$

7. $\dfrac{3}{8} \times \dfrac{2}{3} =$

8. $\dfrac{4}{7} \times \dfrac{2}{4} =$

9. $\dfrac{4}{5} \times \dfrac{1}{2} =$

10. $\dfrac{1}{4} \times \dfrac{1}{8} =$

Dividing Fractions
The four steps for dividing fractions are:

1. Invert (turn upside down) the divisor portion of the problem (the second fraction in the problem).
2. Multiply the two numerators.
3. Multiply the two denominators.
4. Reduce answer to lowest term (fraction or whole number).

EXAMPLE 1.6

$$\frac{2}{4} \div \frac{1}{8} = \frac{2}{4} \times \frac{8}{1} = \frac{16}{4} = 4$$

or

$$\frac{2\,(\text{numerator})}{4\,(\text{denominator})} \div \frac{1\,(\text{numerator})}{8\,(\text{denominator})}$$

$$= \frac{2\,(\text{numerator}) \quad \overset{(\text{inverted fraction})}{\times\ 8\,(\text{numerator})} \quad = 16}{4\,(\text{denominator}) \times 1\,(\text{denominator}) = 4}$$

= 4 (answer reduced to lowest term)

EXAMPLE 1.7

$$\frac{1}{2} \div \frac{2}{4} = \frac{1}{2} \times \frac{4}{2} = \frac{4}{4} = 1$$

or

$$\frac{1\,(\text{numerator})}{2\,(\text{denominator})} \div \frac{2\,(\text{numerator})}{4\,(\text{denominator})}$$

$$= \frac{1\,(\text{numerator}) \quad \overset{(\text{inverted fraction})}{\times\ 4\,(\text{numerator})} \quad = 4}{2\,(\text{denominator}) \times 2\,(\text{denominator}) = 4}$$

= 1 (answer reduced to lowest term)

Exercise 1.3 Dividing Fractions

(See page 24 for answers)

To increase your abilities when working with fractions, divide the following fractions and reduce to the lowest fractional term.

1. $\dfrac{3}{4} \div \dfrac{2}{3} =$

2. $\dfrac{1}{9} \div \dfrac{3}{9} =$

3. $\dfrac{2}{3} \div \dfrac{1}{6} =$

4. $\dfrac{1}{5} \div \dfrac{4}{5} =$

5. $\dfrac{3}{6} \div \dfrac{4}{8} =$

(Exercise continues on page 12)

6. $\dfrac{5}{8} \div \dfrac{5}{8} =$

7. $\dfrac{1}{8} \div \dfrac{2}{3} =$

8. $\dfrac{1}{5} \div \dfrac{1}{2} =$

9. $\dfrac{1}{4} \div \dfrac{1}{2} =$

10. $\dfrac{1}{6} \div \dfrac{1}{3} =$

DECIMALS

Medication orders are often written using decimals, and pharmaceutical manufacturers may use decimals when labeling medications. Therefore, you must understand the learning principles involving decimals and be able to multiply and divide decimals.

- A decimal point is preceded by a zero if not preceded by a number to decrease the chance of an error if the decimal point is missed.

EXAMPLE 1.8

0.25

- A decimal point may be preceded by a number and followed by a number.

EXAMPLE 1.9

1.25

- Numbers to the left of the decimal point are *units, tens, hundreds, thousands,* and *ten-thousands.*
- Numbers to the right of the decimal point are *tenths, hundredths, thousandths,* and *ten-thousandths.*

EXAMPLE 1.10

   0.2 = 2 tenths
  0.05 = 5 hundredths
  0.25 = 25 hundredths
  1.25 = 1 unit and 25 hundredths
110.25 = 110 units and 25 hundredths

Rounding Decimals

- Decimals may be rounded off. If the number to the right of the decimal is greater than or equal to 5, round up to the next number.
- If the number to the right of the decimal is less than 5, delete the remaining numbers.

EXAMPLE 1.11

0.78 = 0.8
0.21 = 0.2

Exercise 1.4   Rounding Decimals
(See page 24 for answers)

Practice rounding off the following decimals to the tenth.

1. 0.75 =
2. 0.88 =
3. 0.44 =
4. 0.23 =
5. 0.67 =
6. 0.27 =
7. 0.98 =
8. 0.92 =
9. 0.64 =
10. 0.250 =

Multiplying Decimals

When multiplying with decimals, the principles of multiplication still apply. The numbers are multiplied in columns, but the number of decimal points are counted and placed in the answer, counting places from right to left.

EXAMPLE 1.12

```
  2.3 (1 decimal point)
×1.5 (1 decimal point)
─────
 115
230
─────
3.45
```

PREVENTING MEDICATION ERRORS

Understanding the importance of a decimal point will assist in preventing **medication errors**. An improper placement of a decimal point can result in a serious medication error. According to the Institute for Safe Medication Practices (ISMP):

Trailing zeros should not be used with whole numbers.

Example: Administer 1 mg of Xanax.

If a decimal point and a zero are placed after the number (1.0 mg), the order could be misread as Administer 10 mg of Xanax.

*Leading zeros should **always** precede a decimal point when the dosage is not a whole number.*

Example: Administer 0.125 mg of Lanoxin.

If a zero is not placed in front of the decimal point the order could be misread as Administer 125 mg of Lanoxin.

Thinking it Through

The answer to the problem before adding decimal points is 345 but when decimal points are correctly added (two decimal points are added to the answer, counting two places from the right to the left) then 3.45 becomes the correct answer.

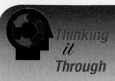

Thinking it Through

Medication orders should not have trailing zeros but you may want to add them when calculating to make sure all placements align.

Exercise 1.5 Multiplying Decimals

(See page 25 for answers)

Practice multiplying the following decimals.

1. 2.5
    × 4.6

2. 1.45
    × 0.25

3. 3.9
    × 0.8

4. 2.56
    × 0.45

5. 10.65
    × 0.05

6. 1.98
    × 3.10

7. 2.75
    × 5.0

8. 5.0
    × 0.45

9. 7.50
    × 0.25

10. 2.5
    × 0.01

Dividing Decimals

When dividing with decimals, the principles of division still apply, except that the dividing number is changed to a whole number by moving the decimal point to the right. The number being divided also changes by accepting the same number of decimal point moves.

EXAMPLE 1.13

$0.5\overline{)0.75}$

Step 1 Move decimal point one place to the right.

Step 2

$$
\begin{array}{r}
1.5 \\
5\overline{)7.5} \\
\underline{5} \\
25 \\
\underline{25} \\
0
\end{array}
$$

● **1.5**

Exercise 1.6 **Dividing Decimals**

(See pages 25–27 for answers)

Practice dividing the following decimals and rounding the answers to the tenth.

1. $3.4\overline{)9.6}$

2. $0.25\overline{)12.50}$

3. $0.56\overline{)18.65}$

4. $0.3\overline{)0.192}$

5. $0.4\overline{)12.43}$

6. $0.5\overline{)12.50}$

7. $0.125\overline{)0.25}$

8. $0.08\overline{)0.085}$

9. $1.5\overline{)22.5}$

10. $5.5\overline{)16.5}$

CONVERTING FRACTIONS TO DECIMALS

When problem solving with dimensional analysis, medication dosage calculation problems may frequently contain both fractions and decimals. Some of you may have fraction phobia and prefer to convert fractions to decimals when solving problems. To convert a fraction to a decimal, divide the numerator portion of the fraction by the denominator portion of the fraction.

When dividing fractions, remember to add a decimal point and a zero if the numerator cannot be divided by the denominator.

PREVENTING MEDICATION ERRORS

Understanding the importance of converting fractions to decimals will assist in preventing **medication errors**. Many medication errors occur because of a simple arithmetic error with dividing. Every nurse should have a calculator to recheck answers for accuracy. If a recheck results in a different answer, the next recheck should include consulting with another nurse or pharmacist.

EXAMPLE 1.14

$$\frac{1}{2} \text{ or } \frac{1 \text{ (numerator)}}{2 \text{ (denominator)}} = 2\overline{)1.0}^{\,0.5\,=\,0.5} \\ \underline{1\,0}$$

EXAMPLE 1.15

$$\frac{3}{4} \text{ or } \frac{3 \text{ (numerator)}}{4 \text{ (denominator)}} = 4\overline{)3.00}^{\,0.75\,=\,0.75} \\ \underline{2\,8} \\ 20 \\ \underline{20}$$

Exercise 1.7   Converting Fractions to Decimals
(See pages 27–28 for answers)

To decrease fraction phobia, practice converting the following fractions to decimals. Remember to follow the rules of rounding.

1. $\dfrac{1}{8} =$

2. $\dfrac{1}{4} =$

3. $\dfrac{2}{5} =$

4. $\dfrac{3}{5} =$

5. $\dfrac{2}{3} =$

6. $\dfrac{6}{8} =$

7. $\dfrac{3}{8} =$

8. $\dfrac{1}{3} =$

9. $\dfrac{3}{6} =$

10. $\dfrac{2}{10} =$

Summary

This chapter has reviewed basic arithmetic that will assist you to successfully implement dimensional analysis as a problem-solving method for medication dosage calculations. To assess your understanding and retention, complete the following practice problems.

Practice Problems for Chapter 1

Arithmetic Review (See pages 28–30 for answers)

Change the following Arabic numbers to Roman numerals.

1. 2 =
2. 4 =
3. 5 =
4. 14 =
5. 19 =
6. 16 =

Change the following Roman numerals to Arabic numbers.

7. VI   =
8. IX   =
9. XII   =
10. XVII =
11. XIX =
12. XXV =

Multiply the following fractions and reduce the answer to the lowest fractional term.

13. $\dfrac{3}{4} \times \dfrac{2}{5} =$

14. $\dfrac{2}{3} \times \dfrac{5}{8} =$

15. $\dfrac{1}{2} \times \dfrac{2}{3} =$

16. $\dfrac{7}{8} \times \dfrac{1}{3} =$

17. $\dfrac{4}{5} \times \dfrac{2}{7} =$

18. $\dfrac{1}{8} \times \dfrac{1}{8} =$

Divide the following fractions and reduce the answer to the lowest fractional term.

19. $\dfrac{1}{2} \div \dfrac{3}{4} =$

20. $\dfrac{1}{3} \div \dfrac{7}{8} =$

21. $\dfrac{1}{5} \div \dfrac{1}{2} =$

22. $\dfrac{4}{8} \div \dfrac{2}{3} =$

23. $\dfrac{1}{3} \div \dfrac{2}{3} =$

24. $\dfrac{3}{4} \div \dfrac{7}{8} =$

Multiply the following decimals.

25. $\begin{array}{r} 6.45 \\ \times\,\underline{1.36} \end{array}$

26. $\begin{array}{r} 3.14 \\ \times\,\underline{2.20} \end{array}$

27. $\begin{array}{r} 16.286 \\ \times\,\underline{0.125} \end{array}$

28. $\begin{array}{r} 1.2 \\ \times\,\underline{0.5} \end{array}$

29. $\begin{array}{r} 7.68 \\ \times\,\underline{0.05} \end{array}$

30. $\begin{array}{r} 0.55 \\ \times\,\underline{0.75} \end{array}$

Divide the following decimals.

31. $0.5\overline{)1.25}$

32. $0.20\overline{)40.80}$

33. $0.125\overline{)0.25}$

34. $0.75\overline{)0.125}$

35. $0.5\overline{)7.30}$

36. $0.3\overline{)0.525}$

(Practice Problems continue on page 20)

Convert the following fractions to decimals and round to the tenth.

37. $\dfrac{1}{2} =$

38. $\dfrac{1}{3} =$

39. $\dfrac{3}{4} =$

40. $\dfrac{2}{3} =$

41. $\dfrac{1}{8} =$

42. $\dfrac{7}{8} =$

Chapter 1 Post-Test

Arithmetic Review

Name _____ Date _____

Converting Between Arabic Numbers and Roman Numerals

1. 4 = _____

2. IX = _____

Multiplying and Dividing Fractions

3. $\dfrac{2}{4} \times \dfrac{1}{2}$ = _____

4. $\dfrac{5}{6} \times \dfrac{3}{4}$ = _____

5. $\dfrac{1}{6} \div \dfrac{1}{3}$ = _____

6. $\dfrac{1}{150} \div \dfrac{1}{2}$ = _____

Converting Fractions to Decimals

7. $\dfrac{1}{2}$ = _____

8. $\dfrac{3}{4}$ = _____

9. $\dfrac{2}{3}$ = _____

Multiplying and Dividing Decimals

10. 0.25×1.25 = _____

11. $0.125 \div 0.25$ = _____

12. 1.5×0.25 = _____

13. $0.125 \div 0.5$ = _____

ANSWER KEY FOR CHAPTER 1: ARITHMETIC REVIEW

Exercise 1.1 **Arabic Numbers and Roman Numerals**

1 1 = I
2 1 + 1 = II
3 1 + 1 + 1 = III
4 5 − 1 = IV
5 5 = V
6 5 + 1 = VI
7 5 + 1 + 1 = VII
8 5 + 1 + 1 + 1 = VIII
9 10 − 1 = IX
10 10 = X
11 10 + 1 = XI
12 10 + 1 + 1 = XII
13 10 + 1 + 1 + 1 = XIII
14 10 + 5 − 1 = XIV
15 10 + 5 = XV
16 10 + 5 + 1 = XVI
17 10 + 5 + 1 + 1 = XVII
18 10 + 5 + 1 + 1 + 1 = XVIII
19 10 + 10 − 1 = XIX
20 10 + 10 = XX
21 50 − 10 + 1 + 1 + 1 = XLIII
22 10 + 10 + 5 − 1 = XXIV
23 50 + 5 = LV
24 10 + 10 + 10 + 1 + 1 = XXXII
25 100 + 1 + 1 = CII
26 100 + 50 = CL
27 50 + 10 + 10 + 5 = LXXV
28 100 − 10 + 1 + 1 = XCII
29 50 + 10 + 5 − 1 = LXIV
30 50 + 10 + 10 − 1 = LXIX
31 II = (1 + 1) = 2
32 IV = (5 − 1) = 4
33 VI = (5 + 1) = 6
34 X = (10) = 10
35 VIII = (5 + 1 + 1 + 1) = 8
36 XIX = (10 − 1 + 10) = 19
37 XX = (10 + 10) = 20
38 XVIII = (10 + 5 + 1 + 1 + 1) = 18
39 I = (1) = 1
40 XV = (10 + 5) = 15
41 III = (1 + 1 + 1) = 3
42 V = (5) = 5
43 IX = (10 − 1) = 9
44 VII = (5 + 1 + 2) = 7
45 XI = (10 + 1) = 11
46 XIV = (10 + 5 − 1) = 14
47 XVI = (10 + 5 + 1) = 16
48 XII = (10 + 1 + 1) = 12
49 XVII = (10 + 5 + 1 + 1) = 17
50 XIII = (10 + 1 + 1 + 1) = 13
51 19 = XIX
52 XII = 12
53 7 = VII
54 IX = 9
55 IV = 4
56 11 = XI
57 VIII = 8
58 16 = XVI
59 XX = 20
60 5 = V
61 I = 1
62 18 = XVIII
63 VI = 6
64 2 = II
65 III = 3
66 10 = X
67 XIII = 13
68 14 = XIV
69 XV = 15
70 17 = XVII

Exercise 1.2 **Multiplying Fractions**

1
$$\frac{3}{4} \times \frac{5}{8} = \frac{3 \times 5 = 15}{4 \times 8 = 32} = \frac{15}{32}$$

2
$$\frac{1}{3} \times \frac{4}{9} = \frac{1 \times 4 = 4}{3 \times 9 = 27} = \frac{4}{27}$$

3

$$\frac{2}{3} \times \frac{4}{5} = \frac{2 \times 4 = 8}{3 \times 5 = 15} = \frac{8}{15}$$

4

$$\frac{3}{4} \times \frac{1}{2} = \frac{3 \times 1 = 3}{4 \times 2 = 8} = \frac{3}{8}$$

5

$$\frac{1}{8} \times \frac{4}{5} = \frac{1 \times 4 = 4 \div 4 = 1}{8 \times 5 = 40 \div 4 = 10} = \frac{1}{10}$$

6

$$\frac{2}{3} \times \frac{5}{8} = \frac{2 \times 5 = 10 \div 2 = 5}{3 \times 8 = 24 \div 2 = 12} = \frac{5}{12}$$

7

$$\frac{3}{8} \times \frac{2}{3} = \frac{3 \times 2 = 6 \div 6 = 1}{8 \times 3 = 24 \div 6 = 4} = \frac{1}{4}$$

8

$$\frac{4}{7} \times \frac{2}{4} = \frac{4 \times 2 = 8 \div 4 = 2}{7 \times 4 = 28 \div 4 = 7} = \frac{2}{7}$$

9

$$\frac{4}{5} \times \frac{1}{2} = \frac{4 \times 1 = 4 \div 2 = 2}{5 \times 2 = 10 \div 2 = 5} = \frac{2}{5}$$

10

$$\frac{1}{4} \times \frac{1}{8} = \frac{1 \times 1 = 1}{4 \times 8 = 32} = \frac{1}{32}$$

Exercise 1.3 Dividing Fractions

1

$$\frac{3}{4} \div \frac{2}{3} = \frac{3}{4} \times \frac{3}{2} \text{ or } \frac{3 \times 3 = 9}{4 \times 2 = 8} = 8\overline{)9} = 1\frac{1}{8}$$

2

$$\frac{1}{9} \div \frac{3}{9} = \frac{1}{9} \times \frac{9}{3} \text{ or } \frac{1 \times 9 = 9 \div 9 = 1}{9 \times 3 = 27 \div 9 = 3} = \frac{1}{3}$$

3

$$\frac{2}{3} \div \frac{1}{6} = \frac{2}{3} \times \frac{6}{1} \text{ or } \frac{2 \times 6 = 12}{3 \times 1 = 3} = 3\overline{)12} = 4$$

4

$$\frac{1}{5} \div \frac{4}{5} = \frac{1}{5} \times \frac{5}{4} \text{ or } \frac{1 \times 5 = 5 \div 5 = 1}{5 \times 4 = 20 \div 5 = 4} = \frac{1}{4}$$

5

$$\frac{3}{6} \div \frac{4}{8} = \frac{3}{6} \times \frac{8}{4} \text{ or } \frac{3 \times 8 = 24}{6 \times 4 = 24} = 24\overline{)24} = 1$$

6

$$\frac{5}{8} \div \frac{5}{8} = \frac{5}{8} \times \frac{8}{5} \text{ or } \frac{5 \times 8 = 40}{8 \times 5 = 40} = 40\overline{)40} = 1$$

7

$$\frac{1}{8} \div \frac{2}{3} = \frac{1}{8} \times \frac{3}{2} \text{ or } \frac{1 \times 3 = 3}{8 \times 2 = 16} = \frac{3}{16}$$

8

$$\frac{1}{5} \div \frac{1}{2} = \frac{1}{5} \times \frac{2}{1} \text{ or } \frac{1 \times 2 = 2}{5 \times 1 = 5} = \frac{2}{5}$$

9

$$\frac{1}{4} \div \frac{1}{2} = \frac{1 \times 2 = 2 \div 2 = 1}{4 \times 1 = 4 \div 2 = 2} = \frac{1}{2}$$

10

$$\frac{1}{6} \div \frac{1}{3} = \frac{1 \times 3 = 3 \div 3 = 1}{6 \times 1 = 6 \div 3 = 2} = \frac{1}{2}$$

Exercise 1.4 Rounding Decimals

1 $0.75 = 0.8$

2 $0.88 = 0.9$

3 $0.44 = 0.4$

4 $0.23 = 0.2$

5 $0.67 = 0.7$

6 $0.27 = 0.3$

7 $0.98 = 1$

8 $0.92 = 0.9$

9 $0.64 = 0.6$

10 $0.250 = 0.3$

Exercise 1.5 Multiplying Decimals

1

2.5 (1 decimal point)
× 4.6 (1 decimal point)
150
1000
1150
11.50 (2 decimal points from the right to left)

2

1.45 (2 decimal points)
× 0.25 (2 decimal points)
725
2900
0000
3625
0.3625 (4 decimal points from right to left)

3

3.9 (1 decimal point)
× 0.8 (1 decimal point)
312
000
312
3.12 (2 decimal points from right to left)

4

2.56 (2 decimal points)
× 0.45 (2 decimal points)
1280
10240
00000
11520
1.1520 (4 decimal points from right to left)

5

10.65 (2 decimal points)
× 0.05 (2 decimal points)
5325
0000
5325
0.5325 (4 decimal points from right to left)

6

1.98 (2 decimal points)
× 3.10 (2 decimal points)
000
1980
59400
61380
6.1380 (4 decimal points from right to left)

7

2.75 (2 decimal points)
× 5.0 (1 decimal point)
000
13750
13750
13.750 (3 decimal points from right to left)

8

5.0 (1 decimal point)
× 0.45 (2 decimal points)
250
2000
0000
2250
2.250 (3 decimal points from right to left)

9

7.50 (2 decimal points)
× 0.25 (2 decimal points)
3750
15000
00000
18750
1.8750 (4 decimal points from right to left)

10

2.5 (1 decimal point)
× 0.01 (2 decimal points)
25
000
0000
0025
0.025 (3 decimal points from right to left)

Exercise 1.6 Dividing Decimals

1

$$3.4\overline{)9.6}$$

(Move decimal points one place to the right)
Answer: 2.82 = 2.8

```
       2.82
  34)96.00
     68
     28 0
     27 2
        80
        68
        12
```

2

$0.25\overline{)12.50}$

(Move decimal points two places to the right)

Answer: 50. = 50

$$25\overline{)1250.} \quad \begin{array}{r} 50. \\ \underline{125} \\ 00 \end{array}$$

3

$0.56\overline{)18.65}$

(Move decimal points two places to the right)

Answer: 33.30 = 33.3

$$56\overline{)1865.00} \quad \begin{array}{r} 33.30 \\ \underline{168} \\ 185 \\ \underline{168} \\ 170 \\ \underline{168} \\ 20 \end{array}$$

4

$0.3\overline{)0.192}$

(Move decimal points one place to the right)

Answer: 0.64 = 0.6

$$3\overline{)01.92} \quad \begin{array}{r} 0.64 \\ \underline{18} \\ 12 \\ \underline{12} \\ 0 \end{array}$$

5

$0.4\overline{)12.43}$

(Move decimal points one place to the right)

Answer: 31.075 = 31.1

$$4\overline{)124.300} \quad \begin{array}{r} 31.075 \\ \underline{12} \\ 04 \\ \underline{4} \\ 030 \\ \underline{28} \\ 20 \\ \underline{20} \\ 0 \end{array}$$

6

$0.5\overline{)12.50}$

(Move decimal points one place to the right)

Answer: 25.0 = 25

$$5\overline{)125.0} \quad \begin{array}{r} 25.0 \\ \underline{10} \\ 25 \\ \underline{25} \\ 0 \end{array}$$

7

$0.125\overline{)0.25}$

(Move decimal points three places to the right)

Answer: 2. = 2

$$125\overline{)250} \quad \begin{array}{r} 2 \\ \underline{250} \\ 0 \end{array}$$

8

$0.08\overline{)0.085}$

(Move decimal points two places to the right)

Answer: 1.0625 = 1.1

$$8\overline{)8.5000} \quad \begin{array}{r} 1.0625 \\ \underline{8} \\ 50 \\ \underline{48} \\ 20 \\ \underline{16} \\ 40 \\ \underline{40} \\ 0 \end{array}$$

9

$1.5\overline{)22.5}$

(Move decimal points one place to the right)

Answer: 15. = 15

$$15.\overline{)225.} \quad \begin{array}{r} 15. \\ \underline{15} \\ 75 \\ \underline{75} \\ 0 \end{array}$$

10

$5.5\overline{)16.5}$

(Move decimal points one place to the right)

Answer: 3. = 3

$$55\overline{)165.}$$
$$\underline{165}$$
$$0$$

with quotient 3. above

| **Exercise 1.7** | **Converting Fractions to Decimals** |

1

$\dfrac{1}{8} = 0.125 = 0.13 = 0.1$

Answer: 0.1

$$8\overline{)1.000}$$
$$\underline{8}$$
$$20$$
$$\underline{16}$$
$$40$$
$$\underline{40}$$
$$0$$

with quotient 0.125 above

2

$\dfrac{1}{4} = 0.25 = 0.3$

Answer: 0.3

$$4\overline{)1.00}$$
$$\underline{8}$$
$$20$$
$$\underline{20}$$
$$0$$

with quotient 0.25 above

3

$\dfrac{2}{5} = 0.4$

Answer: 0.4

$$5\overline{)2.0}$$
$$\underline{20}$$
$$0$$

with quotient 0.4 above

4

$\dfrac{3}{5} = 0.6$

Answer: 0.6

$$5\overline{)3.0}$$
$$\underline{30}$$
$$0$$

with quotient 0.6 above

5

$\dfrac{2}{3} = 0.66 = 0.7$

Answer: 0.7

$$3\overline{)2.00}$$
$$\underline{1\ 8}$$
$$20$$
$$\underline{18}$$
$$2$$

with quotient 0.66 above

6

$\dfrac{6}{8} = 0.75 = 0.8$

Answer: 0.8

$$8\overline{)6.00}$$
$$\underline{56}$$
$$40$$
$$\underline{40}$$
$$0$$

with quotient 0.75 above

7

$\dfrac{3}{8} = 0.375 = 0.38 = 0.4$

Answer: 0.4

$$8\overline{)3.00}$$
$$\underline{24}$$
$$60$$
$$\underline{56}$$
$$40$$
$$\underline{40}$$
$$0$$

with quotient 0.375 above

8

$\dfrac{1}{3} = 0.33 = 0.3$

Answer: 0.3

$$3\overline{)1.00}$$
$$\underline{9}$$
$$10$$
$$\underline{9}$$
$$1$$

with quotient 0.33 above

9

$$\frac{3}{6} = 0.5$$

Answer: 0.5

$$6\overline{)3.0} \quad \frac{0.5}{} $$
$$\underline{30}$$
$$0$$

10

$$\frac{2}{10} = 0.2$$

Answer: 0.2

$$10\overline{)2.0} \quad \frac{0.2}{}$$
$$\underline{20}$$
$$0$$

Practice Problems

1 II

2 IV

3 V

4 XIV

5 XIX

6 XVI

7 6

8 9

9 12

10 17

11 19

12 25

13

$$\frac{3 \times 2 = 6 \div 2 = 3}{4 \times 5 = 20 \div 2 = 10} = \frac{3}{10}$$

14

$$\frac{2 \times 5 = 10 \div 2 = 5}{3 \times 8 = 24 \div 2 = 12} = \frac{5}{12}$$

15

$$\frac{1 \times 2 = 2 \div 2 = 1}{2 \times 3 = 6 \div 2 = 3} = \frac{1}{3}$$

16

$$\frac{7 \times 1 = 7}{8 \times 3 = 24} = \frac{7}{24}$$

17

$$\frac{4 \times 2 = 8}{5 \times 7 = 35} = \frac{8}{35}$$

18

$$\frac{1 \times 1 = 1}{8 \times 8 = 64} = \frac{1}{64}$$

19

$$\frac{1}{2} \div \frac{3}{4} = \frac{1 \times 4 = 4 \div 2 = 2}{2 \times 3 = 6 \div 2 = 3} = \frac{2}{3}$$

20

$$\frac{1}{3} \div \frac{7}{8} = \frac{1 \times 8 = 8}{3 \times 7 = 21} = \frac{8}{21}$$

21

$$\frac{1}{5} \div \frac{1}{2} = \frac{1 \times 2 = 2}{5 \times 1 = 5} = \frac{2}{5}$$

22

$$\frac{4}{8} \div \frac{2}{3} = \frac{4 \times 3 = 12 \div 4 = 3}{8 \times 2 = 16 \div 4 = 4} = \frac{3}{4}$$

23

$$\frac{1}{3} \div \frac{2}{3} = \frac{1 \times 3 = 3 \div 3 = 1}{3 \times 2 = 6 \div 3 = 2} = \frac{1}{2}$$

24

$$\frac{3}{4} \div \frac{7}{8} = \frac{3 \times 8 = 24 \div 4 = 6}{4 \times 7 = 28 \div 4 = 7} = \frac{6}{7}$$

25

6.45 (2 decimal points)

× 1.36 (2 decimal points)

3870

19350

64500

87720

8.7720 (4 decimal points from right to left)

26

3.14 (2 decimal points)

× 2.20 (2 decimal points)

000

6280

62800

69080

6.9080 (4 decimal points from right to left)

27

16.286 (3 decimal points)
× 0.125 (3 decimal points)
81430
325720
1628600
2035750
2.035750 (6 decimal points from right to left)

28

1.2 (1 decimal point)
× 0.5 (1 decimal point)
60
000
060
0.60 (2 decimal points from right to left)

29

7.68 (2 decimal points)
× 0.05 (2 decimal points)
3840
0000
00000
03840
0.3840 (4 decimal points from right to left)

30

0.55 (2 decimal points)
× 0.75 (2 decimal points)
275
3850
00000
000000
0.4125 (4 decimal points from right to left)

31

0.5$\overline{)1.25}$

(Move decimal points one place to the right)
Answer: 2.5

$$
\begin{array}{r}
2.5 \\
5\overline{)12.5} \\
\underline{10} \\
25 \\
\underline{25} \\
0
\end{array}
$$

32

0.20$\overline{)40.80}$

(Move decimal points two places to the right)
Answer: 204. = 204

$$
\begin{array}{r}
204 \\
20\overline{)4080} \\
\underline{40} \\
080 \\
\underline{80} \\
0
\end{array}
$$

33

0.125$\overline{)0.25}$

(Move decimal points three places to the right)
Answer: 2. = 2

$$
\begin{array}{r}
2 \\
125\overline{)250} \\
\underline{250} \\
0
\end{array}
$$

34

0.75$\overline{)0.125}$

(Move decimal points two places to the right)
Answer: 0.166 = 0.17 = 0.2

$$
\begin{array}{r}
0.166 \\
75\overline{)12.500} \\
\underline{75} \\
500 \\
\underline{450} \\
50
\end{array}
$$

35

0.5$\overline{)7.30}$

(Move decimal point one place to the right)
Answer: 14.6

$$
\begin{array}{r}
14.6 \\
5\overline{)73.0} \\
\underline{5} \\
23 \\
\underline{20} \\
30 \\
\underline{30} \\
0
\end{array}
$$

36

0.3)0.525

(Move decimal points one place to the right)

Answer: 1.75 = 1.8

```
      1.75
  3)5.25
      3
      22
      21
      15
      15
       0
```

37 0.5

38 0.33 = 0.3

39 0.75 = 0.8

40 0.66 = 0.7

41 0.125 = 0.13 = 0.1

42 0.875 = 0.88 = 0.9

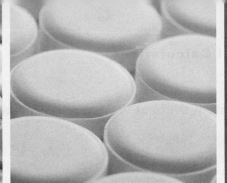

Systems of Measurement and Common Equivalents

Objectives

After completing this chapter, you will successfully be able to:

1. Identify measurements included in the metric, apothecaries', and household systems.

2. Understand abbreviations used in the metric, apothecaries', and household systems.

3. Calculate intake and output necessary for accurate recording in a medical record.

4. Differentiate between Fahrenheit and Celsius thermometers used for monitoring temperature.

5. Differentiate between standard time and military time necessary for accurate recording in a medical record.

Medication calculation need not be difficult if you have a problem-solving method that is easy to understand and implement. In addition, you need to understand common equivalents and units of measurement to visualize all parts of a medication dosage calculation problem. Understanding common equivalents and units of measurement will assist you in preventing **medication errors** related to incorrect dosage.

This chapter will help you to understand the measurement systems used for medication administration. This knowledge is necessary to accurately implement the problem-solving method of dimensional analysis.

SYSTEMS OF MEASUREMENT

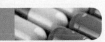

Three systems of measurement are used for medication dosage administration: the metric system, the apothecaries' system, and the household system. To be able to accurately administer medication, you must understand all three of these systems.

The Metric System

The **metric system** is a decimal system of weights and measures based on units of ten in which gram, meter, and liter are the basic units of measurement. However, gram and liter are the only measurements from the metric system that are used in medication administration. The meter is a unit of distance, the gram (abbreviated g or gm) is a unit of weight, and the liter (abbreviated L) is a unit of volume.

The most frequently used metric units of *weight* and their equivalents are summarized in Box 2.1.

Another way to understand the metric units of weight and their equivalents is to visualize the relationship between the measurements and equivalents displayed in Figure 2.1.

The most frequently used metric units for *volume* and their equivalents are summarized in Box 2.2.

Another way to understand the metric units of volume and their equivalents is to visualize the relationship between the measurements and equivalents displayed in Figure 2.2.

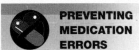

PREVENTING MEDICATION ERRORS

Understanding the three systems of measurement will assist in preventing **medication errors**. Every nurse should have a chart that clearly identifies the conversions between the three systems of measurement to recheck answers for accuracy but it is also the responsibility of the nurse to memorize the equivalents as a chart may not always be available.

BOX 2.1   Metric System Units of Weight and Equivalents

1 kilogram (kg)
1 gram (g)
1 milligram (mg)
1 microgram (mcg)
1 kg = 1000 g
1 g   = 1000 mg
1 mg = 1000 mcg

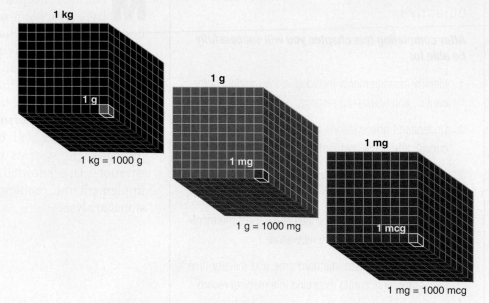

Figure 2.1 Metric system units of weight and equivalents.

BOX 2.2   Metric System Units of Volume and Equivalents

1 liter (L)
1 milliliter (mL)
1 L = 1000 mL

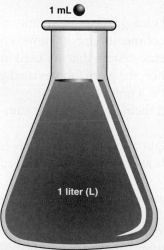

Figure 2.2 Metric system units of volume and equivalents.

The Apothecaries' System

The **apothecaries' system** is a system of measuring and weighing drugs and solutions in which fractions are used to identify parts of the unit of measure. The basic units of measurement in the apothecaries' system include weights and liquid volume. Although the apothecaries' system may not be used in some states, there may be parts of the country where physicians order medications using this system. They may also include Roman numerals in the medication order.

The most frequently used measurements and equivalents within the apothecaries' system's units of *weight* are summarized in Box 2.3, and the most frequently used measurements and equivalents within the apothecaries' system's units of *volume* are summarized in Box 2.4. Figure 2.3 can help you visualize the equivalents for weight and volume.

The Household System

The use of household measurements is considered inaccurate because of the varying sizes of cups, glasses, and eating utensils, and this system generally has been replaced with the metric system. However, as patient care moves away from hospitals, which use the metric system, and into the community, it is once again necessary for the nurse to have an understanding of the household measurement system to be able to use and teach it to clients and families.

The most frequently used measurements and equivalents within the household measurement system are summarized in Box 2.5. Figure 2.4 can help you visualize the equivalents.

BOX 2.3   Apothecaries' System Units of Weight and Equivalents

1 pound (lb)
1 ounce (oz)
1 dram (dr)
1 grain (gr)
1 lb = 16 oz
1 oz = 8 dr
1 dr = 60 gr

BOX 2.4   Apothecaries' System Units of Volume and Equivalents

1 gallon (gal)
1 quart (qt)
1 pint (pt)
1 fluid ounce (fl oz)
1 fluid dram (fl dr)
1 minim (M)
1 gal = 4 qt
1 qt = 2 pt
1 pt = 16 fl oz
1 fl oz = 8 fl dr
1 fl dr = 60 M
1 fl oz = 1 oz
1 fl dr = 1 dr

Weight   **Volume**

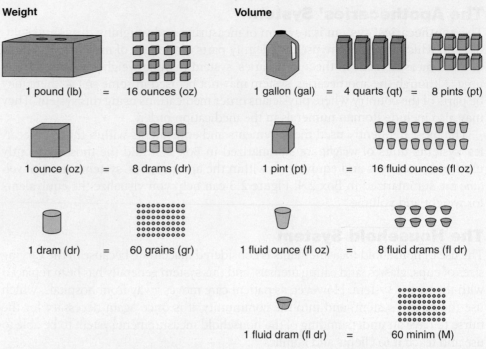

1 pound (lb) = 16 ounces (oz)

1 gallon (gal) = 4 quarts (qt) = 8 pints (pt)

1 ounce (oz) = 8 drams (dr)

1 pint (pt) = 16 fluid ounces (fl oz)

1 dram (dr) = 60 grains (gr)

1 fluid ounce (fl oz) = 8 fluid drams (fl dr)

1 fluid dram (fl dr) = 60 minim (M)

Figure 2.3 Apothecaries' system of equivalents for weight and volume. Please note that the figures are not shown to scale.

BOX 2.5   Household Measurement System and Equivalents

1 cup
1 tablespoon (tbsp or T)
1 teaspoon (tsp or t)
1 drop (gtt)
1 cup   = 8 ounces (oz)
2 Tbsp = 1 oz
3 tsp   = 1 tbsp
1 tsp   = 60 gtt

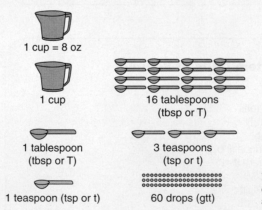

1 cup = 8 oz

1 cup

16 tablespoons
(tbsp or T)

1 tablespoon
(tbsp or T)

3 teaspoons
(tsp or t)

1 teaspoon (tsp or t)

60 drops (gtt)

Figure 2.4 Household measurement system and equivalents for volume. Please note that the figures are not shown to scale.

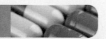

INTAKE AND OUTPUT

Now that you have an understanding of the common equivalents, it is time to utilize that knowledge by calculating the intake from a patient's meal tray. Monitoring the intake of patients is an extremely important nursing function as it provides information regarding fluid retention or fluid loss. If a patient is retaining fluid, the physician or nurse practitioner may need to order a medication to increase the excretion of the fluid as well as limit fluid intake to prevent fluid overload. If a patient is losing fluid, the physician or nurse practitioner may need to increase fluid intake to prevent dehydration. Regardless of the fluid problem, it is the nurse who monitors fluid intake and output to report to the physician or nurse practitioner. Figure 2.5 provides an example of a typical Intake and Output Record.

Intake and Output Record				
Name:				
Date:				
INTAKE		**OUTPUT**		
	Oral		**Voided**	**Catheter**
Breakfast		**Day**		
		Shift		
		0700		
		0800		
AM Snack		0900		
		1000		
		1100		
Lunch		1200		
		1300		
PM Snack		1400		
		Shift		
		Total		
Dinner		**Evening**		
		Shift		
		1500		
		1600		
		1700		
		1800		
Evening Snack		1900		
		2000		
		2100		
		2200		
		Shift		
		Total		
Common Intake Equivalents:		**Night**		
Large Glass	= 240 mL	**Shift**		
Water Glass	= 180 mL	2300		
Juice Glass	= 120 mL	2400		
Coffee Cup	= 240 mL			
Styrofoam Cup	= 180 mL	0100		
Large Milk Carton	= 240 mL	0200		
Small Milk Carton	= 120 mL	0300		
Jell-O Cup	= 120 mL			
Large Soup Bowl	= 200 mL	0400		
Small Soup Bowl	= 100 mL	0500		
Hot Cereal	= 100 mL	0600		
Ice Cream	= 90 mL	**Shift**		
Popsicle	= 80 mL	**Total**		
Pop Can	= 355 mLt			
24-Hour Total Intake		**24-Hour Total Output**		

Figure 2.5 Intake and Output Record.

TEMPERATURE

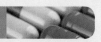

Clients and families are required to monitor temperature changes associated with various medical conditions. Two thermometers may be used for monitoring temperature: a Fahrenheit thermometer or a Celsius thermometer. The nurse must be able to explain both of these systems of measurement when discharging clients and families.

The most frequently used measurements for Celsius and Fahrenheit are summarized in Figure 2.6.

Box 2.6 summarizes a method for converting between Celsius and Fahrenheit or Fahrenheit and Celsius. This easy method requires addition, subtraction, multiplication, or division.

Conversion Chart		
Celsius	to	Fahrenheit
35.0		95.0
35.5		95.9
36.0		96.8
36.5		97.7
37.0		98.6
37.5		99.5
38.0		100.4
38.5		101.3
39.0		102.2
39.5		103.1
40.0		104.0
40.5		104.9
41.0		105.8
41.5		106.7
42.0		107.6

Figure 2.6 Conversion chart for Celsius to Fahrenheit.

BOX 2.6   Temperature Conversion Method

To convert from Fahrenheit to Celsius:
$$°C = (°F - 32) ÷ 1.8$$

To convert from Celsius to Fahrenheit:
$$°F = °C × 1.8 + 32$$

$°C$ = temperature in degrees Celsius
$°F$ = temperature in degrees Fahrenheit

TIME

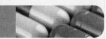

Another conversion that is necessary to learn is the conversion of standard time to military time. Military time has been adopted by all branches of the armed forces, emergency systems, and health care facilities to avoid confusion regarding the

Standard Time	Military Time	Standard Time	Military Time
1:00 am	0100	1:00 pm	12+1 = 1300
1:05 am	0105	1:05 pm	1305
2:00 am	0200	2:00 pm	12+2 = 1400
2:10 am	0210	2:10 pm	1410
3:00 am	0300	3:00 pm	12+3 = 1500
3:15 am	0315	3:15 pm	1515
4:00 am	0400	4:00 pm	12+4 = 1600
4:20 am	0420	4:20 pm	1620
5:00 am	0500	5:00 pm	12+5 = 1700
5:25 am	0525	5:25 pm	1725
6:00 am	0600	6:00 pm	12+6 = 1800
6:30 am	0630	6:30 pm	1830
7:00 am	0700	7:00 pm	12+7 = 1900
7:35 am	0735	7:35 pm	1935
8:00 am	0800	8:00 pm	12+8 = 2000
8:40 am	0840	8:40 pm	2040
9:00 am	0900	9:00 pm	12+9 = 2100
9:45 am	0945	9:45 pm	2145
10:00 am	1000	10:00 pm	12+10 = 2200
10:50 am	1050	10:50 pm	2250
11:00 am	1100	11:00 pm	12+11 = 2300
11:55 am	1155	11:55 pm	2355
12:00 pm (noon)	1200	12:00 am	12+12 = 2400

Figure 2.7 Standard Time and Military Time.

AM (morning) and PM (afternoon/evening) administration of medications. When documenting the administration of medications on the medication administration record (MAR), it is essential that the exact time is noted. Military time uses a 24-hour clock and as the hour hand moves around the clock each hour is clearly identified from 0100 to 1200. After 1200 (noon), the number 12 is added to each number the second time around the clock. Minutes and seconds are recorded the same for standard time and military time but no colon (:) is used to separate the hours and minutes in military time. However, if seconds are to be included in military time then minutes and seconds are separated by a colon (1400:15). Midnight can be referred to as 0000 or 2400 but after midnight the numbers revert to 0100 to 1200. Figure 2.7 displays standard time and military time using a conversion table and Figure 2.8 displays standard time and military time using the face of a clock. Watches are manufactured with standard time and military time visible on the face of a clock to eliminate confusion but learning the conversions is the best method of avoiding errors.

COMMON EQUIVALENTS

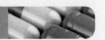

Sometimes it is necessary to convert from one system to another to accurately administer medication. See Table 2.1 for approximate equivalents for weight and Table 2.2 for approximate equivalents for volume.

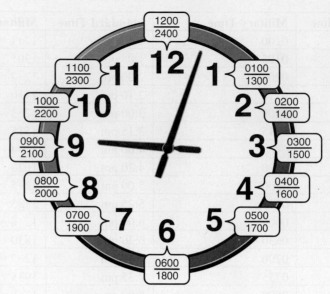

Figure 2.8 Clock with Standard Time and Military Time.

TABLE 2.1	Approximate Equivalents for Weight
Metric	**Apothecaries'**
1 kg (1000 g)	2.2 lb
1 g (1000 mg)	15 gr
60 mg	1 gr

TABLE 2.2	Approximate Equivalents for Volume	
Metric	**Apothecaries'**	**Household**
4000 mL	1 gal (4 qt)	
1 L (1000 mL)	1 qt (2 pt)	
500 mL	1 pt (16 fl oz)	
240 mL	8 oz	1 cup (1 glass)
30 mL	1 oz (8 dr)	2 tbsp
15 mL	½ oz (4 dr)	1 tbsp (3 tsp)
4 mL	1 dr (60 M)	1 tsp (60 gtt)
1 mL	15 M	15 gtt
	1 M	1 gtt

Disclaimer: Converting between measurement systems will often render a different answer depending upon which systems and conversions are being used by the student. The answer to the medication calculation problem will ultimately be the same answer after rounding either up or down (example: 7.5 L or 7.8 L would both be 8 L after rounding up).

Summary

This chapter has reviewed the metric, apothecaries', and household systems of measurement. Calculation of intake and output was explained. This chapter also reviewed Fahrenheit and Celsius as well as standard time and military time. To assess your understanding and retention of these systems of measurement, complete the following practice problems.

Practice Problems for Chapter 2

Systems of Measurement and Common Equivalents

(See pages 45–46 for answers)

Write the correct abbreviation symbols for the following measurements from the metric system:

1. kilogram =   5. liter   =

2. gram   =   6. milliliter =

3. milligram =

4. microgram =

Write the correct abbreviation symbols for the following measurements from the apothecaries' system:

7. pound =   12. quart   =

8. ounce =   13. pint   =

9. dram   =   14. fluid ounce =

10. grain =   15. fluid dram =

11. gallon =   16. minim   =

Write the correct abbreviation symbols for the following measurements from the household system:

17. tablespoon =

18. teaspoon   =

19. drop   =

Identify the correct numerical values for the following measurements:

20. 1 kg = ____ lb

21. 1 kg = ____ g

22. 1 g   = ____ mg

23. 1 mg = ____ mcg

24. 1 g   = ____ gr

(Practice Problems continue on page 40)

Calculate the intake for the following meal trays:

25. Breakfast:

     Coffee Cup = 240 mL (drank ½)

     Water Glass = 180 mL (drank ½ with AM medications)

     Juice Glass = 120 mL (drank all)

     Hot Cereal   = 100 mL (ate ½)

     Total   =

26. Lunch:

     Coffee Cup   = 240 mL (drank all)

     Small Milk Carton = 120 mL (drank all)

     Large Soup Bowl   = 200 mL (ate ½)

     Jell-O Cup   = 120 mL

     Total   =

27. Dinner:

     Coffee Cup   = 240 mL (drank ¼)

     Large Milk Carton = 240 mL (drank ½)

     Ice Cream   = 90 mL (ate all)

     Total   =

28. Coffee Cup   = 240 mL (drank all)

     Juice Glass   = 120 mL (drank ½)

     Hot Cereal   = 100 mL (ate all)

     Total   =

29. Milk Carton   = 120 mL (drank all)

     Soup Bowl   = 100 mL (ate all)

     Jell-O Cup   = 120 mL (ate ½)

     Total   =

Identify the correct numerical values for the following temperatures:

30. 98.6°F   = ____ °C   35. 96.8°F   = ____ °C

31. 39°C   = ____ °F   36. 35°C   = ____ °F

32. 104.9°F = ____ °C   37. 100.4°F = ____ °C

33. 36°C   = ____ °F   38. 39.5°C   = ____ °F

34. 101.3°F = ____ °C

Convert the following Standard Times to Military Time:

39. 1:00 am =   43. midnight =

40. 5:00 pm =   44. 10:15 pm =

41. 3:00 am =   45. 6:00 am   =

42. 8:00 pm =

Convert the following Military Times to Standard Time:

46. 0230 =   50. 2110 =

47. 1600 =   51. 1400 =

48. 0420 =   52. 1630 =

49. 1200 =

Identify the correct numerical values for the following measurements:

53. 1 gr   = ____ mg

54. 1000 mg   = ____ g

55. 1000 mL   = ____ L   = ____ qt

56. 500 mL   = ____ pt

57. 240 mL   = ____ oz

58. 30 mL   = ____ oz = ____ tbsp

59. 15 mL   = ____ oz = ____ tsp

60. 5 mL   = ____ tsp

61. 1 mL   = ____ M   = ____ gtt

62. 2 mL   = ____ gtt

63. 30 gtt   = ____ M   = ____ mL

64. 4 tbsp   = ____ oz = ____ mL

65. 40°C   = ____ °F

66. 1 pt   = ____ fl oz = ____ mL

67. 2 qt   = ____ gal = ____ mL

68. 96.8°F   = ____ °C

69. 2000 g   = ____ kg = ____ lb

70. gr xv   = ____ g   = ____ mg

71. 37.5°C   = ____ °F

72. 1 oz   = ____ dr = ____ mL

73. 32 fl oz = ____ pt = ____ mL

74. 39°C   = ____ °F

75. gr xxx   = ____ g   = ____ mg

76. 240 mL   = ____ oz = ____ cup

77. 99.5°F   = ____ °C

Chapter 2 Post-Test

Systems of Measurement and Common Equivalents

Name _____   Date _____

1. 2.2 lb   = _____ kg
2. 16 fl oz   = _____ pt
3. 1 tsp   = _____ mL
4. 15 gr   = _____ g
5. 1 oz   = _____ mL
6. 1000 mcg   = _____ mg
7. 60 mg   = _____ gr
8. 1 pt   = _____ mL
9. ½ tsp   = _____ mL
10. 1000 mg   = _____ g
11. 1 L   = _____ mL
12. 4 qt   = _____ gal
13. 1 tbsp   = _____ tsp
14. 1 cup   = _____ oz
15. 8 oz   = _____ mL
16. 3 tsp   = _____ mL
17. 15 gtt   = _____ M
18. 1 dr   = _____ mL
19. 15 M   = _____ mL
20. 1000 g   = _____ kg

ANSWER KEY FOR CHAPTER 2: SYSTEMS OF MEASUREMENT AND COMMON EQUIVALENTS

Practice Problems

1	kilogram	= kg
2	gram	= g
3	milligram	= mg
4	microgram	= mcg
5	liter	= L
6	milliliter	= mL
7	pound	= lb
8	ounce	= oz
9	dram	= dr
10	grain	= gr
11	gallon	= gal
12	quart	= qt
13	pint	= pt
14	fluid ounce	= fl oz
15	fluid dram	= fl dr
16	minim	= M
17	tablespoon	= tbsp
18	teaspoon	= tsp
19	drop	= gtt
20	1 kg	= 2.2 lb
21	1 kg	= 1000 g
22	1 g	= 1000 mg
23	1 mg	= 1000 mcg
24	1 g	= 15 gr

25

Breakfast:

Coffee Cup	= 240 mL (drank ½)	120
Water Glass	= 180 mL (drank ½ with AM medications)	90
Juice Glass	= 120 mL (drank all)	120
Hot Cereal	= 100 mL (ate ½)	50
Total	=	380 mL

26

Lunch:

Coffee Cup	= 240 mL (drank all)	240
Small Milk Carton	= 120 mL (drank all)	120
Large Soup Bowl	= 200 mL (ate ½)	100
Jell-O Cup	= 120 mL (ate all)	120
Total	=	580 mL

27

Dinner:

Coffee Cup	= 240 mL (drank ¼)	60
Large Milk Carton	= 240 mL (drank ½)	120
Ice Cream	= 90 mL (ate all)	90
Total	=	270 mL

28

Coffee Cup	= 240 mL (drank all)	240
Juice Glass	= 120 mL (drank ½)	60
Hot Cereal	= 100 mL (ate all)	100
Total	=	400 mL

29

Milk Carton	= 120 mL (drank all)	120
Soup Bowl	= 100 mL (ate all)	100
Jell-O Cup	= 120 mL (ate ½)	60
Total	=	280 mL

30	98.6°F	= 37°C
31	39°C	= 102.2°F
32	104.9°F	= 40.5°C
33	36°C	= 96.8°F
34	101.3°F	= 38.5°C
35	96.8°F	= 36°C
36	35°C	= 95°F
37	100.4°F	= 38°C
38	39.5°C	= 103.1°F

Convert the following Standard Times to Military Time:

39	1:00 am	= 0100
40	5:00 pm	= 1700
41	3:00 am	= 0300
42	8:00 pm	= 2000
43	12:00 am	= 2400
44	10:15 pm	= 2215
45	6:00 am	= 0600

Convert the following Military Times to Standard Time:

46	0230	= 2:30 am
47	1600	= 4:00 pm
48	0420	= 4:20 am
49	1200	= 12:00 pm
50	2110	= 9:10 pm
51	1400	= 2:00 pm
52	1630	= 4:30 pm

Convert the following:

#		
53	1 gr	= 60 mg
54	1000 mg	= 1 g
55	1000 mL	= 1 L = 1 qt
56	500 mL	= 1 pt
57	240 mL	= 8 oz
58	30 mL	= 1 oz = 2 tbsp
59	15 mL	= ½ oz = 3 tsp
60	5 mL	= 1 tsp
61	1 mL	= 15 M = 15 gtt
62	2 mL	= 30 gtt
63	30 gtt	= 30 M = 2 mL
64	4 tbsp	= 2 oz = 60 mL

#		
65	40°C	= 104°F
66	1 pt	= 16 fl oz = 500 mL
67	2 qt	= ½ gal = 2000 mL
68	96.8°F	= 36°C
69	2000 g	= 2 kg = 4.4 lb
70	gr xv	= 1 g = 1000 mg
71	37.5°C	= 99.5°F
72	1 oz	= 8 dr = 30 mL
73	32 fl oz	= 2 pt = 1000 mL
74	39°C	= 102.2°F
75	gr xxx	= 1.8 g = 1800 mg
76	240 mL	= 8 oz = 1 cup
77	99.5°F	= 37.5°C

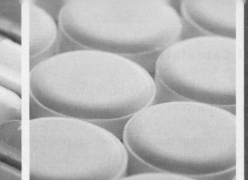

Solving Problems Using Dimensional Analysis

Objectives

After completing this chapter, you will successfully be able to:

1. Define the terms used in dimensional analysis.

2. Explain the step-by-step problem-solving method of dimensional analysis.

3. Solve problems involving common equivalents using dimensional analysis as a problem-solving method.

Dimensional analysis provides a systematic, straightforward way to set up problems and to organize and evaluate data. It is not only easy to learn, but also can reduce **medication errors** when mathematical conversion is required.

Dimensional analysis assists with preventing medication errors by allowing you to visualize all parts of the medication problem and to critically think your way through the problem.

This chapter introduces you to dimensional analysis with a step-by-step explanation of this problem-solving method. The chapter also provides the opportunity to practice solving problems that involve common equivalents.

TERMS USED IN DIMENSIONAL ANALYSIS

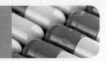

Dimensional analysis is a problem-solving method that can be used whenever two quantities are directly proportional to each other and one quantity must be converted to the other by using a common equivalent, conversion factor, or conversion relation. All medication dosage calculation problems can be solved by dimensional analysis.

It is important to understand the following four terms that provide the basis for dimensional analysis.

- **Given quantity:** the beginning point of the problem
- **Wanted quantity:** the answer to the problem
- **Unit path:** the series of conversions necessary to achieve the answer to the problem
- **Conversion factors:** equivalents necessary to convert between systems of measurement and to allow unwanted units to be canceled from the problem

Each conversion factor is a ratio of units that equals 1.

Dimensional analysis also uses the same terms as fractions: numerators and denominators.

- *Numerator* = the top portion of the problem
- *Denominator* = the bottom portion of the problem

Some problems will have a given quantity and a wanted quantity that contain only numerators. Other problems will have a given quantity and a wanted quantity that contain both a numerator and a denominator. This chapter contains only problems with numerators as the given quantity and the wanted quantity.

Once the beginning point in the problem is identified, then a series of conversions necessary to achieve the answer is established that leads to the problem's solution.

Below is an example of the model that is used in solving problems by the dimensional analysis method. It also demonstrates the correct placement of the basic terms that are used in this method.

Unit Path

| Given Quantity | Conversion Factor for Given Quantity | Conversion Factor for Wanted Quantity | Conversion Computation | Wanted Quantity |

=

THE FIVE STEPS OF DIMENSIONAL ANALYSIS

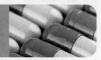

Once the given quantity is identified, the unit path leading to the wanted quantity is established. The problem-solving method of dimensional analysis uses the following five steps.

1. Identify the *given quantity* in the problem.
2. Identify the *wanted quantity* in the problem.
3. Establish the *unit path* from the given quantity to the wanted quantity using equivalents as *conversion factors*.
4. Set up the conversion factors to permit cancellation of unwanted units. Carefully choose each conversion factor and ensure that it is correctly placed in the numerator or denominator portion of the problem to allow the unwanted units to be canceled from the problem.
5. Multiply the numerators, multiply the denominators, and divide the product of the numerators by the product of the denominators to provide the numerical value of the wanted quantity.

The following examples use the five steps to solve problems using dimensional analysis. New information that is added in each step appears in red. Lines show that unwanted units or numbers have been canceled from the unit path. A circle appears around the wanted quantity in the unit path.

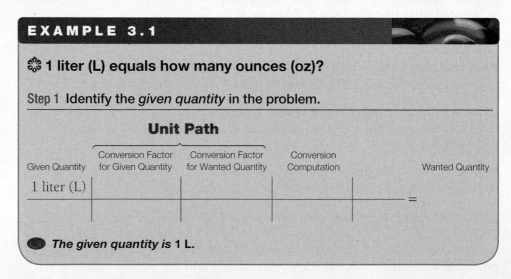

EXAMPLE 3.1

❈ **1 liter (L) equals how many ounces (oz)?**

Step 1 Identify the *given quantity* in the problem.

Unit Path

| Given Quantity | Conversion Factor for Given Quantity | Conversion Factor for Wanted Quantity | Conversion Computation | Wanted Quantity |

1 liter (L)   =

● *The given quantity is* 1 L.

Step 2 Identify the *wanted quantity* in the problem.

Unit Path

Given Quantity	Conversion Factor for Given Quantity	Conversion Factor for Wanted Quantity	Conversion Computation	Wanted Quantity
1 liter (L)				= oz

🔘 *The wanted quantity is the number of* ounces (oz) in 1 L.

Step 3 Establish the *unit path* from the given quantity to the wanted quantity. You must determine what conversion factors are needed to convert the given quantity to the wanted quantity.

🔘 *Given quantity: 1 L   = 1000 mL*
Wanted quantity: 1 oz = 30 mL

Step 4 Write the unit path for the problem so that each unit cancels out the preceding unit until all unwanted units are canceled from the problem except the wanted quantity. *Red lines* indicate that unwanted units or numbers have been canceled.
   The wanted quantity must be within the numerator portion of the problem. A red circle around the wanted quantity demonstrates that the problem is set up correctly.

Unit Path

Given Quantity	Conversion Factor for Given Quantity	Conversion Factor for Wanted Quantity	Conversion Computation	Wanted Quantity
1 liter (L)	1000 mL	1 oz		= oz
	1 liter (L)	30 mL		

Unit Path

Given Quantity	Conversion Factor for Given Quantity	Conversion Factor for Wanted Quantity	Conversion Computation	Wanted Quantity
1 ~~liter (L)~~	1000 ~~mL~~	1 (oz)		= oz
	1 ~~liter (L)~~	30 ~~mL~~		

Step 5 After the unwanted units are canceled from the problem, only the numerical values remain. Multiply the numerators, multiply the denominators, and divide the product of the numerators by the product of the denominators to provide the numerical value for the wanted quantity.
   One (1) times (×) any number equals that number; therefore 1s may be automatically canceled from the problem. Other factors that can be canceled from the problem include like numerical values in the

(Example continues on page 50)

numerator and denominator portion of the problem and the same number of zeroes in the numerator and denominator portion of the problem.

Unit Path

Given Quantity	Conversion Factor for Given Quantity	Conversion Factor for Wanted Quantity	Conversion Computation		Wanted Quantity
~~1 liter (L)~~	1000 ~~mL~~	1 (oz)	1000 × 1	1000	= 33.3 oz
	~~1 liter (L)~~	30 ~~mL~~	30	30	

33.3 oz is the wanted quantity and the answer to the problem.

EXAMPLE 3.2

One gallon (gal) equals how many milliliters (mL)?

Step 1 Identify the given quantity in the problem.

$$\frac{1\text{ gal}}{} =$$

The given quantity is 1 gal.

Step 2 Identify the wanted quantity in the problem.

$$\frac{1\text{ gal}}{} = \text{mL}$$

The wanted quantity is the number of milliliters (mL) in 1 gal.

Step 3 Establish the unit path from the given quantity to the wanted quantity by selecting the equivalents that will be used as conversion factors.

Given quantity: 1 gal = 4 quarts (qt); 1 qt = 1 L
Wanted quantity: 1 L = 1000 mL

Step 4 Write the unit path for the problem so that each unit cancels out (*red lines*) the preceding unit until all unwanted units are canceled from the problem except the wanted quantity, which is circled.

$$\frac{1\ \cancel{\text{gal}}}{} \left| \frac{4\ \text{qt}}{1\ \cancel{\text{gal}}} \right| \frac{1\ \cancel{\text{L}}}{1\ \cancel{\text{qt}}} \left| \frac{1000\ \text{mL}}{1\ \cancel{\text{L}}} \right. = \text{mL}$$

Step 5 After the unwanted units are canceled from the problem, only the numerical values remain. Multiply the numerators, multiply the denominators, and divide the product of the numerators by the product of the denominators to provide the numerical value for the wanted quantity.

$$\frac{\cancel{1\ gal}}{} \left| \frac{4\ qt}{\cancel{1\ gal}} \right| \frac{\cancel{1\ L}}{1\ qt} \left| \frac{1000\ \boxed{mL}}{\cancel{1\ L}} \right| \frac{4 \times 1000}{1} = 4000\ mL$$

● *4000 mL is the wanted quantity and the answer to the problem.*

Exercise 3.1 **Dimensional Analysis**
(See pages 59–61 for answers)

Use dimensional analysis to change the following units of measurement.

1. Problem: 4 mg = How many g?

   Given quantity   =

   Wanted quantity   =

   $$\frac{4\ mg}{} \left| \rule{8cm}{0pt} \right. = \quad\quad g$$

2. Problem: 5000 g = How many kg?

   Given quantity   =

   Wanted quantity   =

   $$\frac{5000\ g}{} \left| \rule{8cm}{0pt} \right. = \quad\quad kg$$

3. Problem: 0.3 L = How many mL?

   Given quantity   =

   Wanted quantity   =

   $$\frac{0.3\ L}{} \left| \rule{8cm}{0pt} \right. = \quad\quad mL$$

4. Problem: 15 mL = How many tsp?

   Given quantity   =

   Wanted quantity   =

   $$\frac{15\ mL}{} \left| \rule{8cm}{0pt} \right. = \quad\quad tsp$$

(Exercise continues on page 52)

5. Problem: 120 lb = How many kg?

   Given quantity   =

   Wanted quantity   =

   $$\frac{120\ lb\ |}{|} = \quad kg$$

6. Problem: 5 gr = How many mg?

   Given quantity   =

   Wanted quantity   =

   $$\frac{5\ gr\ |}{|} = \quad mg$$

7. Problem: 2 g = How many gr?

   Given quantity   =

   Wanted quantity   =

   $$\frac{2\ g\ |}{|} = \quad gr$$

8. Problem: 5 fl dr = How many mL?

   Given quantity   =

   Wanted quantity   =

   $$\frac{5\ fl\ dr\ |}{|} = \quad mL$$

9. Problem: 8 fl dr = How many fl oz?

   Given quantity   =

   Wanted quantity   =

   $$\frac{8\ fl\ dr\ |}{|} = \quad fl\ oz$$

10. Problem: 10 M = How many fl dr?

    Given quantity   =

    Wanted quantity   =

    $$\frac{10\ M\ |}{|} = \quad fl\ dr$$

11. Problem: 35 kg = How many lb?

    Given quantity   =

    Wanted quantity   =

    $$\frac{35\ kg\ |}{|} = \quad lb$$

12. Problem: 10 mL = How many tsp?

    Given quantity =

    Wanted quantity =

    $$\frac{10\ mL\ |\ }{\ \ \ \ \ \ \ \ |\ } = \quad tsp$$

13. Problem: 30 mL = How many tbsp?

    Given quantity =

    Wanted quantity =

    $$\frac{30\ mL\ |\ }{\ \ \ \ \ \ \ \ |\ } = \quad tbsp$$

14. Problem: 0.25 g = How many mg?

    Given quantity =

    Wanted quantity =

    $$\frac{0.25\ g\ |\ }{\ \ \ \ \ \ \ |\ } = \quad mg$$

15. Problem: 350 mcg = How many mg?

    Given quantity =

    Wanted quantity =

    $$\frac{350\ mcg\ |\ }{\ \ \ \ \ \ \ \ \ |\ } = \quad mg$$

16. Problem: 0.75 L = How many mL?

    Given quantity =

    Wanted quantity =

    $$\frac{0.75\ L\ |\ }{\ \ \ \ \ \ \ |\ } = \quad mL$$

17. Problem: 3 hr = How many minutes?

    Given quantity =

    Wanted quantity =

    $$\frac{3\ hr\ |\ }{\ \ \ \ \ |\ } = \quad min$$

18. Problem: 3.5 mL = How many M?

    Given quantity =

    Wanted quantity =

    $$\frac{3.5\ mL\ |\ }{\ \ \ \ \ \ \ |\ } = \quad M$$

(Exercise continues on page 54)

19. Problem: 500 mcg = How many mg?

    Given quantity   =

    Wanted quantity   =

    $$\frac{500 \text{ mcg}}{} = \quad \text{mg}$$

20. Problem: 225 M = How many tsp?

    Given quantity   =

    Wanted quantity   =

    $$\frac{225 \text{ M}}{} = \quad \text{tsp}$$

21. Problem: 2 gal = How many mL?

    Given quantity   =

    Wanted quantity   =

    $$\frac{2 \text{ gal}}{} = \quad \text{mL}$$

22. Problem: 8 pt = How many gal?

    Given quantity   =

    Wanted quantity   =

    $$\frac{8 \text{ pt}}{} = \quad \text{gal}$$

23. Problem: 16 oz = How many mL?

    Given quantity   =

    Wanted quantity   =

    $$\frac{16 \text{ oz}}{} = \quad \text{mL}$$

24. Problem: 2 cup = How many mL?

    Given quantity   =

    Wanted quantity   =

    $$\frac{2 \text{ cup}}{} = \quad \text{mL}$$

25. Problem: 2.5 kg = How many g?

    Given quantity   =

    Wanted quantity   =

    $$\frac{2.5 \text{ kg}}{} = \quad \text{g}$$

Summary

This chapter has introduced you to dimensional analysis with a step-by-step explanation and an opportunity to practice solving problems involving common equivalents. To demonstrate your understanding of dimensional analysis and conversions between systems of measurement, complete the following practice problems.

Practice Problems for Chapter 3

Solving Problems Using Dimensional Analysis
(See pages 61–63 for answers)

1. Problem: $\frac{3}{4}$ mL   = How many M?

2. Problem: gtt XV   = How many M?

3. Problem: $\frac{5}{6}$ gr   = How many mg?

4. Problem: 3 oz   = How many mL?

5. Problem: 0.5 mg   = How many mcg?

6. Problem: 35 gtt   = How many mL?

7. Problem: 3 qt   = How many mL?

8. Problem: 4 gal   = How many qt?

9. Problem: 1.5 cup   = How many mL?

10. Problem: 24 oz   = How many cups?

11. Problem: 132 lb   = How many kg?

12. Problem: 70 kg   = How many lb?

13. Problem: 750 mcg   = How many mg?

14. Problem: 0.5 L   = How many mL?

15. Problem: 1800 g   = How many kg?

16. Problem: 6000 mL   = How many qt?

17. Problem: 180 mL   = How many oz?

18. Problem: 6 dr   = How many mL?

19. Problem: 0.125 mg   = How many mcg?

20. Problem: 90 M   = How many mL?

21. Problem: 145 lb   = How many kg?

22. Problem: $\frac{3}{4}$ gr   = How many mg?

23. Problem: 1500 mg   = How many g?

24. Problem: 3 lb   = How many g?

(Practice Problems continue on page 56)

25. Problem: 0.80 mg   = How many mcg?

26. Problem: $\frac{1}{150}$ gr   = How many mg?

27. Problem: $\frac{1}{300}$ gr   = How many mg?

28. Problem: 30 mg   = How many gr?

29. Problem: 45 gr   = How many g?

30. Problem: 15 mg   = How many mcg?

Chapter 3 Post-Test

Solving Problems Using Dimensional Analysis

Name _____   Date _____

Use dimensional analysis to solve the following conversion problems:

1. 2045 g   = How many lb?
2. 0.004 g   = How many mcg?
3. 6 tsp   = How many dr?
4. 0.5 L   = How many pt?
5. How many L in 250 oz?
6. How many tbsp in 30 mL?
7. How many minims in 60 mL?
8. How many oz in 1800 g?
9. 300 mg   = How many gr?
10. How many mg in gr ¼?
11. 20 mL   = How many M?
12. How many mcg in 0.75 mg?
13. 1.5 pt   = How many mL?
14. How many lb in 84 kg?
15. How many kg in 165 lb?
16. 6500 mcg = How many mg?
17. 24 fl oz   = How many mL?
18. 1.89 L   = How many mL?
19. How many gal in 64 fl oz?
20. 0.5 L   = How many mL?
21. 140 lb   = How many kg?
22. 1.7 g   = How many mg?
23. 16 oz   = How many mL?
24. 850 mcg   = How many mg?
25. 4 qt   = How many mL?
26. 30 kg   = How many lb?
27. 2 cups   = How many oz?
28. 450 mg   = How many g?
29. 3200 mL   = How many L?
30. 5.5 g   = How many mcg?

ANSWER KEY FOR CHAPTER 3: SOLVING PROBLEMS USING DIMENSIONAL ANALYSIS

Exercise 3.1   Dimensional Analysis

1

Problem:	4 mg = How many g?
Given quantity	= 4 mg
Wanted quantity	= g
Conversion factor	= 1 g = 1000 mg

$$\frac{4 \text{ mg}}{} \left| \frac{1 \text{ g}}{1000 \text{ mg}} \right| \frac{4 \times 1}{1000} \right| \frac{4}{1000} = 0.004 \text{ g}$$

2

Problem:	5000 g = How many kg?
Given quantity	= 5000 g
Wanted quantity	= kg
Conversion factor	= 1 kg = 1000 g

$$\frac{5000 \text{ g}}{} \left| \frac{1 \text{ kg}}{1000 \text{ g}} \right| \frac{5 \times 1}{1} \right| \frac{5}{1} = 5 \text{ kg}$$

3

Problem:	0.3 L = How many mL?
Given quantity	= 0.3 L
Wanted quantity	= mL
Conversion factor	= 1 L = 1000 mL

$$\frac{0.3 \text{ L}}{} \left| \frac{1000 \text{ mL}}{1 \text{ L}} \right| \frac{0.3 \times 1000}{1} \right| \frac{300}{1} = 300 \text{ mL}$$

4

Problem:	15 mL = How many tsp?
Given quantity	= 15 mL
Wanted quantity	= tsp
Conversion factor	= 1 tsp = 5 mL

$$\frac{15 \text{ mL}}{} \left| \frac{1 \text{ tsp}}{5 \text{ mL}} \right| \frac{15 \times 1}{5} \right| \frac{15}{5} = 3 \text{ tsp}$$

5

Problem:	120 lb = How many kg?
Given quantity	= 120 lb
Wanted quantity	= kg
Conversion factor	= 2.2 lb = 1 kg

$$\frac{120 \text{ lb}}{} \left| \frac{1 \text{ kg}}{2.2 \text{ lb}} \right| \frac{120 \times 1}{2.2} \right| \frac{120}{2.2} = 54.5 \text{ kg}$$

6

Problem:	5 gr = How many mg?
Given quantity	= 5 gr
Wanted quantity	= mg
Conversion factor	= 1 gr = 60 mg

$$\frac{5 \text{ gr}}{} \left| \frac{60 \text{ mg}}{1 \text{ gr}} \right| \frac{5 \times 60}{1} \right| \frac{300}{1} = 300 \text{ mg}$$

7

Problem:	2 g = How many gr?
Given quantity	= 2 g
Wanted quantity	= gr
Conversion factor	= 1 g = 15 gr

$$\frac{2 \text{ g}}{} \left| \frac{15 \text{ gr}}{1 \text{ g}} \right| \frac{2 \times 15}{1} \right| \frac{30}{1} = 30 \text{ gr}$$

8

Problem:	5 fl dr = How many mL?
Given quantity	= 5 fl dr
Wanted quantity	= mL
Conversion factor	= 1 fl dr = 5 mL

$$\frac{5 \text{ fl dr}}{} \left| \frac{5 \text{ mL}}{1 \text{ fl dr}} \right| \frac{5 \times 5}{1} \right| \frac{25}{1} = 25 \text{ mL}$$

9

Problem:	8 fl dr = How many fl oz?
Given quantity	= 8 fl dr
Wanted quantity	= fl oz
Conversion factor	= 1 fl dr = 5 mL
Conversion factor	= 1 fl oz = 30 mL

$$\frac{8 \text{ fl dr}}{} \left| \frac{5 \text{ mL}}{1 \text{ fl dr}} \right| \frac{1 \text{ fl oz}}{30 \text{ mL}} \right| \frac{8 \times 5 \times 1}{1 \times 30} \right| \frac{40}{30} = 1.3 \text{ fl oz}$$

10

Problem:	10 M = How many fl dr?
Given quantity	= M
Wanted quantity	= fl dr
Conversion factor	= 1 mL = 15 M
Conversion factor	= 1 fl dr = 5 mL

$$\frac{10 \text{ M}}{} \left| \frac{1 \text{ mL}}{15 \text{ M}} \right| \frac{1 \text{ fl dr}}{5 \text{ mL}} \right| \frac{10 \times 1 \times 1}{15 \times 5} \right| \frac{10}{75} = 0.13 \text{ fl dr}$$

11

Problem:	35 kg = How many lb?
Given quantity	= 35 kg
Wanted quantity	= lb
Conversion factor	= 1 kg = 2.2 lb

$$\frac{35 \text{ kg}}{} \left| \frac{2.2 \text{ lb}}{1 \text{ kg}} \right| \frac{35 \times 2.2}{1} \right| \frac{77}{1} = 77 \text{ lb}$$

12

Problem:	10 mL = How many tsp?
Given quantity	= 10 mL
Wanted quantity	= tsp
Conversion factor	= 1 tsp = 5 mL

$$\frac{10 \text{ mL}}{} \left| \frac{5 \text{ tsp}}{5 \text{ mL}} \right| \frac{10 \times 1}{5} \right| \frac{10}{5} = 2 \text{ tsp}$$

13

Problem:	30 mL = How many tbsp?
Given quantity	= 30 mL
Wanted quantity	= tbsp
Conversion factor	= 1 tbsp = 15 mL

$$\frac{30\ \text{mL} \quad | \quad 1\ \text{(tbsp)} \quad | \quad 30 \times 1 \quad | \quad 30}{\qquad\qquad | \quad 15\ \text{mL} \quad | \quad 15 \quad | \quad 15} = 2\ \text{tbsp}$$

14

Problem:	0.25 g = How many mg?
Given quantity	= 0.25 g
Wanted quantity	= mg
Conversion factor	= 1 g = 1000 mg

$$\frac{0.25\ \text{g} \quad | \quad 1000\ \text{(mg)} \quad | \quad 0.25 \times 1000 \quad | \quad 250}{\qquad\qquad | \quad 1\ \text{g} \quad | \quad 1 \quad | \quad 1} = 250\ \text{mg}$$

15

Problem:	350 mcg = How many mg?
Given quantity	= 350 mcg
Wanted quantity	= mg
Conversion factor	= 1 mg = 1000 mcg

$$\frac{350\ \text{mcg} \quad | \quad 1\ \text{(mg)} \quad | \quad 350 \times 1 \quad | \quad 350}{\qquad\qquad | \quad 1000\ \text{mcg} \quad | \quad 1000 \quad | \quad 1000} = 0.35\ \text{mg}$$

16

Problem:	0.75 L = How many mL?
Given quantity	= 0.75 L
Wanted quantity	= mL
Conversion factor	= 1 L = 1000 mL

$$\frac{0.75\ \text{L} \quad | \quad 1000\ \text{(mL)} \quad | \quad 0.75 \times 1000 \quad | \quad 750}{\qquad\qquad | \quad 1\ \text{L} \quad | \quad 1 \quad | \quad 1} = 750\ \text{mL}$$

17

Problem:	3 hr = How many minutes?
Given quantity	= 3 hr
Wanted quantity	= minutes
Conversion factor	= 1 hr = 60 min

$$\frac{3\ \text{hr} \quad | \quad 60\ \text{(min)} \quad | \quad 3 \times 60 \quad | \quad 180}{\qquad\qquad | \quad 1\ \text{hr} \quad | \quad 1 \quad | \quad 1} = 180\ \text{min}$$

18

Problem:	3.5 mL = How many M?
Given quantity	= 3.5 mL
Wanted quantity	= M
Conversion factor	= 1 mL = 15 M

$$\frac{3.5\ \text{mL} \quad | \quad 15\ \text{(M)} \quad | \quad 3.5 \times 15 \quad | \quad 52.5}{\qquad\qquad | \quad 1\ \text{mL} \quad | \quad 1 \quad | \quad 1} = 52.5\ \text{M}$$

19

Problem:	500 mcg = How many mg?
Given quantity	= 500 mcg
Wanted quantity	= mg
Conversion factor	= 1 mg = 1000 mcg

$$\frac{500\ \text{mcg} \quad | \quad 1\ \text{(mg)} \quad | \quad 500 \times 1 \quad | \quad 500}{\qquad\qquad | \quad 1000\ \text{mcg} \quad | \quad 1000 \quad | \quad 1000} = 0.5\ \text{mg}$$

20

Problem:	225 M = How many tsp?
Given quantity	= 225 M
Wanted quantity	= tsp
Conversion factor	= 1 mL = 15 M
Conversion factor	= 1 tsp = 5 mL

$$\frac{225\ \text{M} \quad | \quad 1\ \text{mL} \quad | \quad 1\ \text{(tsp)} \quad | \quad 225 \times 1 \times 1 \quad | \quad 225}{\qquad\quad | \quad 15\ \text{M} \quad | \quad 5\ \text{mL} \quad | \quad 15 \times 5 \quad | \quad 75} = 3\ \text{tsp}$$

21

Problem:	2 gal = How many mL?
Given quantity	= gal
Wanted quantity	= mL
Conversion factor	= 1 gal = 4000 mL

$$\frac{2\ \text{gal} \quad | \quad 4000\ \text{(mL)} \quad | \quad 2 \times 4000 \quad | \quad 8000}{\qquad\quad | \quad 1\ \text{gal} \quad | \quad 1 \quad | \quad 1} = 8000\ \text{mL}$$

22

Problem:	8 pt = How man gal?
Given quantity	= pt
Wanted quantity	= gal
Conversion factor	= 1 qt = 2 pt
Conversion factor	= 1 gal = 4 qt

$$\frac{8\ \text{pt} \quad | \quad 1\ \text{qt} \quad | \quad 1\ \text{(gal)} \quad | \quad 8 \times 1 \times 1 \quad | \quad 8}{\qquad\quad | \quad 2\ \text{pt} \quad | \quad 4\ \text{qt} \quad | \quad 2 \times 4 \quad | \quad 8} = 1\ \text{gal}$$

23

Problem:	16 oz = How many mL?
Given quantity	= oz
Wanted quantity	= mL
Conversion factor	= 1 oz = 30 mL

$$\frac{16\ \text{oz} \quad | \quad 30\ \text{(mL)} \quad | \quad 16 \times 30 \quad | \quad 480}{\qquad\quad | \quad 1\ \text{oz} \quad | \quad 1 \quad | \quad 1} = 480\ \text{mL}$$

24

Problem:	2 cup = How many mL?
Given quantity	= cup
Wanted quantity	= mL
Conversion factor	= 1 cup = 8 oz
Conversion factor	= 8 oz = 240 mL

$$\frac{2\ \text{cup} \quad | \quad 8\ \text{oz} \quad | \quad 240\ \text{(mL)} \quad | \quad 2 \times 8 \times 240 \quad | \quad 3840}{\qquad\quad | \quad 1\ \text{cup} \quad | \quad 8\ \text{oz} \quad | \quad 1 \times 8 \quad | \quad 8} = 480\ \text{mL}$$

25

Problem: 2.5 kg = How many g?
Given quantity   = kg
Wanted quantity   = g
Conversion factor   = 1 kg = 1000 g

$$\frac{2.5 \text{ kg} \mid 1000 \text{ ⓖ} \mid 2.5 \times 1000 \mid 2500}{1 \text{ kg} \mid 1 \mid 1} = 2500 \text{ g}$$

Practice Problems

1

Problem: $\frac{3}{4}$ mL = How many M?
Given quantity   = $\frac{3}{4}$ mL
Wanted quantity   = M
Conversion factor   = 1 mL = 15 M

$$\frac{\frac{3}{4} \text{ mL} \mid 15 \text{ Ⓜ} \mid \frac{3}{4} \times 15 \mid \frac{3}{4} \times \frac{15}{1} \mid \frac{45}{4} \mid 11.25 \text{ M}}{1 \text{ mL} \mid 1 \mid 1 \mid 1 \mid 1} = 11.25 \text{ M} = 11.3 \text{ M} = 11 \text{ M}$$

2

Problem: gtt XV = How many M?
Given quantity   = 15 gtt
Wanted quantity   = M
Conversion factor   = 1 gtt = 1 M

$$\frac{15 \text{ gtt} \mid 1 \text{ Ⓜ} \mid 15}{1 \text{ gtt}} = 15 \text{ M}$$

3

Problem: $\frac{5}{6}$ gr = How many mg?
Given quantity   = $\frac{5}{6}$ gr
Wanted quantity   = mg
Conversion factor   = 1 gr = 60 mg

$$\frac{\frac{5}{6} \text{ gr} \mid 60 \text{ ⓜⓖ} \mid \frac{5}{6} \times 60 \mid \frac{5}{6} \times \frac{60}{1} \mid \frac{300}{6} \mid 50}{1 \text{ gr} \mid 1 \mid 1 \mid 1 \mid 1} = 50 \text{ mg}$$

4

Problem: How many mL in 3 oz?
Given quantity   = 3 oz
Wanted quantity   = mL
Conversion factor   = 1 oz = 30 mL

$$\frac{3 \text{ oz} \mid 30 \text{ ⓜⓛ} \mid 3 \times 30 \mid 90}{1 \text{ oz} \mid 1 \mid 1} = 90 \text{ mL}$$

5

Problem: 0.5 mg = How many mcg?
Given quantity   = 0.5 mg
Wanted quantity   = mcg
Conversion factor   = 1 mg = 1000 mcg

$$\frac{0.5 \text{ mg} \mid 1000 \text{ ⓜⓒⓖ} \mid 0.5 \times 1000 \mid 500}{1 \text{ mg} \mid 1 \mid 1} = 500 \text{ mcg}$$

6

Problem: 35 gtt = How many mL?
Given quantity   = 35 gtt
Wanted quantity   = mL
Conversion factor   = 1 gtt = 1 M
Conversion factor   = 15 M = 1 mL

$$\frac{35 \text{ gtt} \mid 1 \text{ M} \mid 1 \text{ ⓜⓛ} \mid 35 \times 1 \times 1 \mid 35}{1 \text{ gtt} \mid 15 \text{ M} \mid 1 \times 15 \mid 15} = 2.3 \text{ mL}$$

7

Problem: How many mL in 3 qt?
Given quantity   = 3 qt
Wanted quantity   = mL
Conversion factor   = 1 qt = 1000 mL

$$\frac{3 \text{ qt} \mid 1000 \text{ ⓜⓛ} \mid 3 \times 1000 \mid 3000}{1 \text{ qt} \mid 1 \mid 1} = 3000 \text{ mL}$$

8

Problem: 4 gal = How many qt?
Given quantity   = 4 gal
Wanted quantity   = qt
Conversion factor   = 1 gal = 4 qt

$$\frac{4 \text{ gal} \mid 4 \text{ ⓠⓣ} \mid 4 \times 4 \mid 16}{1 \text{ gal} \mid 1 \mid 1} = 16 \text{ qt}$$

9

Problem: 1.5 cup = How many mL?
Given quantity   = 1.5 cup
Wanted quantity   = mL
Conversion factor   = 1 cup = 240 mL

$$\frac{1.5 \text{ cup} \mid 240 \text{ ⓜⓛ} \mid 1.5 \times 240 \mid 360}{1 \text{ cup} \mid 1 \mid 1} = 360 \text{ mL}$$

10

Problem: 24 oz = How many cups?
Given quantity   = 24 oz
Wanted quantity   = cups
Conversion factor   = 1 cup = 8 oz

$$\frac{24 \text{ oz} \mid 1 \text{ ⓒⓤⓟ} \mid 24 \times 1 \mid 24}{8 \text{ oz} \mid 8 \mid 8} = 3 \text{ cups}$$

11

Problem: 132 lb = How many kg?
Given quantity   = 132 lb
Wanted quantity   = kg
Conversion factor   = 2.2 lb = 1 kg

$$\frac{132 \text{ lb} \mid 1 \text{ ⓚⓖ} \mid 132 \times 1 \mid 132}{2.2 \text{ lb} \mid 2.2 \mid 2.2} = 60 \text{ kg}$$

12

Problem: 70 kg = How many lb?
Given quantity   = 70 kg
Wanted quantity   = lb
Conversion factor   = 1 kg = 2.2 lb

$$\frac{70 \text{ kg}}{} \left| \frac{2.2 \text{ (lb)}}{1 \text{ kg}} \right| \frac{70 \times 2.2}{1} \left| \frac{154}{1} \right. = 154 \text{ lb}$$

13

Problem: 750 mcg = How many mg?
Given quantity   = 750 mcg
Wanted quantity   = mg
Conversion factor   = 1000 mcg = 1 mg

$$\frac{750 \text{ mcg}}{} \left| \frac{1 \text{ (mg)}}{1000 \text{ mcg}} \right| \frac{75 \times 1}{100} \left| \frac{75}{100} \right. = 0.75 \text{ mg}$$

14

Problem: 0.5 L = How many mL?
Given quantity   = 0.5 L
Wanted quantity   = mL
Conversion factor   = 1 L = 1000 mL

$$\frac{0.5 \text{ L}}{} \left| \frac{1000 \text{ (mL)}}{1 \text{ L}} \right| \frac{0.5 \times 1000}{1} \left| \frac{500}{1} \right. = 500 \text{ mL}$$

15

Problem: 1800 g = How many kg?
Given quantity   = 1800 g
Wanted quantity   = kg
Conversion factor   = 1000 g = 1 kg

$$\frac{1800 \text{ g}}{} \left| \frac{1 \text{ (kg)}}{1000 \text{ g}} \right| \frac{18 \times 1}{10} \left| \frac{18}{10} \right. = 1.8 \text{ kg}$$

16

Problem: How many qt in 6000 mL?
Given quantity   = 6000 mL
Wanted quantity   = qt
Conversion factor   = 1000 mL = 1 qt

$$\frac{6000 \text{ mL}}{} \left| \frac{1 \text{ (qt)}}{1000 \text{ mL}} \right| \frac{6000 \times 1}{1000} \left| \frac{6000}{1000} \right. = 6 \text{ qt}$$

17

Problem: 180 mL = How many oz?
Given quantity   = 180 mL
Wanted quantity   = oz
Conversion factor   = 30 mL = 1 oz

$$\frac{180 \text{ mL}}{} \left| \frac{1 \text{ (oz)}}{30 \text{ mL}} \right| \frac{18 \times 1}{3} \left| \frac{18}{3} \right. = 6 \text{ oz}$$

18

Problem: 6 dr = How many mL?
Given quantity   = 6 dr
Wanted quantity   = mL
Conversion factor   = 1 dr = 5 mL

$$\frac{6 \text{ dr}}{} \left| \frac{5 \text{ (mL)}}{1 \text{ dr}} \right| \frac{6 \times 5}{1} \left| \frac{30}{1} \right. = 30 \text{ mL}$$

19

Problem: 0.125 mg = How many mcg?
Given quantity   = 0.125 mg
Wanted quantity   = mcg
Conversion factor   = 1 mg = 1000 mcg

$$\frac{0.125 \text{ mg}}{} \left| \frac{1000 \text{ (mcg)}}{1 \text{ mg}} \right| \frac{0.125 \times 1000}{1} \left| \frac{125}{1} \right. = 125 \text{ mcg}$$

20

Problem: How many mL in 90 M?
Given quantity   = 90 M
Wanted quantity   = mL
Conversion factor   = 1 mL = 15 M

$$\frac{90 \text{ M}}{} \left| \frac{1 \text{ (mL)}}{15 \text{ M}} \right| \frac{90 \times 1}{15} \left| \frac{90}{15} \right. = 6 \text{ mL}$$

21

Problem: 145 lb = How many kg?
Given quantity   = 145 lb
Wanted quantity   = kg
Conversion factor   = 1 kg = 2.2 lb

$$\frac{145 \text{ lb}}{} \left| \frac{1 \text{ (kg)}}{2.2 \text{ lb}} \right| \frac{145 \times 1}{2.2} \left| \frac{145}{2.2} \right. = 65.9 \text{ kg}$$

22

Problem: $\frac{3}{4}$ gr = How many mg?
Given quantity   = $\frac{3}{4}$ gr
Wanted quantity   = mg
Conversion factor   = 1 gr = 60 mg

$$\frac{\frac{3}{4} \text{ gr}}{} \left| \frac{60 \text{ (mg)}}{1 \text{ gr}} \right| \frac{\frac{3}{4} \times \frac{60}{1}}{1} \left| \frac{\frac{180}{4}}{1} \right| \frac{45}{1} = 45 \text{ mg}$$

23

Problem: How many g in 1500 mg?
Given quantity   = 1500 mg
Wanted quantity   = g
Conversion factor   = 1 g = 1000 mg

$$\frac{1500 \text{ mg}}{} \left| \frac{1 \text{ (g)}}{1000 \text{ mg}} \right| \frac{1500 \times 1}{1000} \left| \frac{1500}{1000} \right. = 1.5 \text{ g}$$

24

Problem: 3 lb = How many g?
Given quantity   = 3 lb
Wanted quantity   = g
Conversion factor   = 2.2 lb = 1 kg = 1000 g

$$\frac{3 \text{ lb}}{} \left| \frac{1000 \text{ (g)}}{2.2 \text{ lb}} \right| \frac{3 \times 1000}{2.2} \left| \frac{3000}{2.2} \right. = 1363.6 \text{ g}$$

25

Problem: 0.80 mg = How many mcg?
Given quantity   = 0.80 mg
Wanted quantity   = mcg
Conversion factor   = 1 mg = 1000 mcg

$$\frac{0.80 \text{ mg}}{} \left| \frac{1000 \text{ (mcg)}}{1 \text{ mg}} \right| \frac{0.80 \times 1000}{1} \left| \frac{800}{1} \right. = 800 \text{ mcg}$$

26

Problem: $\frac{1}{150}$ gr = How many mg?

Given quantity = $\frac{1}{150}$ gr

Wanted quantity = mg

Conversion factor = 1 gr = 60 mg

$$\frac{\frac{1}{150} \text{ gr}}{} \left| \frac{60 \text{ (mg)}}{1 \text{ gr}} \right| \frac{\frac{1}{150} \times \frac{60}{1}}{1} \left| \frac{\frac{60}{150}}{1} \right| \frac{0.4}{1} = 0.4 \text{ mg}$$

27

Problem: $\frac{1}{300}$ gr = How many mg?

Given quantity = $\frac{1}{300}$ gr

Wanted quantity = mg

Conversion factor = 1 gr = 60 mg

$$\frac{\frac{1}{300} \text{ gr}}{} \left| \frac{60 \text{ (mg)}}{1 \text{ gr}} \right| \frac{\frac{1}{300} \times \frac{60}{1}}{1} \left| \frac{\frac{60}{300}}{1} \right| \frac{0.2}{1} = 0.2 \text{ mg}$$

28

Problem: How many gr in 30 mg?

Given quantity = 30 mg

Wanted quantity = gr

Conversion factor = 1 gr = 60 mg

$$\frac{30 \text{ mg}}{} \left| \frac{1 \text{ (gr)}}{60 \text{ mg}} \right| \frac{30 \times 1}{60} \left| \frac{30}{60} \right| = 1/2 \text{ gr}$$

29

Problem: How many g in 45 gr?

Given quantity = 45 gr

Wanted quantity = g

Conversion factor = 1 g = 15 gr

$$\frac{45 \text{ gr}}{} \left| \frac{1 \text{ (g)}}{15 \text{ gr}} \right| \frac{45 \times 1}{15} \left| \frac{45}{15} \right| = 3 \text{ g}$$

30

Problem: 15 mg = How many mcg?

Given quantity = 15 mg

Wanted quantity = mcg

Conversion factor = 1 mg = 1000 mcg

$$\frac{15 \text{ mg}}{} \left| \frac{1000 \text{ (mcg)}}{1 \text{ mg}} \right| \frac{15 \times 1000}{1} \left| \frac{15000}{1} \right| = 15000 \text{ mcg}$$

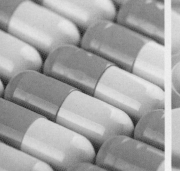
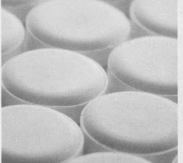

 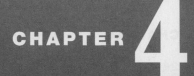
One-Factor Medication Problems

Objectives

After completing this chapter, you will successfully be able to:

1. Interpret medication orders correctly, based on the six rights of medication administration.

2. Identify components from a drug label that are needed for accurate medication administration and documentation.

3. Describe the different routes of medication administration: tablets and capsules, liquids given by medicine cup or syringe, and parenteral injections using different types of syringes.

4. Calculate medication problems accurately from the one-factor–given quantity to the one-factor–wanted quantity using the sequential or random method of dimensional analysis.

For accurate administration of medication, the six rights of medication administration form the foundation of communication between the person writing the medication order and the person reading the medication order.

The physician or nurse practitioner writes a medication order using the six rights, and the nurse administers the medication to the patient based on the six rights. There may be a slight variation in the way each person writes a medication order, but information pertaining to the six rights should be included in the medication order to ensure safe administration by the nurse and the prevention of **medication errors**.

To calculate the change from a one-factor-given quantity to a one-factor-wanted quantity using dimensional analysis, it is necessary to have a clear understanding of the six rights of medication administration. This chapter teaches you to interpret medication orders correctly and to calculate medication problems accurately using dimensional analysis.

INTERPRETATION OF MEDICATION ORDERS

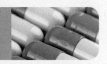

Physicians and nurse practitioners order medications using the **six rights** of medication administration, including the:

1. Right **patient**
2. Right **drug**
3. Right **dosage**
4. Right **route**
5. Right **time**
6. Right **documentation**

Right Patient

Many medication errors can be prevented by correctly identifying the **right patient**. Patients in the hospital setting wear identification bands, whereas other facilities may use a photograph to identify the **right patient**.

Regardless of the identification method, the medication order must correspond to the identification of the patient. Checking identification and asking patients to state their names assists in reducing medication errors. It is also important to "listen" to the patient. If the patient states, "I don't take a blue pill," go back and check the medication order for correctness.

Right Drug

Medications can be ordered using their **trade name** or **generic name**.
Examples:

1. Tagamet® or cimetidine
2. Cipro® or ciprofloxacin hydrochloride

It is the responsibility of the nurse to look up a medication before administration to ensure that the **right drug** is being administered.

It is the responsibility of the nurse to know the classification of the drug being administered and that the drug corresponds with the patient diagnosis. Many drugs have similar names.
Example:

1. Celebrex® (an anti-inflammatory)
2. Celexa® (an antidepressant)

It is also the responsibility of the nurse to know the side effects of the drug being administered. The nurse must be aware of any patient allergies before medication administration to ensure safety of the patient. Allergies should be clearly recorded on medication records or a patient should wear an allergy bracelet.

Because it is impossible to know all medications, the nurse can use a nursing drug reference to look up medications to ensure accuracy and prevent medication errors.

Right Dosage

Medications are available in different dosages. It is the responsibility of the nurse to ensure that the **right dosage** is administered. The pharmacy may supply the exact dosage ordered or the dosage may need to be converted using a common equivalent or calculated based on the weight of the patient. If the medication must be reconstituted, the correct diluent must be used for reconstitution. If a patient is to receive a tablet but has difficulty swallowing, the nurse must obtain an order to have the medication changed to an elixir. Medication orders are to be administered exactly in the dosage ordered. A nursing drug reference assists with preventing medication errors by supplying information regarding the dosages of medications that can be safely administered to a patient based on age and weight.

Right Route

Medications may be administered by different routes including oral (tablets, capsules, or liquid), parenteral (intradermal, subcutaneous, intramuscular, or intravenous), or cutaneous (skin and mucous membranes). Improper medication administration techniques (crushing an enteric-coated tablet, opening a capsule, or giving an injection using the wrong route) are considered medication errors. A nursing drug reference provides information regarding the routes that can be safely used to administer medication and eliminate medication errors. It is the responsibility of the nurse to use this information to safely administer the medication to the patient using the **right route**.

Right Time

Medications are ordered and need to be administered at specific times to ensure the effective absorption of the medication. Failure to administer a medication on time or failure to document the administration of a medication is a medication error of omission. Some medications are ordered before meals (ac), after meals (pc), or at bedtime. Other medications may be ordered based on frequency of time (once a day [qd],

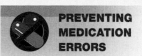

PREVENTING MEDICATION ERRORS

Medication errors can be prevented by carefully adhering to these **six rights,** understanding the important concepts that apply to each right, and utilizing a nursing drug reference to provide accurate information for each medication administered.

Once you are able to interpret the important components of a medication order, you can perform accurate calculations for the correct dosage using dimensional analysis. If you cannot correctly interpret the components of a medication order (illegible prescription order), call the physician or nurse practitioner for clarification to prevent **medication errors.**

twice a day [bid], three times a day [tid], or four times a day [qid]). A nursing drug reference provides the nurse with the appropriate information to ensure that the medication is effectively and safely administered to eliminate a medication error based on adsorption. Most facilities allow a window of administration that is usually 30 minutes before or 30 minutes after the prescribed time. It is the responsibility of the nurse to use this information to safely administer the medication to the patient at the **right time**.

Once you are able to interpret the important components of an order for medication, you can perform accurate calculations for the correct drug dosage by using dimensional analysis.

Right Documentation

Documentation is the sixth "right of medication administration" and should be completed as soon as possible after the administration of the medication. Documentation is an important right that can prevent medication errors related to over- or under-medication. The general rule of documentation is "if you didn't chart it…you didn't do it"; therefore, medication should never be charted before administration of the medication. Documentation should follow medication administration and include documentation regarding refusals, delays, and responses (including adverse effects) of medication administration.

Exercise 4.1   Interpretation of Medication Orders

(See page 107 for answers)

In the following medication orders, identify the six rights of medication administration.

1. Give gr 10 aspirin to Mrs. Anna Clark orally every 4 hours as needed for fever.

   a. Right patient   _____

   b. Right drug   _____

   c. Right dosage   _____

   d. Right route   _____

   e. Right time   _____

   f. Right documentation   _____

2. Administer PO to Mr. William Smith, Advil (ibuprofen) 400 mg every 6 hours for arthritis.

   a. Right patient   _____

   b. Right drug   _____

   c. Right dosage   _____

   d. Right route   _____

   e. Right time   _____

   f. Right documentation   _____

3. Tylenol (acetaminophen) gr 10 PO every 4 hours for Mr. Thomas Jones prn for headache.

a. Right patient   _____

b. Right drug   _____

c. Right dosage   _____

d. Right route   _____

e. Right time   _____

f. Right documentation   _____

Medication Administration Record

A Medication Administration Record or MAR is a document used to chart the administration of medication. In an effort to reduce medication errors related to misinterpretation of handwriting, many health care facilities are now using an Electronic Medication Administration Record or eMAR. Documentation must occur on the MAR after the administration of a medication as well as if a medication is not administered. If a medication is not administered, the reason that the medication was not administered must also be written on the MAR. A sample MAR will provide an opportunity to practice the sixth right of medication administration using Exercise 4.2.

Exercise 4.2   Medication Administration Record

(Answers in Exercise 4.1 f, p. 107)

Name	Medication	Date/ Time/ Route	Reason/ Effects	Initials
Mrs. Anna Clark ID# _____ Allergies: _____	Aspirin 10 gr orally every 4 hours as needed			
Mr. William Smith ID# _____ Allergies: _____	Advil (Ibuprofen) 400 mg PO every 6 hours			
Mr. Thomas Jones ID# _____ Allergies: _____	Tylenol (acetamino-phen) 10 gr PO every 4 hours PRN			

(Exercise continues on page 68)

Initials		Staff Signature			

Name	Medication	Date/ Time/ Route	Reason/ Effects		Initials

Initials		Staff Signature			

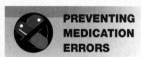

PREVENTING MEDICATION ERRORS

The **given quantity** is the **doctor's order** and should contain all **six rights** of the medication order, except documentation.

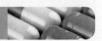

ONE-FACTOR MEDICATION PROBLEMS

Medication problems can be easily solved using the five steps of dimensional analysis:

- The first step in interpreting any physician's order for medication is to identify the **given quantity** or the exact dosage that the physician ordered.
- The second step is to identify the **wanted quantity** or the answer to the medication problem.
- The third step is to establish the **unit path** from the given quantity to the wanted quantity, using equivalents as **conversion factors** to complete the problem. Identification of the available dosage of medicine (dose on hand) is considered part of the unit path.
- The fourth step is to set up the problem to cancel out unwanted units.
- The fifth step is to multiply the numerators, multiply the denominators, and divide the product of the numerators by the product of the denominators to provide the numerical value of the **wanted quantity** or answer to the problem.

You may choose to implement either the **sequential method** or the **random method** of dimensional analysis.

The **sequential method** of dimensional analysis requires ordering and reorganizing the conversion factors into the unit path in a logical, sequential method. The sequential method requires identification of the given quantity followed by the appropriate conversion factors to allow logical progression and cancellation toward the wanted quantity, keeping in mind correct placement for cancellation. The sequential method is based on a logical process and placement of factors into the unit path. Examples 4.1 to 4.3 demonstrate the use of the sequential method of dimensional analysis.

The **random method** of dimensional analysis allows for indiscriminate placement of conversion factors into the unit path in an arbitrary, random method. The random method requires identification of the given quantity and the wanted quantity but permits individualized placement of the conversion factors into the unit path. The random method focuses on the correct placement of the conversion factor (dose on hand) in the unit path to correspond with the answer (wanted quantity). If the wanted quantity is tablets, then tablets must be in the numerator position in the unit path with the dosage in the denominator position. The random method allows for canceling of conversion factors without regard to logical, sequential placement of the conversion factors. Example 4.4 demonstrates the use of the random method of dimensional analysis.

Below is an example of a one-factor problem showing the placement of components used in dimensional analysis.

Unit Path

Given Quantity	Conversion Factor for Given Quantity	Conversion Computation	Wanted Quantity
10 gr	tablets	10	
	5 gr	5	= 2 tablets
	Conversion Factor for Wanted Quantity		

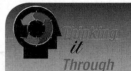

EXAMPLE 4.1

The physician orders gr 10 aspirin orally every 4 hours, as needed for fever. The unit dose of medication on hand is gr 5 per tablet (5 gr/tab).

❀ **How many tablets will you administer?**

Given quantity   = 10 gr
Wanted quantity   = tablets
Dose on hand   = gr/tablet

Step 1 Identify the *given quantity* (the physician's order).

Unit Path

Given Quantity	Conversion Factor for Given Quantity	Conversion Computation	Wanted Quantity
10 gr			=
	Conversion Factor for Wanted Quantity		

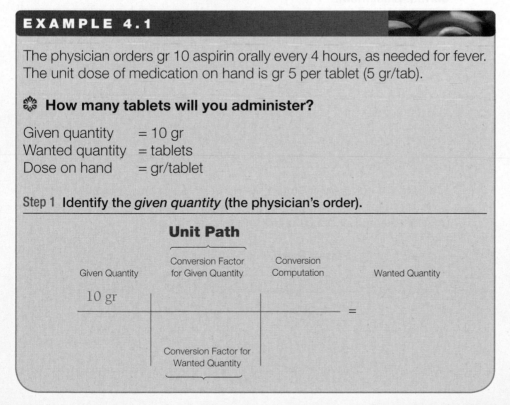

Thinking it Through

Both *10 gr* and *tablets* are numerators without a denominator. This is called a **one-factor** medication problem because the given quantity and the wanted quantity contain only numerators.

The dose on hand (5 gr/tablet) is an equivalent that is used as a conversion factor and is factored into the unit path.

The unwanted units (gr) can be canceled from the problem leaving the wanted quantity (tablets) in the numerator.

(Example continues on page 70)

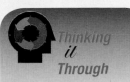

Thinking it Through

The **sequential method** of dimensional analysis has been used to factor in the dose on hand, which allows the previous unit (given quantity) to be canceled. When using the sequential method, the conversion factor that is factored in always cancels out the preceding unit.

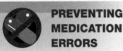

PREVENTING MEDICATION ERRORS

When preparing to administer more than two tablets or capsules to a patient, always recalculate the answer to ensure the correct answer and prevent **medication errors**. Rarely does a patient receive more than two tablets or capsules of a medication. If more than two tablets or capsules are being administered, a different dosage of the medication should be discussed with the pharmacist.

Step 2 Identify the *wanted quantity* (the answer to the problem).

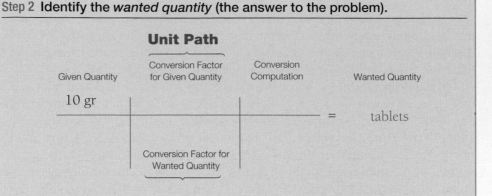

Unit Path

Given Quantity	Conversion Factor for Given Quantity	Conversion Computation	Wanted Quantity

10 gr

= tablets

Conversion Factor for Wanted Quantity

Step 3 Establish the unit path from the given quantity to the wanted quantity using equivalents as conversion factors.

Unit Path

Given Quantity	Conversion Factor for Given Quantity	Conversion Computation	Wanted Quantity

$$\frac{10 \text{ gr} \quad | \quad \text{tablets}}{5 \text{ gr}} = \text{tablets}$$

Conversion Factor for Wanted Quantity

Step 4 Set up the problem to allow cancellation of unwanted units and circle the wanted quantity within the unit path to demonstrate correct placement.

Unit Path

Given Quantity	Conversion Factor for Given Quantity	Conversion Computation	Wanted Quantity

$$\frac{10 \text{ gr} \quad | \quad \text{(tablets)}}{5 \text{ gr}} = \text{tablets}$$

Conversion Factor for Wanted Quantity

Step 5 Multiply the numerators, multiply the denominators, and divide the product of the numerators by the product of the denominators to provide the numerical value for the wanted quantity.

Unit Path

Given Quantity	Conversion Factor for Given Quantity	Conversion Computation	Wanted Quantity

$$\frac{10 \text{ gr} \quad | \quad \text{(tablets)} \quad | \quad 10}{5 \text{ gr} \quad | \quad 5} = 2 \text{ tablets}$$

Conversion Factor for Wanted Quantity

● *2 tablets is the wanted quantity and the answer to the problem.*

EXAMPLE 4.2

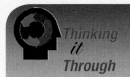

Administer PO Advil (ibuprofen) 400 mg every 6 hours for arthritis. The dosage on hand is 200 mg/tablet.

❁ **How many tablets will you give?**

Given quantity   = 400 mg
Wanted quantity = tablets
Dose on hand   = 200 mg/tablet

Step 1 Identify the *given quantity.*

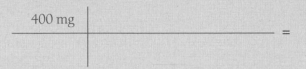

$$\frac{400 \text{ mg}}{} \quad =$$

Step 2 Identify the *wanted quantity.*

$$\frac{400 \text{ mg}}{} \quad = \text{tablets}$$

Step 3 Establish the unit path from the given quantity to the wanted quantity using equivalents as conversion factors.

$$\frac{400 \text{ mg}}{} \left| \frac{\text{tablet}}{200 \text{ mg}} \right. = \text{tablets}$$

Step 4 Set up the problem to allow cancellation of unwanted units and circle the wanted quantity within the unit path to demonstrate correct placement.

$$\frac{400 \ \cancel{\text{mg}}}{} \left| \frac{\text{(tablet)}}{200 \ \cancel{\text{mg}}} \right. = \text{tablets}$$

Step 5 Multiply the numerators, multiply the denominators, and divide the product of the numerators by the product of the denominators to provide the numerical value of the wanted quantity.

$$\frac{400 \ \cancel{\text{mg}}}{} \left| \frac{\text{(tablet)}}{200 \ \cancel{\text{mg}}} \right| \frac{4}{2} = 2 \text{ tablets}$$

● ***2 tablets is the wanted quantity and the answer to the problem.***

Thinking
it
Through

The **sequential method** of dimensional analysis has been used to set up the problem. The unwanted units (mg) have been canceled from the unit path by correctly factoring in the dose on hand (200 mg/tablet). The same number of zeroes has also been canceled from the numerator and denominator.

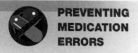

Principles of Rounding

If an answer does not result in a whole number, but instead a decimal in the tenths (4.7) or hundredths (4.75), the answer can be rounded up or down to allow for administration of the medication. Some medications may not require rounding when the exact amount of medication calculated needs to be administered.

If the tablets are scored, a half of the tablet can be administered. If a tablet is not scored, a decision must be made by the nurse whether to give one or two tablets. If a liquid medication to be administered involves decimals, then the nurse must make a decision regarding the amount of medication to be given.

If the number following the decimal is 5 or greater, then the number is rounded up.

Example in the tenths: 4.7 → 5
Example in the hundredths: 4.75 → 4.8

If the number following the decimal is less than 5, then the number is rounded down.

Example in the tenths: 4.4 → 4
Example in the hundredths: 4.42 → 4.4

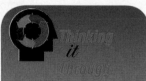

Thinking it Through

The **sequential method** of dimensional analysis has been used. The unwanted unit (gr) has been canceled by factoring in a conversion factor (1 gr = 60 mg).

The dose on hand (325 mg/caplet) is factored into the unit path, which allows the unwanted unit (mg) to be canceled.

The remaining unit (caplet) is in the numerator and correctly correlates with the wanted quantity in the numerator.

EXAMPLE 4.3

Administer Tylenol (acetaminophen) gr 10 PO every 4 hours for headache. The unit dose of medication on hand is 325 mg per caplet.

❧ **How many caplets will you give?**

Given quantity   = 10 gr
Wanted quantity   = caplets
Dose on hand   = 325 mg/caplet

Step 1   Identify the *given quantity*.

$$\frac{10 \text{ gr}}{} \quad = $$

Step 2   Identify the *wanted quantity*.

$$\frac{10 \text{ gr}}{} \quad = \text{caplets}$$

Step 3   Establish the *unit path* from the given quantity to the wanted quantity using equivalents as conversion factors.

$$\frac{10 \text{ gr}}{} \Bigg| \frac{60 \text{ mg}}{1 \text{ gr}} \Bigg| \frac{\text{caplet}}{325 \text{ mg}} = \text{caplets}$$

Step 4 Set up the problem to allow cancellation of unwanted units and circle the wanted quantity within the unit path to demonstrate correct placement.

$$\frac{10 \text{ gr}}{} \cdot \frac{60 \text{ mg}}{1 \text{ gr}} \cdot \frac{\text{caplet}}{325 \text{ mg}} = \text{caplets}$$

Step 5 Multiply the numerators, multiply the denominators, and divide the product of the numerators by the product of the denominators to provide the numerical value of the wanted quantity.

$$\frac{10 \text{ gr}}{} \cdot \frac{60 \text{ mg}}{1 \text{ gr}} \cdot \frac{\text{caplet}}{325 \text{ mg}} \cdot \frac{10 \times 60}{1 \times 325} \cdot \frac{600}{325} = 1.8 \text{ caplets}$$

1.8 caplets is the wanted quantity and the answer to the problem, but, by using the rounding rule, 2 caplets would be given.

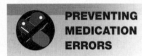

PREVENTING MEDICATION ERRORS

Following the principles of rounding, two caplets would be given as the correct dosage of medication.

Dimensional analysis is a problem-solving method that uses critical thinking, not a specific formula. Therefore, the important concept to remember is that *all* unwanted units must be canceled from the unit path. The **random method** of dimensional analysis can also be used when solving medication problems. When using the random method of dimensional analysis, the focus is on the correct placement of the conversion factor. It must correlate with the wanted quantity in the numerator portion of the unit path, without considering the preceding units.

EXAMPLE 4.4

The random method of dimensional analysis will be used to calculate the answer for Example 4.4.

Step 1 Identify the *given quantity*.

$$\frac{10 \text{ gr}}{} = $$

Step 2 Identify the *wanted quantity*.

$$\frac{10 \text{ gr}}{} = \text{caplet}$$

(Example continues on page 74)

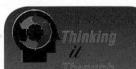

Thinking it Through

When using the random method, the focus is on the correct placement of the conversion factor to correspond with the wanted quantity. The problem is set up correctly as long as the dose on hand (caplet) correlates with the wanted quantity (caplet), both in the numerator.

A conversion factor (1 gr = 60 mg) is factored into the problem to cancel out the unwanted units (gr and mg). The remaining unit (caplet) correlates with the wanted quantity.

Step 3 Establish the *unit path* from the given quantity to the wanted quantity using equivalents as conversion factors.

$$\frac{10 \text{ gr} \quad | \quad \text{caplet}}{| \quad 325 \text{ mg}} = \text{caplet}$$

Step 4 Set up the problem to allow cancellation of unwanted units and circle the wanted quantity within the unit path to demonstrate correct placement.

$$\frac{10 \text{ gr} \quad | \quad \boxed{\text{caplet}} \quad | \quad 60 \text{ mg}}{| \quad 325 \text{ mg} \quad | \quad 1 \text{ gr}} = \text{caplet}$$

Step 5 Multiply the numerators, multiply the denominators, and divide the product of the numerators by the product of the denominators to provide the numerical value of the wanted quantity.

$$\frac{10 \text{ gr} \quad | \quad \boxed{\text{caplet}} \quad | \quad 60 \text{ mg} \quad | \quad 10 \times 60 \quad | \quad 600}{| \quad 325 \text{ mg} \quad | \quad 1 \text{ gr} \quad | \quad 325 \times 1 \quad | \quad 325} = 1.8 \text{ caplets}$$

⬤ *1.8 caplets is the wanted quantity and the answer to the problem, but, by using the rounding rule, 2 caplets would be given.*

Exercise 4.3   One-Factor Medication Problems
(See page 107 for answers)

1. The physician orders Achromycin (tetracycline) 0.25 g PO every 12 hours for acne. The dosage of medication on hand is 250 mg per capsule.

   ▶ **How many capsules will you give?** _____

2. Administer phenobarbital gr ½ PO tid for sedation. The dosage on hand is 15 mg/tablet.

   ▶ **How many tablets will you give?** _____

3. Give 0.5 g Diuril PO bid for hypertension. Unit dose is 500 mg per tablet.

   ▶ **How many tablets will you give?** _____

4. Order: Restoril 0.03 g PO at bedtime for sedation. Supply: Restoril 30-mg capsules.

   ▶ **How many capsules will you give?** _____

5. Order: Thorazine gr ½ PO tid for singultus. Supply: Thorazine 30-mg capsules.

   ▶ **How many capsules will you give?** _____

COMPONENTS OF A DRUG LABEL

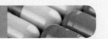

All medications (stock and unit dose) are labeled with a drug label that includes specific information to assist in the accurate administration of the medication.

Identifying the Components

Information on the drug label includes:

- Name of the drug, including the trade name (name given by the pharmaceutical company identified with a trademark symbol) and the generic name (chemical name given to the drug)
- Dosage of medication (the amount of medication in each tablet, capsule, or liquid)
- Form of medication (tablet, capsule, or liquid)
- Expiration date (how long the medication will remain stable and safe to administer)
- Lot number or batch number (the manufacturer's batch series for this medication)
- Manufacturer (the pharmaceutical company that produced the medication)

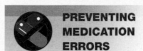
PREVENTING MEDICATION ERRORS

Before administering any medication, the nurse should check the expiration date on the label. Administering a medication that has expired would be considered a **medication error**.

EXAMPLE 4.5

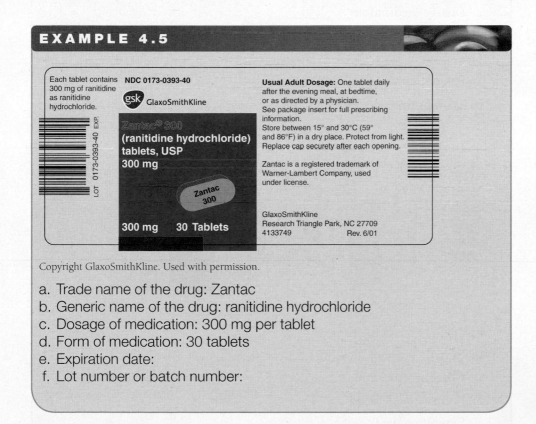

Each tablet contains 300 mg of ranitidine as ranitidine hydrochloride.

NDC 0173-0393-40

gsk GlaxoSmithKline

Zantac® 300
(ranitidine hydrochloride) tablets, USP
300 mg

Zantac 300

300 mg   30 Tablets

LOT 0173-0393-40 EXP.

Usual Adult Dosage: One tablet daily after the evening meal, at bedtime, or as directed by a physician.
See package insert for full prescribing information.
Store between 15° and 30°C (59° and 86°F) in a dry place. Protect from light. Replace cap securely after each opening.

Zantac is a registered trademark of Warner-Lambert Company, used under license.

GlaxoSmithKline
Research Triangle Park, NC 27709
4133749   Rev. 6/01

Copyright GlaxoSmithKline. Used with permission.

a. Trade name of the drug: Zantac
b. Generic name of the drug: ranitidine hydrochloride
c. Dosage of medication: 300 mg per tablet
d. Form of medication: 30 tablets
e. Expiration date:
f. Lot number or batch number:

Exercise 4.4   Identifying the Components of Drug Labels

(See pages 107–108 for answers)

1.

DESCRIPTION: Each tablet contains ciprofloxacin hydrochloride equivalent to 500 mg of ciprofloxacin.
DOSAGE: See accompanying literature for complete information on dosage and administration.
RECOMMENDED STORAGE: Store below 86°F (30°C).
Batch:
Expires:

851310   NDC 0026-8513-51

CIPRO®

(ciprofloxacin hydrochloride)

Equivalent to
500 mg ciprofloxacin
100 Tablets

Caution: Federal (USA) law prohibits dispensing without a prescription.

Bayer

Bayer Corporation
Pharmaceutical Division
400 Morgan Lane
West Haven, CT 06516

4743
©1995 Bayer Corporation
Printed in USA
PL500002
6505-01-333-4154
3 0026-8513-51 0

Courtesy of Bayer Corporation Pharmaceutical Division.

a. Trade name of the drug _____

b. Generic name of the drug _____

c. Dosage medication _____

d. Form of medication _____

e. Expiration date _____

f. Batch number _____

g. Manufacturer _____

2.

Store at 15° to 25°C (59° to 77°F) and protect from moisture.
Do not use if printed safety seal under cap is broken or missing.
Dispense in a tight container as defined in the USP.
See prescribing information for dosage information.

100 Tablets   NDC 0173-0949-55

ZOVIRAX® (acyclovir)
Tablets

Each tablet contains

400 mg

R_x only

gsk GlaxoSmithKline

GlaxoSmithKline
Research Triangle Park, NC 27709
Made in India
10000000076613   Rev. 1/10

3 0173-0949-55 4
A076613

Copyright GlaxoSmithKline. Used with permission.

a. Trade name of the drug _____

b. Generic name of the drug _____

c. Dosage medication _____

d. Form of medication _____

e. Expiration date _____

f. Batch number _____

g. Manufacturer _____

3.

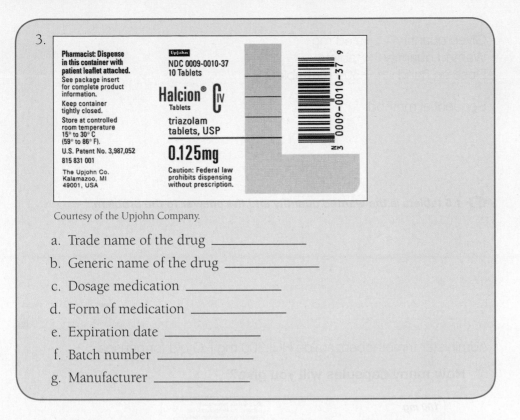

Courtesy of the Upjohn Company.

a. Trade name of the drug _____

b. Generic name of the drug _____

c. Dosage medication _____

d. Form of medication _____

e. Expiration date _____

f. Batch number _____

g. Manufacturer _____

Solving Problems With Components of Drug Labels

Once you are able to identify the components of a drug label, you can use critical thinking to solve problems with dimensional analysis.

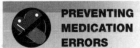

EXAMPLE 4.6

The physician orders Cipro 750 mg PO every 12 hours for a bacterial infection.

❈ **How many tablets will you give?**

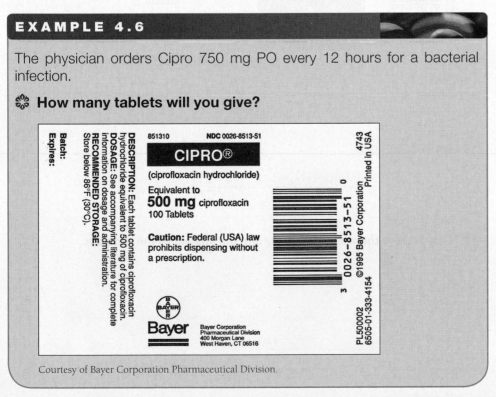

Courtesy of Bayer Corporation Pharmaceutical Division.

PREVENTING MEDICATION ERRORS

The wanted quantity and the answer to the problem is 1.5 tablets. A scored tablet can be cut in half, allowing the exact dosage to be administered. To prevent medication errors, always check with a pharmacist before altering the form of any medication.

(Example continues on page 78)

Given quantity = 750 mg
Wanted quantity = tablets
Dose on hand = 500 mg/tablet

Sequential method:

$$\frac{750 \text{ mg} \quad \boxed{\text{tablet}} \quad 75}{500 \text{ mg} \quad | \quad 50} = 1.5 \text{ tablets}$$

● **1.5 tablets is the wanted quantity and the answer to the problem.**

EXAMPLE 4.7

Administer trimethobenzamide HCl 200 mg PO qid for nausea.

❀ **How many capsules will you give?**

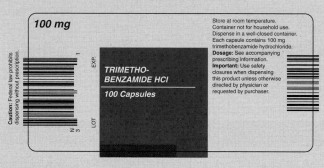

100 mg

Store at room temperature.
Container not for household use.
Dispense in a well-closed container.
Each capsule contains 100 mg
trimethobenzamide hydrochloride.
Dosage: See accompanying
prescribing information.
Important: Use safety
closures when dispensing
this product unless otherwise
directed by physician or
requested by purchaser.

Caution: Federal law prohibits
dispensing without prescription.

EXP.

LOT

**TRIMETHO-
BENZAMIDE HCl**

100 Capsules

Given quantity = 200 mg
Wanted quantity = capsules
Dose on hand = 100 mg/capsules

Sequential method:

$$\frac{200 \text{ mg} \quad \boxed{\text{capsules}} \quad 2}{100 \text{ mg} \quad | \quad 1} = 2 \text{ capsules}$$

● **2 capsules is the wanted quantity and the answer to the problem.**

EXAMPLE 4.8

Order: Halcion 0.25 mg PO at bedtime prn.

✺ **How many tablets will you give?**

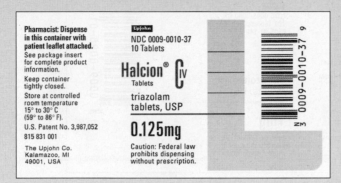

Pharmacist: Dispense in this container with patient leaflet attached.
See package insert for complete product information.
Keep container tightly closed.
Store at controlled room temperature 15° to 30° C (59° to 86° F).
U.S. Patent No. 3,987,052
815 831 001
The Upjohn Co.
Kalamazoo, MI
49001, USA

Upjohn
NDC 0009-0010-37
10 Tablets

Halcion® C IV
Tablets
triazolam tablets, USP

0.125mg

Caution: Federal law prohibits dispensing without prescription.

Courtesy of the Upjohn Company.

Given quantity   = 0.25 mg
Wanted quantity = tablets
Dose on hand   = 0.125 mg/tablet

Sequential method:

$$\frac{0.25 \text{ mg}}{} \left| \frac{\text{tablet}}{0.125 \text{ mg}} \right| \frac{0.25}{0.125} = 2 \text{ tablets}$$

● **2 tablets is the wanted quantity and the answer to the problem.**

Exercise 4.5 **Problems With Components of Drug Labels**

(See page 108 for answers)

1. Order: methylphenidate 10 mg PO before breakfast and lunch for attention-deficit hyperactivity disorder (ADHD)

▶ **How many tablets will you give?** _____

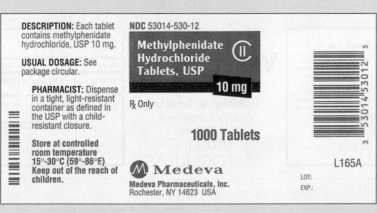

DESCRIPTION: Each tablet contains methylphenidate hydrochloride, USP 10 mg.

USUAL DOSAGE: See package circular.

PHARMACIST: Dispense in a tight, light-resistant container as defined in the USP with a child-resistant closure.

Store at controlled room temperature 15°-30°C (59°-86°F) Keep out of the reach of children.

NDC 53014-530-12

Methylphenidate Hydrochloride Tablets, USP C II
10 mg
℞ Only

1000 Tablets

Ⓜ **Medeva**
Medeva Pharmaceuticals, Inc.
Rochester, NY 14623 USA

L165A

LOT:
EXP.:

Courtesy of Medeva Pharmaceuticals.

(Exercise continues on page 80)

2. Order: Xanax 500 mcg PO bid for anxiety

▶ **How many tablets will you give?** _____

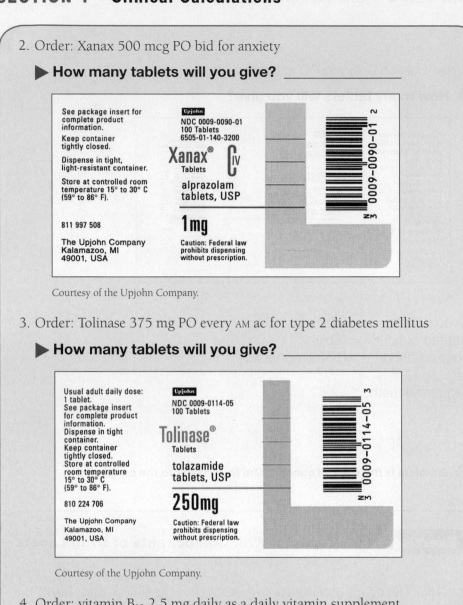

See package insert for complete product information.

Keep container tightly closed.

Dispense in tight, light-resistant container.

Store at controlled room temperature 15° to 30° C (59° to 86° F).

811 997 508

The Upjohn Company
Kalamazoo, MI
49001, USA

Upjohn
NDC 0009-0090-01
100 Tablets
6505-01-140-3200

Xanax® C IV
Tablets

alprazolam
tablets, USP

1mg

Caution: Federal law prohibits dispensing without prescription.

0009-0090-01 2

Courtesy of the Upjohn Company.

3. Order: Tolinase 375 mg PO every AM ac for type 2 diabetes mellitus

▶ **How many tablets will you give?** _____

Usual adult daily dose: 1 tablet.
See package insert for complete product information.
Dispense in tight container.
Keep container tightly closed.
Store at controlled room temperature 15° to 30° C (59° to 86° F).

810 224 706

The Upjohn Company
Kalamazoo, MI
49001, USA

Upjohn
NDC 0009-0114-05
100 Tablets

Tolinase®
Tablets

tolazamide
tablets, USP

250mg

Caution: Federal law prohibits dispensing without prescription.

0009-0114-05 3

Courtesy of the Upjohn Company.

4. Order: vitamin B_{12} 2.5 mg daily as a daily vitamin supplement

▶ **How many tablets will you give?** _____

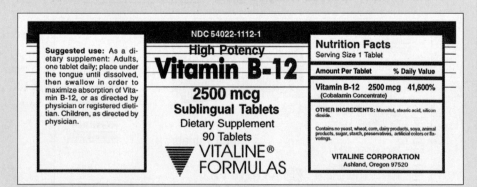

Suggested use: As a dietary supplement: Adults, one tablet daily; place under the tongue until dissolved, then swallow in order to maximize absorption of Vitamin B-12, or as directed by physician or registered dietitian. Children, as directed by physician.

NDC 54022-1112-1

High Potency
Vitamin B-12

2500 mcg
Sublingual Tablets
Dietary Supplement
90 Tablets

▼ **VITALINE®**
FORMULAS

Nutrition Facts
Serving Size 1 Tablet

Amount Per Tablet	% Daily Value
Vitamin B-12 2500 mcg 41,600%	
(Cobalamin Concentrate)	

OTHER INGREDIENTS: Mannitol, stearic acid, silicon dioxide.

Contains no yeast, wheat, corn, dairy products, soya, animal products, sugar, starch, preservatives, artificial colors or flavorings.

VITALINE CORPORATION
Ashland, Oregon 97520

Courtesy of Vitaline Corporation.

5. Order: trimethobenzamide HCl 250 mg PO qid prn for nausea

▶ **How many capsules will you give?** _____

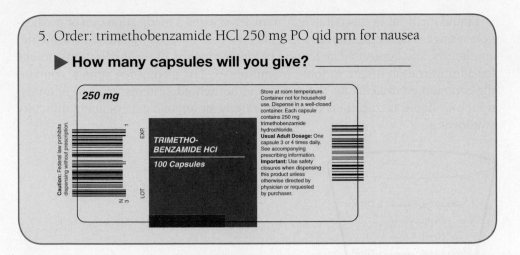

250 mg

TRIMETHO-
BENZAMIDE HCl

100 Capsules

Store at room temperature.
Container not for household
use. Dispense in a well-closed
container. Each capsule
contains 250 mg
trimethobenzamide
hydrochloride.
Usual Adult Dosage: One
capsule 3 or 4 times daily.
See accompanying
prescribing information.
Important: Use safety
closures when dispensing
this product unless
otherwise directed by
physician or requested
by purchaser.

ADMINISTERING MEDICATION BY DIFFERENT ROUTES

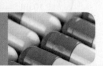

Medication may be administered by various routes, including oral, parenteral, or intravenous, involving tablets, capsules, caplets or liquid.

Enteral Medications

Oral (PO) medications are administered using tablets, caplets, capsules, or liquid. Tablets and caplets may be scored, which permits a more accurate administration when one fourth or one half of a tablet must be given.

Tablets and caplets may also be enteric coated, which allows the medication to bypass disintegration in the stomach to decrease irritation, and then later break down in the small intestine for absorption. Enteric-coated tablets and caplets should never be crushed, because such medications irritate the stomach.

Capsules are usually of the time-release type, and these should never be crushed or opened because the medication would be immediately released into the system, instead of being released slowly over time.

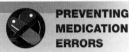
PREVENTING MEDICATION ERRORS

Crushing enteric-coated tablets and caplets would be considered a **medication error** because the nurse did not administer the medication using the **right route**. The patient could suffer erosion of the esophagus or stomach resulting in a bleeding ulcer. **Aspirin** is an example of a medication that is enteric-coated to prevent erosion of gastrointestinal tissue.

PREVENTING MEDICATION ERRORS

Opening capsules and adding the medication to applesauce or pudding would also be considered a **medication error** because the nurse did not administer the medication using the **right route**. The patient could receive an incorrect dosage of the medication as the medication quickly enters the gastrointestinal system.

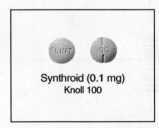

Synthroid (0.1 mg)
Knoll 100

Tablets: note scored tablet on right.

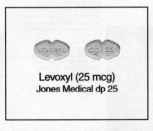

Levoxyl (25 mcg)
Jones Medical dp 25

Caplets: note scored caplet on right.

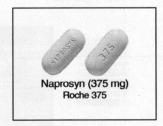

Naprosyn (375 mg)
Roche 375

Enteric-coated caplets.

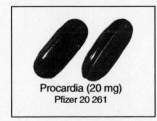

Procardia (20 mg)
Pfizer 20 261

Capsules.

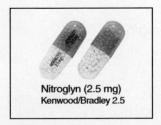

Nitroglyn (2.5 mg)
Kenwood/Bradley 2.5

Controlled-release capsules.

Liquid medication is accurately administered using a medication cup or medication syringe. The medication cup contains the common equivalents for the metric, apothecary, and household systems to permit adaptation of the medication's dosage for administration under various circumstances. The medication syringe contains the common equivalents for the metric and household systems to allow administration of liquid medications to infants, elderly, or anyone experiencing difficulty swallowing.

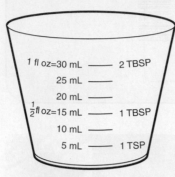

1 fl oz=30 mL ——— 2 TBSP
25 mL ———
20 mL ———
$\frac{1}{2}$ fl oz=15 mL ——— 1 TBSP
10 mL ———
5 mL ——— 1 TSP

Medication cup

Medication syringe

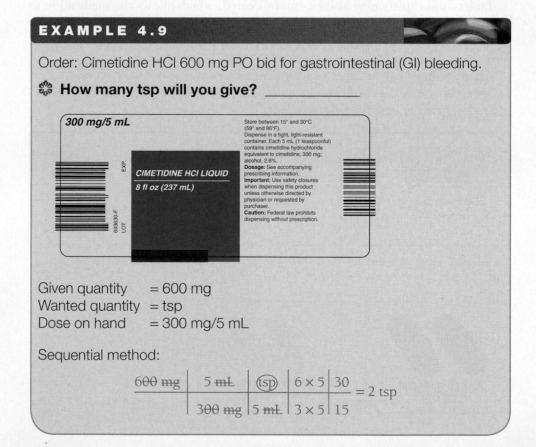

EXAMPLE 4.9

Order: Cimetidine HCl 600 mg PO bid for gastrointestinal (GI) bleeding.

❀ **How many tsp will you give?** _____

300 mg/5 mL

CIMETIDINE HCl LIQUID
8 fl oz (237 mL)

Store between 15° and 30°C (59° and 86°F).
Dispense in a tight, light-resistant container. Each 5 mL (1 teaspoonful) contains cimetidine hydrochloride equivalent to cimetidine, 300 mg; alcohol, 2.8%.
Dosage: See accompanying prescribing information.
Important: Use safety closures when dispensing this product unless otherwise directed by physician or requested by purchaser.
Caution: Federal law prohibits dispensing without prescription.

Given quantity   = 600 mg
Wanted quantity   = tsp
Dose on hand   = 300 mg/5 mL

Sequential method:

$$\frac{600\ \text{mg}}{} \quad \frac{5\ \text{mL}}{300\ \text{mg}} \quad \frac{\text{tsp}}{5\ \text{mL}} \quad \frac{6 \times 5}{3 \times 5} \quad \frac{30}{15} = 2\ \text{tsp}$$

● **2 tsp is the wanted quantity and the answer to the problem.**

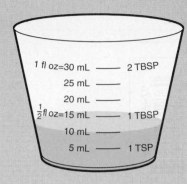

EXAMPLE 4.10

Order: Prochlorperazine 10 mg PO qid for psychomotor agitation.

✿ **How many mL will you give?** _____

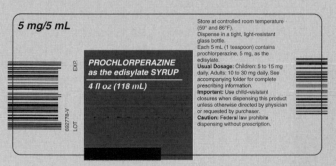

5 mg/5 mL

Store at controlled room temperature (59° and 86°F).
Dispense in a tight, light-resistant glass bottle.
Each 5 mL (1 teaspoon) contains prochlorperazine, 5 mg, as the edisylate.
Usual Dosage: Children: 5 to 15 mg daily. Adults: 10 to 30 mg daily. See accompanying folder for complete prescribing information.
Important: Use child-resistant closures when dispensing this product unless otherwise directed by physician or requested by purchaser.
Caution: Federal law prohibits dispensing without prescription.

PROCHLORPERAZINE
as the edisylate SYRUP
4 fl oz (118 mL)

Given quantity   = 10 mg
Wanted quantity   = mL
Dose on hand   = 5 mg/5 mL

Sequential method:

$$\frac{10 \text{ mg}}{} \cdot \frac{5 \text{ mL}}{5 \text{ mg}} \cdot \frac{10}{} = 10 \text{ mL}$$

● **10 mL is the wanted quantity and the answer to the problem.**

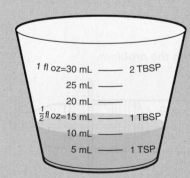

EXAMPLE 4.11

Order: Tegretol 100 mg PO qid for convulsions.

�֍ **How many tsp will you give?** _____

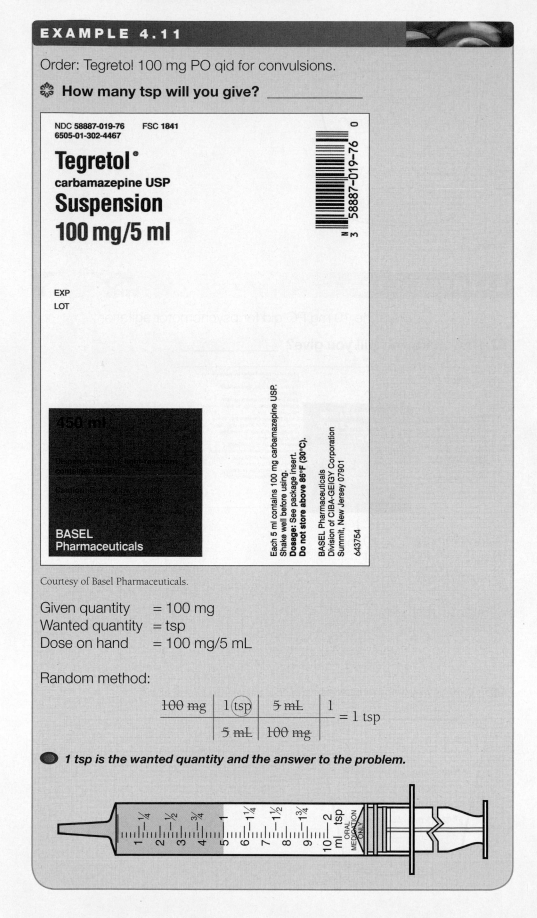

NDC 58887-019-76   FSC 1841
6505-01-302-4467

Tegretol®
carbamazepine USP
Suspension
100 mg/5 ml

EXP

LOT

450 ml

Dispense in tight, light-resistant
container (USP).

Caution: Federal law prohibits
dispensing without prescription.

BASEL
Pharmaceuticals

Each 5 ml contains 100 mg carbamazepine USP.
Shake well before using.
Dosage: See package insert.
Do not store above 86°F (30°C).

BASEL Pharmaceuticals
Division of CIBA-GEIGY Corporation
Summit, New Jersey 07901

643754

Courtesy of Basel Pharmaceuticals.

Given quantity   = 100 mg
Wanted quantity   = tsp
Dose on hand   = 100 mg/5 mL

Random method:

$$\frac{\cancel{100\ mg}}{} \left| \frac{1\ \text{(tsp)}}{5\ \cancel{mL}} \right| \frac{5\ \cancel{mL}}{100\ \cancel{mg}} \left| \frac{1}{} \right. = 1\ \text{tsp}$$

⬤ *1 tsp is the wanted quantity and the answer to the problem.*

Exercise 4.6 **Administering Enteral Medications**

(See page 108 for answers)

1. Order: phenobarbital gr ½ PO daily for convulsions

   On hand: 20 mg/5 mL

   ▶ **How many mL will you give?** _____

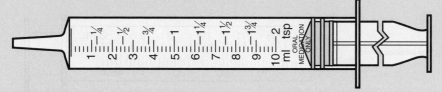

2. Order: Zantac 0.15 g PO bid for ulcers

   On hand: 15 mg/mL

   ▶ **How many tsp will you give?** _____

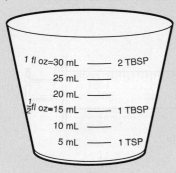

3. Order: Dilaudid 3 mg PO every 3 hours prn for pain

   On hand: Dilaudid Liquid 1 mg/mL

   ▶ **How many mL will you give?** _____

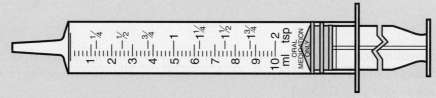

4. Order: lactulose 20 g PO tid for hepatic encephalopathy

   On hand: lactulose 10 g/15 mL

   ▶ **How many oz will you give?** _____

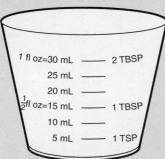

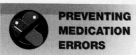
Parenteral Medications

Medications may also be ordered by the physician for the parenteral route of administration, including subcutaneous (SQ), intramuscular (IM), and intravenous (IV). Parenteral medications are sterile solutions obtained from vials or ampules and are administered using a syringe or prefilled syringes. The three syringes most often used are:

1. 3-mL syringe (used for a variety of medications requiring administration of doses from 0.2 to 3 mL).

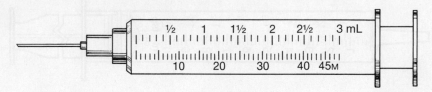

3-mL syringe

2. Insulin syringe (used specifically to administer insulin). Two types are illustrated below. **A.** 0.5-mL low-dose syringe for U-100 insulin and **B.** 1-mL syringe for U-100 insulin.

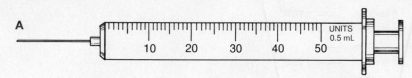

0.5-mL low-dose syringe

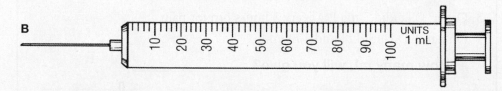

1-mL syringe

3. Tuberculin syringe (used for a variety of medications requiring administration of doses from 0.1 to 1 mL). Marked in hundredths to allow for rounding or exact dosage (e.g., 0.75 mL).

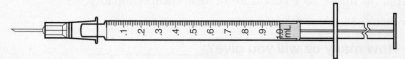

Tuberculin syringe

EXAMPLE 4.12

Order: Trimethobenzamide 100 mg IM qid for nausea.

✿ **How many mL will you give?** _____

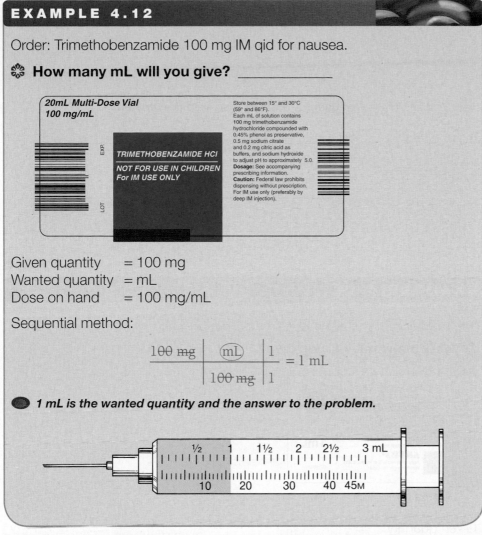

Given quantity   = 100 mg
Wanted quantity = mL
Dose on hand   = 100 mg/mL

Sequential method:

$$\frac{100\ \text{mg}}{} \quad \frac{\boxed{\text{mL}}}{100\ \text{mg}} \quad \frac{1}{1} = 1\ \text{mL}$$

⬤ *1 mL is the wanted quantity and the answer to the problem.*

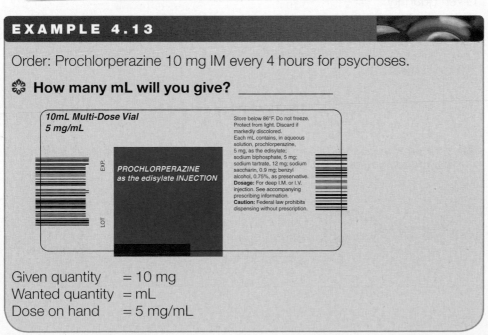

EXAMPLE 4.13

Order: Prochlorperazine 10 mg IM every 4 hours for psychoses.

✿ **How many mL will you give?** _____

10mL Multi-Dose Vial
5 mg/mL

PROCHLORPERAZINE
as the edisylate INJECTION

Store below 86°F. Do not freeze.
Protect from light. Discard if
markedly discolored.
Each mL contains, in aqueous
solution, prochlorperazine,
5 mg, as the edisylate;
sodium biphosphate, 5 mg;
sodium tartrate, 12 mg; sodium
saccharin, 0.9 mg; benzyl
alcohol, 0.75%, as preservative.
Dosage: For deep I.M. or I.V.
injection. See accompanying
prescribing information.
Caution: Federal law prohibits
dispensing without prescription.

Given quantity   = 10 mg
Wanted quantity = mL
Dose on hand   = 5 mg/mL

(Example continues on page 88)

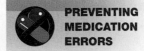

PREVENTING MEDICATION ERRORS

The nurse needs to be familiar with the different types of anticoagulants (heparin, Warfarin, and Coumadin) to ensure patient safety and prevent **medication errors**. The nurse needs to know which laboratory value to monitor (PT, PTT, INR) and which antidote (protamine sulfate or vitamin K) to have available for emergencies.

Heparin is an anticoagulant that is used to decrease the clotting ability of the blood and help prevent harmful clots from forming in the blood vessels. Although heparin is commonly referred to as a blood thinner, it does not dissolve blood clots that have already formed. Heparin may help prevent blood clots from becoming larger and causing more serious problems to the heart or lungs.

Heparin is administered using a tuberculin syringe, which is calibrated from 0.1 to 1 mL. This allows for more accurate administration of medication dosages of less than 1 mL.

Sequential method:

$$\frac{10\ \text{mg}}{} \left|\ \frac{\boxed{\text{mL}}}{5\ \text{mg}}\ \right|\ \frac{10}{5} = 2\ \text{mL}$$

⬤ *2 mL is the wanted quantity and the answer to the problem.*

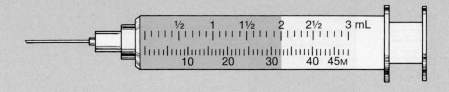

EXAMPLE 4.14

Order: morphine sulfate, $\frac{1}{4}$ gr every 4 hours prn for pain.

✻ **How many mL will you give?** _____

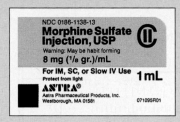

NDC 0186-1138-13
**Morphine Sulfate
Injection, USP** Ⓒ
Warning: May be habit forming
8 mg (¹/₈ gr.)/mL
For IM, SC, or Slow IV Use **1 mL**
Protect from light
ANTRA®
Astra Pharmaceutical Products, Inc.
Westborough, MA 01581   071095R01

Courtesy of Astra Pharmaceutical Products.

Given quantity $= \frac{1}{4}$ gr
Wanted quantity $=$ mL
Dose on hand $= 8$ mg/mL or $\frac{1}{8}$ gr/mL

Random method:

$$\frac{\frac{1}{4}\ \text{gr}}{8\ \text{mg}}\ \left|\ \frac{\boxed{\text{mL}}}{1\ \text{gr}}\ \right|\ \frac{60\ \text{mg}}{8 \times 1}\ \left|\ \frac{\frac{1}{4} \times \frac{60}{1}}{8}\ \right|\ \frac{\frac{60}{4}}{8}\ \right|\ \frac{15}{8} = 1.87\ \text{mL or } 1.9\ \text{mL}$$

⬤ *1.87 mL is the wanted quantity and the answer to the problem, but, by using the rounding rule, 1.9 mL would be given.*

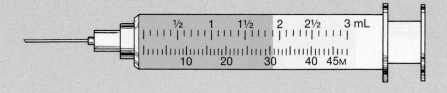

EXAMPLE 4.15

Order: NPH human insulin 20 units SQ every AM for type 1 diabetes mellitus.

❁ **How many units will you give?** _____

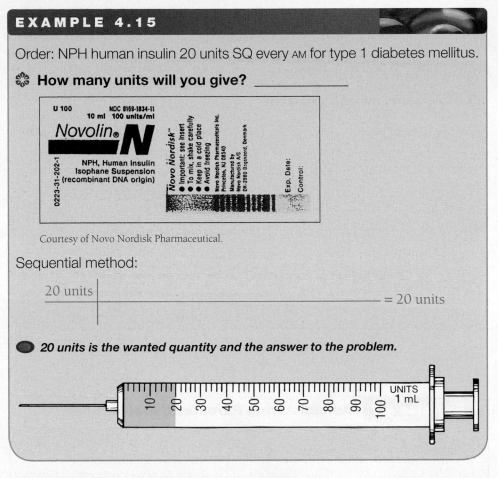

Courtesy of Novo Nordisk Pharmaceutical.

Sequential method:

$$\frac{20 \text{ units}}{} \text{————————————} = 20 \text{ units}$$

⬤ *20 units is the wanted quantity and the answer to the problem.*

EXAMPLE 4.16

Order: NPH human insulin 45 units SQ every AM for type 1 diabetes mellitus.

❁ **How many units will you give?** _____

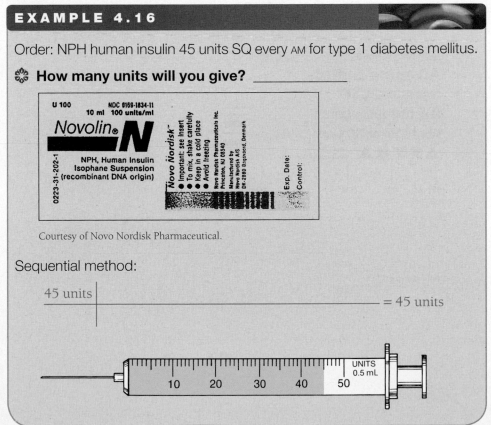

Courtesy of Novo Nordisk Pharmaceutical.

Sequential method:

$$\frac{45 \text{ units}}{} \text{————————————} = 45 \text{ units}$$

EXAMPLE 4.17

Order: heparin 5000 units SQ bid for prevention of thrombi.

On hand: heparin 10,000 units/mL.

❀ **How many mL will you give?** _____

Sequential method:

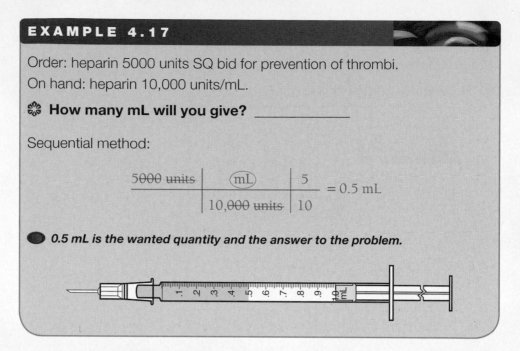

$$\frac{5000\ \text{units}}{} \times \frac{\text{mL}}{10{,}000\ \text{units}} \times \frac{5}{10} = 0.5\ \text{mL}$$

● *0.5 mL is the wanted quantity and the answer to the problem.*

Exercise 4.7   Administering Parenteral Medications

(See page 109 for answers)

1. Order: atropine sulfate 300 mcg IM for preoperative medication.

   ▶ **How many mL will you give?** _____

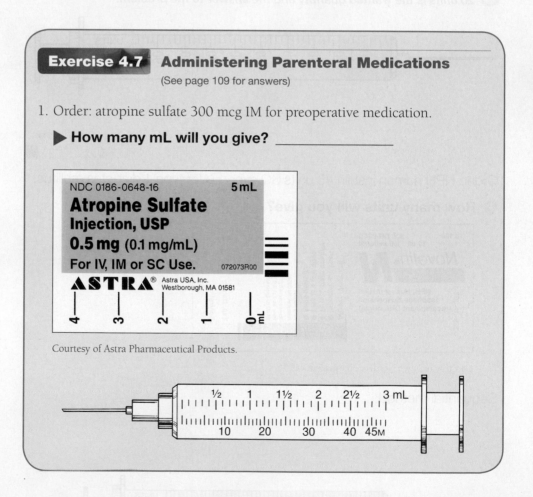

NDC 0186-0648-16   5 mL

Atropine Sulfate
Injection, USP
0.5 mg (0.1 mg/mL)
For IV, IM or SC Use.   072073R00

ASTRA® Astra USA, Inc.
Westborough, MA 01581

4   3   2   1   0 mL

Courtesy of Astra Pharmaceutical Products.

2. Order: hydromorphone 3 mg IM every 4 hours for pain.

▶ **How many mL will you give?** _____

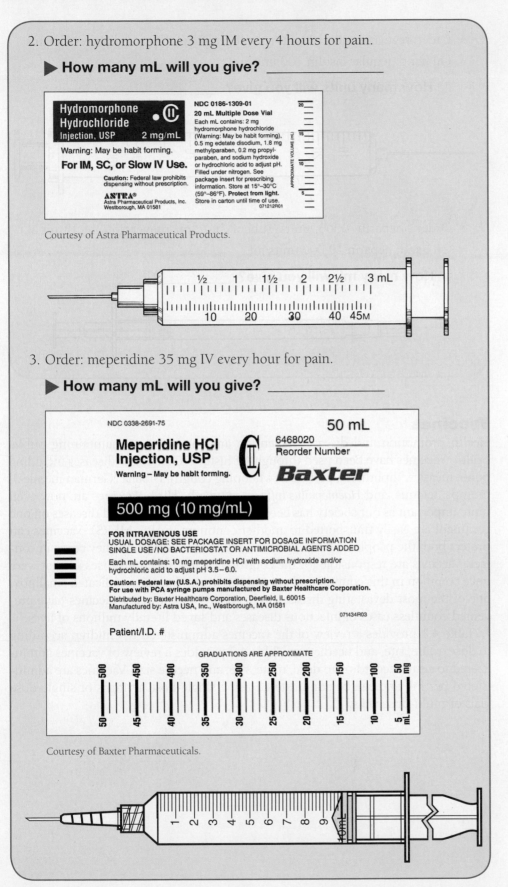

Courtesy of Astra Pharmaceutical Products.

3. Order: meperidine 35 mg IV every hour for pain.

▶ **How many mL will you give?** _____

Courtesy of Baxter Pharmaceuticals.

(Exercise continues on page 92)

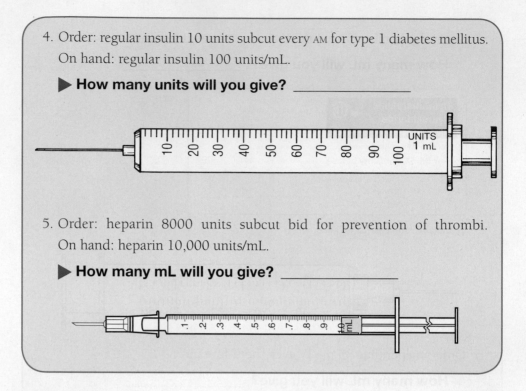

4. Order: regular insulin 10 units subcut every AM for type 1 diabetes mellitus. On hand: regular insulin 100 units/mL.

▶ **How many units will you give?** _____

5. Order: heparin 8000 units subcut bid for prevention of thrombi. On hand: heparin 10,000 units/mL.

▶ **How many mL will you give?** _____

Vaccines

Health promotion and disease prevention are important to maintaining public health. Vaccines have been used throughout history to eradicate diseases including polio, measles, diphtheria, pertussis (whooping cough), rubella (German measles), mumps, tetanus, and *Haemophilus influenzae* type b (Hib). Vaccines are now even more important as our society has become increasingly mobile and diseases on one continent are easily transported to another continent (SARS, MERS). Vaccines can protect both the people who receive them and those with whom they come in contact. Vaccines are responsible for the control of many infectious diseases that were once common in this country and around the world. Vaccine eradicated smallpox, one of the most devastating diseases in history. Over the years vaccines have prevented countless cases of infectious diseases and saved literally millions of lives.

Table 4.1 provides a review of the vaccines administered to children according to dose, route, site, and needle size. Table 4.2 provides a review of vaccines administered to adults according to dose, route, site, and needle size. Vaccines are administered per mL and can be administered using single-dose syringes or single-dose vials or multi-dose vials.

TABLE 4.1	Administering Vaccines to Children: Dose, Route, Site, and Needle Size

Vaccine	Dose	Route
Diphtheria, Tetanus, Pertussis (DTaP, DT, Tdap, Td)	0.5 mL	IM
Haemophilus influenzae **type b** (Hib)	0.5 mL	IM
Hepatitis A (HepA)	≤18 yrs; 0.5 mL	IM
	≥19 yrs; 1.0 mL	
Hepatitis B (HepB) *Persons 11–15 yrs may be given Recombivax HB (Merck) 1.0 mL adult formulation on a 2-dose schedule.*	<19yrs: 0.5 mL ≥20 yrs: 1.0 mL	IM
Human papillomavirus (HPV)	0.5 mL	IM
Influenza, live attenuated (LAIV)	0.2 mL	Intranasal spray
Influenza, trivalent inactivated (TIV)	6–35 mos: 0.25 mL	IM
	≥3 yrs: 0.5 mL	
TIV: Fluzone intradermal (18–64 yrs)	0.1 mL	ID
Measles, Mumps, Rubella (MMR)	0.5 mL	SC
Meningococcal conjugate (MCV)	0.5 mL	IM
Meningococcal polysaccharide (MPSV)	0.5 mL	SC
Pneumococcal conjugate (PCV)	0.5 mL	IM
Pneumococcal polysaccharide (PPSV)	0.5 mL	IM or SC
Polio, inactivated (IPV)	0.5 mL	IM or SC
Rotavirus (RV)	Rotarix: 1.0 mL	Oral
	Rotateq: 2.0 mL	
Varicella (Var)	0.5 mL	SC
Zoster (Zos)	0.65 mL	SC
Combination Vaccines		
DTaP-HepB-IPV (Pediarix) DTaP-IPV/Hib (Pentacel) DTaP-IPV (Kinrix) Hib-HepB (Comvax)	0.5 mL	IM
MMRV (ProQuad)	≤12 yrs: 0.5 mL	SC
HepA-HepB (Twinrix)	≥18 yrs: 1.0 mL	IM

Injection Site and Needle Size

Subcutaneous (SC) injection
Use a 23–25-gauge needle. Choose the injection site that is appropriate to the person's age and body mass.

Age	Needle Length	Injection Site
Infants (1–12 mos)	⅝"	Fatty tissue over anterolateral thigh muscle
Children 12 mos or older, adolescents, and adults	⅝"	Fatty tissue over anterolateral thigh muscle or fatty tissue over triceps

Intramuscular (IM) injection
Use a 22–25-gauge needle. Choose the injection site and needle length appropriate to the person's age and body mass.

Age	Needle Length	Injection Site
Newborns (first 28 days)	⅝"*	Anterolateral thigh muscle
Infants (1–12 mos)	1"	Anterolateral thigh muscle
Toddlers (1–2 yrs)	1–1¼" ⅝–1"*	Anterolateral thigh muscle or deltoid muscle of arm
Children and teens (3–18 yrs)	⅝–1"* 1"–1¼"	Deltoid muscle of arm or anterolateral thigh muscle
Adults 19 yrs or older		
Male or female less than 130 lb	⅝–1"*	Deltoid muscle of arm
Female 130–200 lb Male 130–260 lb	1–1½"	Deltoid muscle of arm
Female 200+ lb Male 260+ lb	1½"	Deltoid muscle of arm

*A ⅝"-needle may be used for patients weighing less than 130 lb (<60 kg) for IM injection in the deltoid muscle only if the skin is stretched tight, the subcutaneous tissue is not bunched, and the injection is made at a 90-degree angle.

Intramuscular (IM) injection	Subcutaneous (SC) injection	Intradermal (ID) administration of Fluzone ID vaccine	Intranasal (IN) administration of FluMist (LAIV) vaccine

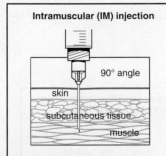
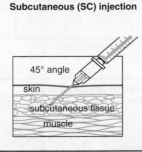
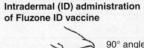
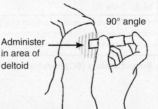
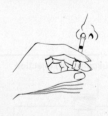

Please note: Always refer to the package insert included with each biologic for complete vaccine administration information. CDC's Advisory Committee on Immunization Practices (ACIP) recommendations for the particular vaccine should be reviewed as well (see www.immunize.org/acip).

Technical content reviewed by the Centers for Disease Control and Prevention

www.immunize.org/catg.d/p3085.pdf • Item #P3085 (7/12)

Acquired from www.immunize.org on May 14, 2014. We thank the Immunization Action Coalition.

TABLE 4.2   **Administering Vaccines to Adults: Dose, Route, Site, and Needle Size**

Vaccine	Dose	Route
Hepatitis A (HepA)	≤18 yrs: 0.5 mL	IM
	≥19 yrs: 1.0 mL	
Hepatitis B (HepB)	≤19 yrs: 0.5 mL	IM
	≥20 yrs: 1.0 mL	
HepA-HepB (Twinrix)	≥18 yrs: 1.0 mL	IM
Human papillomavirus (HPV)	0.5 mL	IM
Influenza, live attenuated (LAIV)	0.2 mL (0.1 mL into each nostril)	Intranasal spray
Influenza, trivalent inactivated (TIV), including Fluzone High-Dose	0.5 mL	IM
Influenza (TIV) Fluzone Intradermal, for ages 18 through 64 yrs	0.1 mL	Intradermal
Measles, Mumps, Rubella (MMR)	0.5 mL	SC
Meningococcal conjugate (MCV4)	0.5 mL	IM
Meningococcal polysaccharide (MPSV4)	0.5 mL	SC
Pneumococcal conjugate (PCV13)	0.5 mL	IM
Pneumococcal polysaccharide (PPSV)	0.5 mL	IM
		SC
Tetanus, Diphtheria (Td) with Pertussis (Tdap)	0.5 mL	IM
Varicella (VAR)	0.5 mL	SC
Zoster (Zos)	0.65 mL	SC

Injection Site and Needle Size

Subcutaneous (SC) injection

Use a 23–25-gauge, ⅝" needle. Inject in fatty tissue over triceps.

Intramuscular (IM) injection

Use a 22–25-gauge needle. Inject in deltoid muscle of arm. Choose the needle length as indicated below:

Gender/Weight	Needle Length
Male or female less than 130 lb	⅝"*–1"
Female 130–200 lb	1–1½"
Male 130–260 lb	
Female 200+ lb	1½"
Male 260+ lb	

*A ⅝" needle may be used for patients weighing less than 130 lb (<60 kg) for IM injection in the deltoid muscle only if the subcutaneous tissue is not bunched and the injection is made at a 90-degree angle.

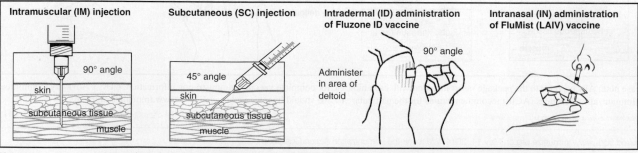

Intramuscular (IM) injection — 90° angle, skin, subcutaneous tissue, muscle

Subcutaneous (SC) injection — 45° angle, skin, subcutaneous tissue, muscle

Intradermal (ID) administration of Fluzone ID vaccine — 90° angle, Administer in area of deltoid

Intranasal (IN) administration of FluMist (LAIV) vaccine

Note: Always refer to the package insert included with each biologic for complete vaccine administration information. CDC's Advisory Committee on Immunization Practices (ACIP) recommendations for the particular vaccine should be reviewed as well. Access the ACIP recommendations at www.immunize.org/acip.

Technical content reviewed by the Centers for Disease Control and Prevention   www.immunize.org/catg.d/p3084.pdf • Item #P3084 (7/12)

Acquired from www.immunize.org on May 14, 2014. We thank the Immunization Action Coalition.

Exercise 4.8   Administering Vaccines

(See page 109 for answers)

Refer to Table 4.1 on p. 93 and then answer the following questions.

1. Identify how many mLs of Diphtheria, Tetanus, Pertussis will be given to a child and via which route.

    _____ mL _____ route

2. Identify how many mLs of Influenza, trivalent inactivated (TIV) will be given to an infant who is 24 months old and via which route.

    _____ mL _____ route

3. Identify how many mLs of Measles, Mumps, Rubella (MMR) will be given to a child and via which route.

    _____ mL _____ route

4. Identify how many mLs of Varicella will be given to a child and via which route.

    _____ mL _____ route

Refer to Table 4.2 and then answer the following questions.

5. Identify how many mLs of Hepatitis A (HepA) will be given to a 21-year-old college student and via which route.

    _____ mL _____ route

6. Identify how many mLs of Human papillomavirus (HPV) will be given to a 25-year-old college student and via which route.

    _____ mL _____ route

7. Identify how many mLs of Measles, Mumps, Rubella (MMR) will be given and via which route.

    _____ mL _____ route

8. Identify how many mLs of Influenza (TIV) Fluzone will be given to a 45-year-old and via which route.

    _____ mL _____ route

Summary

This chapter has taught you to interpret medication orders and drug labels and to calculate one-factor medication problems using dimensional analysis. To demonstrate your ability to interpret correctly and calculate accurately, complete the following practice problems.

Practice Problems for Chapter 4

One-Factor Medication Problems (See pages 109–111 for answers)

1. The physician orders Tigan 0.2 g IM qid for nausea. The dosage of medication on hand is a multiple-dose vial labeled 100 mg/mL.

   ✳ **How many mL will you give?** _____

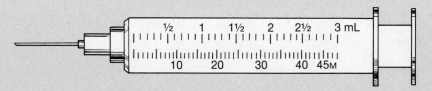

2. A physician orders Thorazine 50 mg tid prn for singultus. The dose on hand is Thorazine 25-mg tablets.

   ✳ **How many tablets will you give?** _____

3. Order: Orinase 1 g PO bid for type 2 diabetes mellitus.

   ✳ **How many tablets will you give?** _____

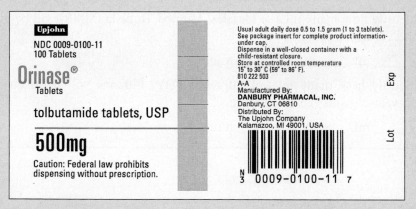

Courtesy of the Upjohn Company.

4. Order: Persantine 50 mg PO qid for prevention of thromboembolism.

❋ **How many tablets will you give?** _____

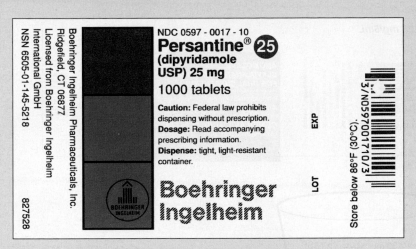

Courtesy of Boehringer Ingelheim Pharmaceuticals.

5. Order: NPH insulin 56 units SQ every AM for type 1 diabetes mellitus.
On hand: NPH insulin 100 units/mL

❋ **How many units will you give?** _____

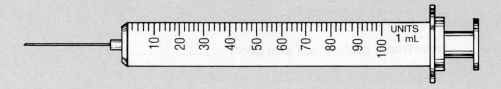

6. Order: heparin 7500 units SQ bid for prevention of thrombi.
On hand: heparin 10,000 units/mL

❋ **How many mL will you give?** _____

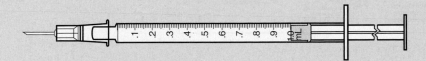

(Practice Problems continue on page 98)

7. Order: Amoxicillin/clavulanate potassium 500 mg PO every 8 hours for infection.

   ✳ **How many mL will you give?** _____

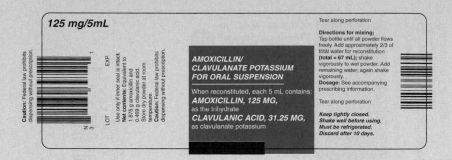

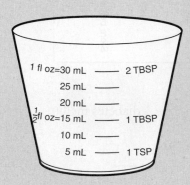

8. Order: Zaroxolyn 5 mg PO every AM for hypertension.

   ✳ **How many tablets will you give?** _____

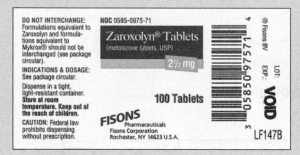

Courtesy of Fisons Pharmaceuticals.

9. Order: methylphenidate (Ritalin) 10 mg PO tid for attention-deficit hyperactivity disorder (ADHD).

   ✳ **How many tablets will you give?** _____

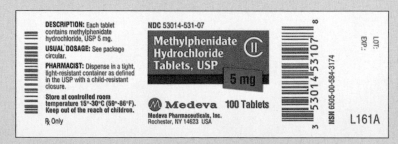

Courtesy of Medeva Pharmaceuticals.

10. Order: meperidine 50 mg IM every 3 hours prn for pain.
    On hand: meperidine 100 mg/mL

    ❋ **How many mL will you give?** _____

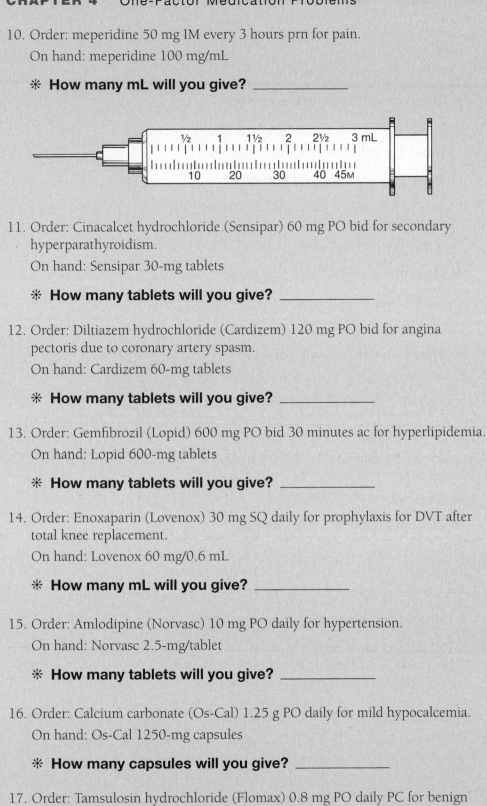

11. Order: Cinacalcet hydrochloride (Sensipar) 60 mg PO bid for secondary hyperparathyroidism.
    On hand: Sensipar 30-mg tablets

    ❋ **How many tablets will you give?** _____

12. Order: Diltiazem hydrochloride (Cardizem) 120 mg PO bid for angina pectoris due to coronary artery spasm.
    On hand: Cardizem 60-mg tablets

    ❋ **How many tablets will you give?** _____

13. Order: Gemfibrozil (Lopid) 600 mg PO bid 30 minutes ac for hyperlipidemia.
    On hand: Lopid 600-mg tablets

    ❋ **How many tablets will you give?** _____

14. Order: Enoxaparin (Lovenox) 30 mg SQ daily for prophylaxis for DVT after total knee replacement.
    On hand: Lovenox 60 mg/0.6 mL

    ❋ **How many mL will you give?** _____

15. Order: Amlodipine (Norvasc) 10 mg PO daily for hypertension.
    On hand: Norvasc 2.5-mg/tablet

    ❋ **How many tablets will you give?** _____

16. Order: Calcium carbonate (Os-Cal) 1.25 g PO daily for mild hypocalcemia.
    On hand: Os-Cal 1250-mg capsules

    ❋ **How many capsules will you give?** _____

17. Order: Tamsulosin hydrochloride (Flomax) 0.8 mg PO daily PC for benign prostatic hypertrophy.
    On hand: Flomax 0.4-mg capsules

    ❋ **How many capsules will you give?** _____

18. Order: Ropinirole hydrochloride (Requip) 1.5 mg PO daily for Parkinson's disease.

    On hand: Requip 0.5-mg tablets

    ✳ **How many tablets will you give?** _____

19. Order: Lisinopril (Prinivil) 5 mg PO daily for hypertension.

    On hand: Prinivil 2.5-mg tablets

    ✳ **How many tablets will you give?** _____

20. Order: Metformin hydrochloride (Glucophage) 1000 mg PO daily for type 2 diabetes.

    On hand: Glucophage 500-mg tablets

    ✳ **How many tablets will you give?** _____

21. Order: Flublok 0.5 mL influenza vaccine IM for 20 year old.

    Supply: Flublok 0.5-mL/dose vial

    ✳ **How many doses will you give?** _____

22. Order: Abiraterone (Zytiga) 1000 mg PO every day with Prednisone 5 mg PO every 12 hours for prostate cancer.

    Supply: Abiraterone 250-mg tablets

    ✳ **How many tablets will you give?** _____

23. Order: L-tryptophan (Tryptophan) 1 g PO 20 minutes before bedtime for insomnia.

    Supply: L-tryptophan 500-mg capsules

    ✳ **How many capsules will you give?** _____

24. Order: Prolia (Denosumab) 60 mg SC every 6 months for osteoporosis. Supplement with calcium 1000 mg/day and vitamin D 400 IU/day.

    Supply: Prolia 60 mg in 1-mL prefilled syringe

    ✳ **How many mL will you give?** _____

25. Order: Tocilizumab (Actemra) 162 mg SC every other week for rheumatoid arthritis for patients weighing under 100 kg and 162 mg SC every week for patients weighing over 100 kg.

    Supply: Tocilizumab 162 mg/0.9 mL-prefilled syringe

    Patient weight: 110 lb

    ✳ **How much does the patient weigh in kg?** _____

    ✳ **How often will the patient receive the SC injection?** _____

    ✳ **How many mL will you give?** _____

Chapter 4 Post-Test

One-Factor Medication Problems

Name _____   Date _____

1. Order: Micronase 1.25 mg PO daily for non-insulin-dependent diabetes mellitus

   ✳ **How many tablets will you give?** _____

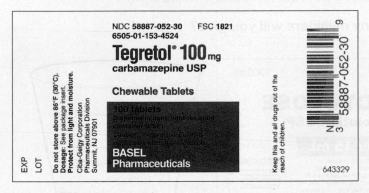

> See package insert for complete product information.
>
> Dispense in tight, light-resistant container.
>
> Keep container tightly closed.
>
> Store at controlled room temperature 15° to 30° C (59° to 86° F).
>
> 812 372 405
>
> The Upjohn Co. Kalamazoo, MI 49001, USA
>
> **Upjohn**
> NDC 0009-0141-01
> 100 Tablets
> 6505-01-216-6289
> **Micronase®**
> Tablets
> glyburide tablets
> **2.5mg**
> Caution: Federal law prohibits dispensing without prescription.

Courtesy of the Upjohn Company.

2. Order: Tegretol 50 mg PO qid for seizures

   ✳ **How many tablets will you give?** _____

> NDC 58887-052-30   FSC 1821
> 6505-01-153-4524
> **Tegretol® 100 mg**
> carbamazepine USP
>
> **Chewable Tablets**
>
> 100 tablets
> Dispense in tight, light-resistant container (USP).
> Caution: Federal law prohibits dispensing without prescription.
> **BASEL Pharmaceuticals**
>
> Do not store above 86°F (30°C).
> Dosage: See package insert.
> Protect from light and moisture.
> Ciba-Geigy Corporation
> Pharmaceuticals Division
> Summit, NJ 07901
> EXP   LOT
>
> Keep this and all drugs out of the reach of children.
> 643329
>
> 3 58887-052-30 9

Courtesy of Basel Pharmaceuticals.

(Post-Test continues on page 102)

3. Order: acetaminophen 240 mg PO every 4 hours prn for moderate pain

❋ **How many milliliters will you give?** _____

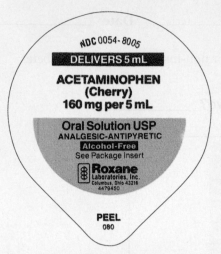

NDC 0054-8005

DELIVERS 5 mL

ACETAMINOPHEN
(Cherry)
160 mg per 5 mL

Oral Solution USP
ANALGESIC-ANTIPYRETIC
Alcohol-Free
See Package Insert

Ⓡ **Roxane**
Laboratories, Inc.
Columbus, Ohio 43216
4479450

PEEL
080

Courtesy of Roxane Laboratories, Inc.

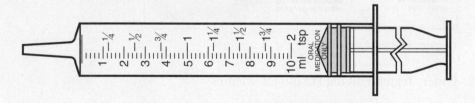

4. Order: lactulose 30 g PO qid for hepatic encephalopathy

❋ **How many milliliters will you give?** _____

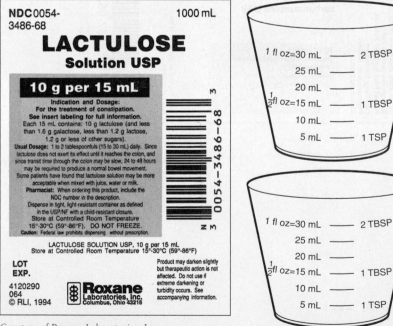

NDC 0054-
3486-68   1000 mL

LACTULOSE
Solution USP

10 g per 15 mL

Indication and Dosage:
For the treatment of constipation.
See insert labeling for full information.
Each 15 mL contains: 10 g lactulose (and less
than 1.6 g galactose, less than 1.2 g lactose,
1.2 g or less of other sugars).
Usual Dosage: 1 to 2 tablespoonfuls (15 to 30 mL) daily. Since
lactulose does not exert its effect until it reaches the colon, and
since transit time through the colon may be slow, 24 to 48 hours
may be required to produce a normal bowel movement.
Some patients have found that lactulose solution may be more
acceptable when mixed with juice, water or milk.
Pharmacist: When ordering this product, include the
NDC number in the description.
Dispense in tight, light-resistant container as defined
in the USP/NF with a child-resistant closure.
Store at Controlled Room Temperature
15°-30°C (59°-86°F). DO NOT FREEZE.
Caution: Federal law prohibits dispensing without prescription.

LACTULOSE SOLUTION USP, 10 g per 15 mL.
Store at Controlled Room Temperature 15°-30°C (59°-86°F)

LOT
EXP.

4120290
064
© RLI, 1994

Ⓡ **Roxane**
Laboratories, Inc.
Columbus, Ohio 43216

Product may darken slightly
but therapeutic action is not
affected. Do not use if
extreme darkening or
turbidity occurs. See
accompanying information.

3 0054-3486-68 3

1 fl oz=30 mL ——— 2 TBSP
25 mL ———
20 mL ———
½ fl oz=15 mL ——— 1 TBSP
10 mL ———
5 mL ——— 1 TSP

1 fl oz=30 mL ——— 2 TBSP
25 mL ———
20 mL ———
½ fl oz=15 mL ——— 1 TBSP
10 mL ———
5 mL ——— 1 TSP

Courtesy of Roxane Laboratories, Inc.

5. Order: Cimetidine HCl 300 mg PO qid for short-term treatment of active ulcers

   ✳ **How many teaspoons will you give?** _____

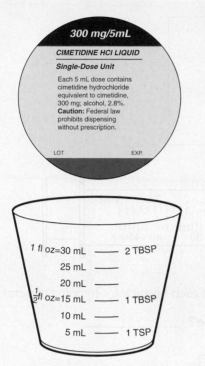

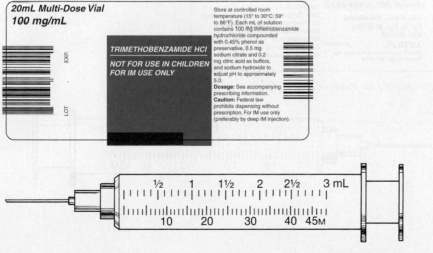

6. Order: Trimethobenzamide HCl 0.2 g IM tid prn for nausea

   ✳ **How many milliliters will you give?** _____

(Post-Test continues on page 104)

7. Order: hydromorphone 3 mg IM every 3 hours for pain

❋ **How many milliliters will you give?** _____

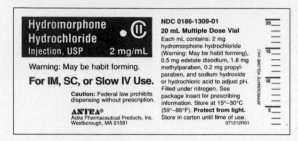

NDC 0186-1309-01
20 mL Multiple Dose Vial
Each mL contains: 2 mg
hydromorphone hydrochloride
(Warning: May be habit forming),
0.5 mg edetate disodium, 1.8 mg
methylparaben, 0.2 mg propyl-
paraben, and sodium hydroxide
or hydrochloric acid to adjust pH.
Filled under nitrogen. See
package insert for prescribing
information. Store at 15°–30°C
(59°–86°F). Protect from light.
Store in carton until time of use.
071212R01

Hydromorphone
Hydrochloride
Injection, USP   2 mg/mL

Warning: May be habit forming.

For IM, SC, or Slow IV Use.

Caution: Federal law prohibits
dispensing without prescription.

ASTRA®
Astra Pharmaceutical Products, Inc.
Westborough, MA 01581

Courtesy of Astra Pharmaceutical Products.

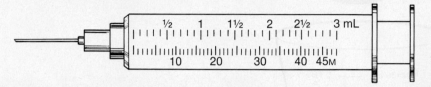

8. Order: magnesium sulfate 1000 mg IM in each buttock for hypomagnesemia

❋ **How many milliliters will you give?** _____

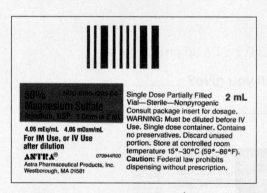

50%
Magnesium Sulfate
Injection, USP   1 Gram in 2 mL

4.06 mEq/mL   4.06 mOsm/mL
**For IM Use, or IV Use
after dilution**
ASTRA®   070944R00
Astra Pharmaceutical Products, Inc.
Westborough, MA 01581

Single Dose Partially Filled
Vial—Sterile—Nonpyrogenic   **2 mL**
Consult package insert for dosage.
WARNING: Must be diluted before IV
Use. Single dose container. Contains
no preservatives. Discard unused
portion. Store at controlled room
temperature 15°–30°C (59°–86°F).
Caution: Federal law prohibits
dispensing without prescription.

Courtesy of Astra Pharmaceutical Products.

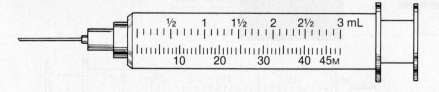

9. Order: naloxone HCl 200 mcg IV stat for respiratory depression

   ❋ **How many milliliters will you give?** _____

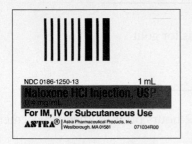

Courtesy of Astra Pharmaceutical
Products.

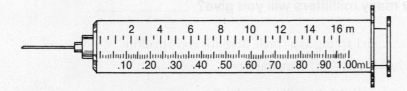

10. Order: Solu-Medrol 40 mg IM daily for autoimmune disorder

    ❋ **How many milliliters will you give?** _____

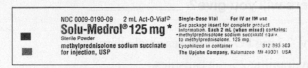

Courtesy of the Upjohn Company.

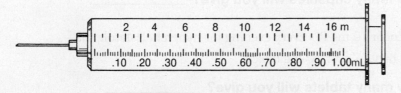

11. Order: Coumadin 7.5 mg once daily for DVT post-op hip replacement

    Dose on hand: Coumadin 2.5-mg tablets

    ❋ **How many tablets will you give?** _____

12. Order: 500 mL to infuse at 50 mL/hr. The infusion started at 7 AM.

    ❋ **What time will the infusion end?** _____

13. Order: Nexium 40 mg once daily for GERD

    Dose on hand: Nexium 20-mg tablets

    ❋ **How many tablets will you give?** _____

(Post-Test continues on page 106)

14. Order: Xanax 0.25-mg tablets prn for anxiety
    Dose on hand: Xanax 0.5-mg scored tablets

    ✴ **How many tablets will you give?** _____

15. Order: Colchicine 0.5 mg PO tid prophylaxis for gout
    Dose on hand: Colchicine 0.5-mg tablets

    ✴ **How many tablets will you give?** _____

16. Order: Lovenox 30 mg SC injection every 12 hours prior to knee replacement surgery
    Dose on hand: Multiple-dose vial 300 mg/3 mL

    ✴ **How many milliliters will you give?** _____

17. Order: Bisacodyl 15 mg as a single dose for constipation
    Dose on hand: Bisacodyl 5-mg/tablets

    ✴ **How many tablets will you give?** _____

18. Order: Acetaminophen 325 mg PO q6h pain
    Dose on hand: Acetaminophen solution 100 mg/mL

    ✴ **How many milliliters will you give?** _____

19. Order: Diphenhydramine 25 mg PO q4h for seasonal allergies
    Dose on hand: Diphenhydramine 25-mg capsules

    ✴ **How many capsules will you give?** _____

20. Order: Zocor 10 mg PO every evening for hypercholesterolemia
    Dose on hand: Zocor 10-mg tablets

    ✴ **How many tablets will you give?** _____

ANSWER KEY FOR CHAPTER 4: ONE-FACTOR MEDICATION PROBLEMS

Exercise 4.1 **Interpretation of Medication Orders**

1

a. Right patient   Mrs. A. Clark
b. Right drug   Aspirin for fever
c. Right dosage   gr 10
d. Right route   orally (PO)
e. Right time   every 4 hr as needed (prn)
f. Right documentation: The patient's name, the drug, the dosage, the route administered, and the date and time administered should be charted on the Medication Administration Record (MAR). Aspirin is a prn medication and therefore the reason the drug was administered; the effects following administration of the drug should also be charted on the MAR. The nurse's signature and initials should appear on the MAR.

2

a. Right patient   Mr. W. Smith
b. Right drug   Advil (ibuprofen) for arthritis
c. Right dosage   400 mg
d. Right route   PO (orally)
e. Right time   every 6 hr
f. Right documentation: The patient's name, the drug, the dosage, the route administered, and the date and time administered should be charted on the Medication Administration Record (MAR). Advil is a regularly scheduled medication and the reason for the drug administration is listed as arthritis. The nurse's signature and initials should appear on the MAR.

3

a. Right patient   Mr. T. Jones
b. Right drug   Tylenol (acetaminophen) for headache
c. Right dosage   gr 10
d. Right route   PO (orally)
e. Right time   every 4 hr prn
f. Right documentation: The patient's name, the drug, the dosage, the route administered, and the date and time administered should be charted on the Medication Administration Record (MAR). Tylenol is a prn medication and therefore the reason the drug was administered; the effects following administration of the drug should also be charted. The nurse's signature and initials should appear on the MAR.

Exercise 4.3 **One-Factor Medication Problems**

1

Sequential method:

$$\frac{0.25\ g\ \mid\ 1000\ mg\ \mid\ \boxed{capsule}\ \mid\ 0.25\times100\ \mid\ 25}{1\ g\ \mid\ 250\ mg\ \mid\ 1\times25\ \mid\ 25}=1\ capsule$$

Random method:

$$\frac{0.25\ g\ \mid\ \boxed{capsule}\ \mid\ 1000\ mg\ \mid\ 0.25\times100\ \mid\ 25}{250\ mg\ \mid\ 1\ g\ \mid\ 25\times1\ \mid\ 25}=1\ capsule$$

2

Sequential method:

$$\frac{\frac{1}{2}\ gr\ \mid\ 60\ mg\ \mid\ \boxed{tablet}\ \mid\ \frac{1}{2}\times\frac{60}{1}\ \mid\ \frac{60}{2}\ \mid\ 30}{1\ gr\ \mid\ 15\ mg\ \mid\ 1\times15\ \mid\ 15\ \mid\ 15}=2\ tablets$$

Random method:

$$\frac{\frac{1}{2}\ gr\ \mid\ \boxed{tablet}\ \mid\ 60\ mg\ \mid\ \frac{1}{2}\times\frac{60}{1}\ \mid\ \frac{60}{2}\ \mid\ 30}{15\ mg\ \mid\ 1\ gr\ \mid\ 15\times1\ \mid\ 15\ \mid\ 15}=2\ tablets$$

3

Sequential method:

$$\frac{0.5\ g\ \mid\ 1000\ mg\ \mid\ \boxed{tablet}\ \mid\ 0.5\times10\ \mid\ 5}{1\ g\ \mid\ 500\ mg\ \mid\ 1\times5\ \mid\ 5}=1\ tablet$$

Random method:

$$\frac{0.5\ g\ \mid\ \boxed{tablet}\ \mid\ 1000\ mg\ \mid\ 0.5\times10\ \mid\ 5}{500\ mg\ \mid\ 1\ g\ \mid\ 5\times1\ \mid\ 5}=1\ tablet$$

4

Sequential method:

$$\frac{0.03\ g\ \mid\ 1000\ mg\ \mid\ \boxed{capsules}\ \mid\ 0.03\times100\ \mid\ 3}{1\ g\ \mid\ 30\ mg\ \mid\ 1\times3\ \mid\ 3}=1\ capsule$$

Random method:

$$\frac{0.03\ g\ \mid\ \boxed{capsules}\ \mid\ 1000\ mg\ \mid\ 0.03\times100\ \mid\ 3}{30\ mg\ \mid\ 1\ g\ \mid\ 3\times1\ \mid\ 3}=1\ capsule$$

5

Sequential method:

$$\frac{\frac{1}{2}\ gr\ \mid\ 60\ mg\ \mid\ \boxed{capsules}\ \mid\ \frac{1}{2}\times\frac{60}{1}\ \mid\ \frac{60}{2}\ \mid\ 30}{1\ gr\ \mid\ 30\ mg\ \mid\ 1\times30\ \mid\ 30\ \mid\ 30}=1\ capsule$$

Random method:

$$\frac{\frac{1}{2}\ gr\ \mid\ \boxed{capsules}\ \mid\ 60\ mg\ \mid\ \frac{1}{2}\times\frac{60}{1}\ \mid\ \frac{60}{2}\ \mid\ 30}{30\ mg\ \mid\ 1\ gr\ \mid\ 30\times1\ \mid\ 30\ \mid\ 30}=1\ capsule$$

Exercise 4.4 **Identifying the Components of Drug Labels**

1

a. Cipro
b. Ciprofloxacin hydrochloride
c. 500 mg per tablet

d. 100 tablets
e. *Not listed on the label
f. *Not listed on the label
g. Bayer Corporation, Pharmaceutical Division

2

a. Zovirax
b. acyclovir
c. 400 mg per capsule
d. 100 tablets
e. *Not listed on the label
f. *Not listed on the label
g. GlaxoSmithKline

3

a. Halcion
b. Triazolam
c. 0.125 mg per tablet
d. 10 tablets
e. *Not listed on the label
f. *Not listed on the label
g. The Upjohn Company

Exercise 4.5   **Problems With Components of Drug Labels**

1

Sequential method:

$$\frac{10 \text{ mg}}{} \left|\frac{\text{tablet}}{10 \text{ mg}}\right| \frac{10}{10} = 1 \text{ tablet}$$

2

Random method:

$$\frac{500 \text{ mcg}}{} \left|\frac{\text{tablet}}{1 \text{ mg}}\right| \frac{1 \text{ mg}}{1000 \text{ mcg}} \left|\frac{5}{10}\right| = \frac{1}{2} \text{ tablet}$$

3

Sequential method:

$$\frac{375 \text{ mg}}{} \left|\frac{\text{tablet}}{250 \text{ mg}}\right| \frac{375}{250} = 1\frac{1}{2} \text{ tablets}$$

4

Random method:

$$\frac{2.5 \text{ mg}}{} \left|\frac{\text{tablet}}{2500 \text{ mcg}}\right| \frac{1000 \text{ mcg}}{1 \text{ mg}} \left|\frac{2.5 \times 10}{25 \times 1}\right| \frac{25}{25} = 1 \text{ tablet}$$

5

Sequential method:

$$\frac{250 \text{ mg}}{} \left|\frac{\text{capsule}}{250 \text{ mg}}\right| \frac{25}{25} = 1 \text{ capsule}$$

Exercise 4.6   **Administering Enteral Medications**

1

Random method:

$$\frac{\frac{1}{2} \text{ gr}}{} \left|\frac{5 \text{ mL}}{20 \text{ mg}}\right| \frac{60 \text{ mg}}{1 \text{ gr}} \left|\frac{\frac{1}{2} \times \frac{5}{1} \times \frac{6}{1}}{2 \times 1}\right| \frac{30}{2} \left|\frac{15}{2}\right| = 7.5 \text{ mL}$$

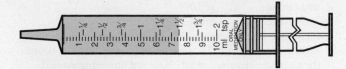

2

Sequential method:

$$\frac{0.15 \text{ g}}{} \left|\frac{1000 \text{ mg}}{1 \text{ g}}\right| \frac{\text{mL}}{15 \text{ mg}} \left|\frac{\frac{1}{4} \text{ tsp}}{5 \text{ mL}}\right| \frac{0.15 \times 1000}{15 \times 5} \left|\frac{150}{75}\right| = 2 \text{ tsp}$$

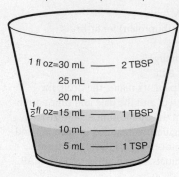

3

Sequential method:

$$\frac{3 \text{ mg}}{} \left|\frac{\text{mL}}{1 \text{ mg}}\right| \frac{3}{1} = 3 \text{ mL}$$

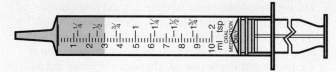

4

Sequential method:

$$\frac{20 \text{ g}}{} \left|\frac{15 \text{ mL}}{10 \text{ g}}\right| \frac{1 \text{ oz}}{30 \text{ mL}} \left|\frac{2 \times 15 \times 1}{1 \times 30}\right| \frac{30}{30} = 1 \text{ oz}$$

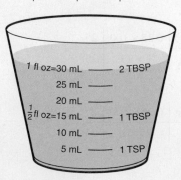

Exercise 4.7 Administering Parenteral Medications

1

Random method:

$$\frac{300 \text{ mcg}}{} \left| \frac{\text{mL}}{0.1 \text{ mg}} \right| \frac{1 \text{ mg}}{1000 \text{ mcg}} \left| \frac{3 \times 1}{0.1 \times 10} \right| \frac{3}{1} = 3 \text{ mL}$$

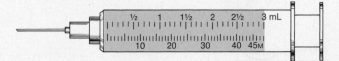

2

Sequential method:

$$\frac{3 \text{ mg}}{} \left| \frac{\text{mL}}{2 \text{ mg}} \right| \frac{3}{2} = 1.5 \text{ mL}$$

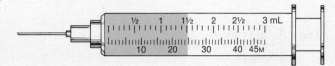

3

Sequential method:

$$\frac{35 \text{ mg}}{} \left| \frac{\text{mL}}{10 \text{ mg}} \right| \frac{35}{10} = 3.5 \text{ mL}$$

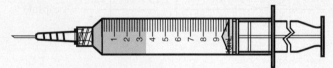

4

Sequential method:

$$\frac{10 \text{ units}}{} = 10 \text{ units}$$

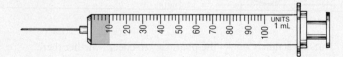

5

Sequential method:

$$\frac{8000 \text{ units}}{} \left| \frac{\text{mL}}{10,000 \text{ units}} \right| \frac{8}{10} = 0.8 \text{ mL}$$

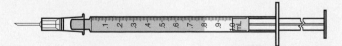

Exercise 4.8 Administering Vaccines

Using Table 4.1

1

0.5 mL Intramuscular

2

0.25 mL Intramuscular

3

0.5 mL Subcutaneous

4

0.5 mL Subcutaneous

Using Table 4.2

5

1.0 mL Intramuscular

6

0.5 mL Intramuscular

7

0.5 mL Subcutaneous

8

0.1 mL Intradermal

Practice Problems

1

Random method:

$$\frac{0.2 \text{ g}}{} \left| \frac{\text{mL}}{100 \text{ mg}} \right| \frac{1000 \text{ mg}}{1 \text{ g}} \left| \frac{0.2 \times 10}{1 \times 1} \right| \frac{2}{1} = 2 \text{ mL}$$

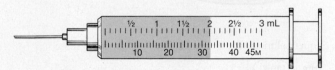

2

Sequential method:

$$\frac{50 \text{ mg}}{} \left| \frac{\text{tablet}}{25 \text{ mg}} \right| \frac{50}{25} = 2 \text{ tablets}$$

3

Random method:

$$\frac{1 \text{ g}}{} \left| \frac{\text{tablet}}{500 \text{ mg}} \right| \frac{1000 \text{ mg}}{1 \text{ g}} \left| \frac{1 \times 10}{5 \times 1} \right| \frac{10}{5} = 2 \text{ tablets}$$

4

Random method:

$$\frac{50 \text{ mg}}{} \left| \frac{\text{tablet}}{25 \text{ mg}} \right| \frac{50}{25} = 2 \text{ tablets}$$

5

Sequential method:

$$\frac{56 \text{ units}}{} \bigg| = 56 \text{ units}$$

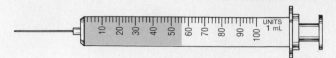

6

Sequential method:

$$\frac{7500 \text{ units}}{10000 \text{ units}} \bigg| \frac{\text{mL}}{} \bigg| \frac{75}{100} = 0.75 \text{ mL}$$

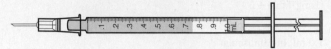

7

Sequential method:

$$\frac{500 \text{ mg}}{125 \text{ mg}} \bigg| \frac{5 \text{ mL}}{} \bigg| \frac{500 \times 5}{125} \bigg| \frac{2500}{125} = 20 \text{ mL}$$

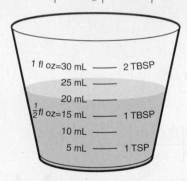

8

Sequential method:

$$\frac{5 \text{ mg}}{2.5 \text{ mg}} \bigg| \frac{\text{tablet}}{} \bigg| \frac{5}{2.5} = 2 \text{ tablets}$$

9

Sequential method:

$$\frac{10 \text{ mg}}{5 \text{ mg}} \bigg| \frac{\text{tablet}}{} \bigg| \frac{10}{5} = 2 \text{ tablets}$$

10

Sequential method:

$$\frac{50 \text{ mg}}{100 \text{ mg}} \bigg| \frac{\text{mL}}{} \bigg| \frac{5}{10} = 0.5 \text{ mL}$$

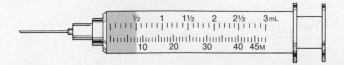

11

$$\frac{60 \text{ mg}}{30 \text{ mg}} \bigg| \frac{\text{tablet}}{} \bigg| \frac{6}{3} = 2 \text{ tablets}$$

12

$$\frac{120 \text{ mg}}{60 \text{ mg}} \bigg| \frac{\text{tablet}}{} \bigg| \frac{12}{6} = 2 \text{ tablets}$$

13

$$\frac{600 \text{ mg}}{600 \text{ mg}} \bigg| \frac{\text{tablet}}{} \bigg| \frac{6}{6} = 1 \text{ tablet}$$

14

$$\frac{30 \text{ mg}}{60 \text{ mg}} \bigg| \frac{0.6 \text{ mL}}{} \bigg| \frac{3 \times 0.6}{6} \bigg| \frac{1.8}{6} = 0.3 \text{ mL}$$

15

$$\frac{10 \text{ mg}}{2.5 \text{ mg}} \bigg| \frac{\text{tablet}}{} \bigg| \frac{10}{2.5} = 4 \text{ tablets}$$

Nursing action: Contact the pharmacy to check whether there is a different dosage so that four tablets would not have to be given. Tablets are available as 5-mg and 10-mg tablets.

16

$$\frac{1.25 \text{ g}}{1250 \text{ mg}} \bigg| \frac{\text{capsule}}{} \bigg| \frac{1000 \text{ mg}}{1 \text{ g}} \bigg| \frac{1.25 \times 100}{125 \times 1} \bigg| \frac{125}{125} = 1 \text{ capsule}$$

17

$$\frac{0.8 \text{ mg}}{0.4 \text{ mg}} \bigg| \frac{\text{capsule}}{} \bigg| \frac{0.8}{0.4} = 2 \text{ capsules}$$

18

$$\frac{1.5 \text{ mg}}{0.5 \text{ mg}} \bigg| \frac{\text{tablet}}{} \bigg| \frac{1.5}{0.5} = 3 \text{ tablets}$$

Nursing action: Contact the pharmacy to check whether there is a different dosage so that three tablets would not have to be given. Tablets are available as 1-mg tablets.

19

$$\frac{5 \text{ mg}}{2.5 \text{ mg}} \bigg| \frac{\text{tablet}}{} \bigg| \frac{5}{2.5} = 2 \text{ tablets}$$

20

$$\frac{1000 \text{ mg}}{500 \text{ mg}} \bigg| \frac{\text{tablet}}{} \bigg| \frac{10}{5} = 2 \text{ tablets}$$

21

Sequential method:

$$\frac{0.5 \text{ mL}}{} \left| \frac{1 \text{ dose}}{0.5 \text{ mL}} \right| \frac{0.5 \times 1}{0.5} \left| \frac{0.5}{0.5} \right. = 1 \text{ dose}$$

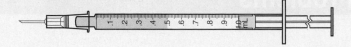

22

Sequential method:

$$\frac{1000 \text{ mg}}{} \left| \frac{\text{tablet}}{250 \text{ mg}} \right| \frac{100}{25} = 4 \text{ tablets}$$

Nursing action: Contact pharmacy to check whether there is a different dosage so that four tablets would not have to be given. Abiraterone (Zytiga) only comes in 250-mg tablets.

23

Random method:

$$\frac{1 \text{ g}}{} \left| \frac{\text{capsule}}{500 \text{ mg}} \right| \frac{1000 \text{ mg}}{1 \text{ g}} \left| \frac{10}{5} \right. = 2 \text{ capsules}$$

24

Sequential method:

$$\frac{60 \text{ mg}}{} \left| \frac{1 \text{ mL}}{60 \text{ mg}} \right| \frac{1}{} = 1 \text{ mL}$$

25

Sequential method:

$$\frac{110 \text{ lb}}{} \left| \frac{1 \text{ kg}}{2.2 \text{ lb}} \right| \frac{110 \times 1}{2.2} \left| \frac{110}{2.2} \right. = 50 \text{ kg}$$

Every other week

$$\frac{162 \text{ mg}}{} \left| \frac{0.9 \text{ mL}}{162 \text{ mg}} \right| \frac{0.9}{} = 0.9 \text{ mL}$$

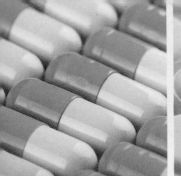
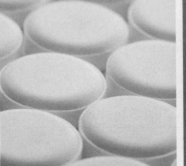

Two-Factor Medication Problems

Objectives

After completing this chapter, you will successfully be able to:

1. Solve two-factor–given quantity to one-factor–wanted quantity medication problems involving a specific amount of medication ordered based on the weight of the patient.

2. Calculate medication problems requiring reconstitution of medications by using information from a nursing drug reference, label, or package insert.

3. Solve two-factor–given quantity to two-factor–wanted quantity medication problems involving a specific amount of fluid to be delivered over limited time using an intravenous pump delivering milliliters per hour (mL/hr).

4. Solve two-factor–given quantity to two-factor–wanted quantity medication problems involving a specific amount of fluid to be delivered over a limited time using different types of intravenous tubing that deliver drops per minute (gtt/min) based on a specific *drop factor*.

Although medications are ordered by physicians or nurse practitioners and administered by nurses using the "six rights of medication administration," other factors must be considered when administering certain medications or intravenous (IV) fluids.

The **weight** of the patient often must be factored into a medication problem when determining how much medication can safely be given to an infant or a child or an elderly patient.

The dosage of medication available may be in a powdered form that needs **reconstitution** to a liquid form before parenteral or IV administration.

Also, the length of **time** over which medication or IV fluids can be given plays an important role in the safe administration of IV therapy.

To be able to calculate a two-factor–given quantity to one-factor– or two-factor–wanted quantity medication problem, it is important to understand all factors that may need to be considered in some medication problems. With use of dimensional analysis, this chapter will teach you to calculate medication problems involving the weight of the patient, the reconstitution of medications from powder to liquid form, and the amount of time over which medications or IV fluids can be safely administered.

MEDICATION PROBLEMS INVOLVING WEIGHT

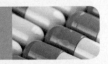

When solving problems with dimensional analysis, you can use either the *sequential method* or the *random method* to calculate two-factor–given quantity medication problems. The **given quantity** (the physician's order) contains two parts including a **numerator** (dosage of medication) and a **denominator** (the weight of the patient). This type of medication problem is called a *two-factor* medication problem because the *given quantity* now contains two parts (a numerator and a denominator) instead of just one part (a numerator).

Example 5.1 demonstrates the problem-solving method showing placement of basic terms used in dimensional analysis, applied to a two-factor medication problem involving weight.

Unit Path

Given Quantity	Conversion Factor for Given Quantity (Numerator)	Conversion Factor for Given Quantity (Denominator)		Conversion Computation	Wanted Quantity	
$\dfrac{2.5 \text{ mg}}{\text{kg}}$	$\dfrac{\text{mL}}{40 \text{ mg}}$	$\dfrac{1 \text{ kg}}{2.2 \text{ lb}}$	60 lb	$\dfrac{2.5 \times 1 \times 6}{4.22}$	$\dfrac{15}{8.8}$	$= 1.7 \text{ mL}$

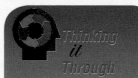

EXAMPLE 5.1

The physician orders gentamicin 2.5 mg/kg IV (intravenous) every 8 hours for infection. The vial of medication is labeled 40 mg/mL. The child weighs 60 lb.

❋ **How many milliliters will you give?** _____

Given quantity   = 2.5 mg/kg
Wanted quantity = mL
Dose on hand   = 40 mg/mL
Weight   = 60 lb

Sequential method:

Step 1 Identify the two-factor–given quantity (the physician's order).

Unit Path

Given Quantity	Conversion Factor for Given Quantity (Numerator)	Conversion Factor for Given Quantity (Denominator)	Conversion Computation	Wanted Quantity
$\dfrac{2.5 \text{ mg}}{\text{kg}}$				$= \text{mL}$

Step 2

Unit Path

Given Quantity	Conversion Factor for Given Quantity (Numerator)	Conversion Factor for Given Quantity (Denominator)	Conversion Computation	Wanted Quantity
$\dfrac{2.5 \text{ mg}}{\text{kg}}$	$\dfrac{\text{mL}}{40 \text{ mg}}$			$= \text{mL}$

Step 3

Unit Path

Given Quantity	Conversion Factor for Given Quantity (Numerator)	Conversion Factor for Given Quantity (Denominator)	Conversion Computation	Wanted Quantity
$\dfrac{2.5 \text{ mg}}{\text{kg}}$	$\dfrac{\text{mL}}{40 \text{ mg}}$	$\dfrac{1 \text{ kg}}{2.2 \text{ lb}}$		$= \text{mL}$

(Example continues on page 114)

Thinking it Through

The two-factor–given quantity has been set up with a numerator (2.5 mg) and a denominator (kg) leading across the unit path to a one-factor–wanted quantity with only a numerator (mL).

The *dose on hand* (40 mg/mL) has been factored in to cancel out the preceding unwanted unit (mg). The wanted unit (mL) is in the numerator and corresponds with the one-factor–wanted quantity (mL).

A *conversion factor* (1 kg = 2.2 lb) is factored into the unit path to cancel out the preceding unwanted unit (kg).

The *weight* is finally factored in to cancel out the preceding unwanted unit (lb) in the denominator. All unwanted units are canceled and only the wanted unit (mL) remains and corresponds with the wanted quantity (mL). Multiply the numerators, multiply the denominators, and divide the product of the numerators by the product of the denominators to provide the numerical value.

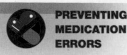

PREVENTING MEDICATION ERRORS

One of the most frequent **medication errors** is the error made with the conversion of weight.

The weight conversion [1 kg = 2.2 lb] is often incorrectly written [1 lb = 2.2 kg].

Remember that you would rather tell someone your weight in kilograms as it is a much smaller number [1 kg = 2.2 lb or, put in more realistic terms, 90.9 kg = 200 lb].

Step 4

Unit Path

Given Quantity	Conversion Factor for Given Quantity (Numerator)	Conversion Factor for Given Quantity (Denominator)		Conversion Computation	Wanted Quantity
$\dfrac{2.5\ \text{mg}}{\text{kg}}$	$\dfrac{\text{mL}}{40\ \text{mg}}$	$\dfrac{1\ \text{kg}}{2.2\ \text{lb}}$	$60\ \text{lb}$		$= \text{mL}$

Step 5

Unit Path

Given Quantity	Conversion Factor for Given Quantity (Numerator)	Conversion Factor for Given Quantity (Denominator)		Conversion Computation	Wanted Quantity
$\dfrac{2.5\ \text{mg}}{\text{kg}}$	$\dfrac{\text{mL}}{40\ \text{mg}}$	$\dfrac{1\ \text{kg}}{2.2\ \text{lb}}$	$60\ \text{lb}$	$\dfrac{2.5 \times 1 \times 6}{4 \times 2.2} \quad \dfrac{15}{8.8}$	$= 1.7\ \text{mL}$

 1.7 mL is the wanted quantity and the answer to the problem.

Dimensional analysis is a problem-solving method that uses critical thinking. When implementing the *random method* of dimensional analysis, the medication problem can be set up in a number of different ways. The focus is on the correct placement of conversion factors to cancel out all unwanted units. The wanted unit is placed in the numerator to correctly correspond with the wanted quantity.

$$\frac{2.5\ \text{mg}}{\text{kg}} \left| \frac{1\ \text{kg}}{2.2\ \text{lb}} \right| 60\ \text{lb} \left| \frac{\text{mL}}{40\ \text{mg}} \right| \frac{2.5 \times 1 \times 6}{2.2 \times 4} \quad \frac{15}{8.8} = 1.7\ \text{mL}$$

Exercise 5.1   **Pediatric Medication Problems Involving Weight**

(See page 145 for answers)

1. Order: Furosemide 1 mg/kg IV bid for hypercalcemia. The child weighs 45 lb.

   ▶ **How many milliliters will you give?** _____

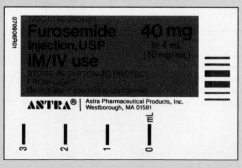

Courtesy of Astra Pharmaceutical Products.

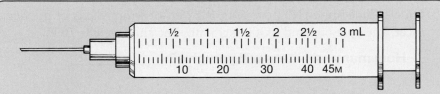

2. Order: atropine sulfate 0.01 mg/kg IV stat for bradycardia. The child weighs 20 lb.

▶ **How many milliliters will you give?** _____

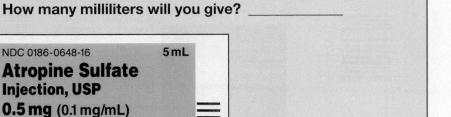

Courtesy of Astra Pharmaceutical Products.

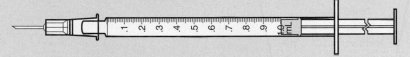

3. Order: phenergan 0.5 mg/kg IV every 4 hours prn for nausea. The dose on hand is 25 mg/mL. The child weighs 45 lb.

▶ **How many milliliters will you give?** _____

4. Order: morphine 50 mcg/kg IV every 4 hours prn for pain. The child weighs 75 lb.

▶ **How many milliliters will you give?** _____

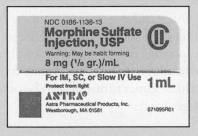

Courtesy of Astra Pharmaceutical Products.

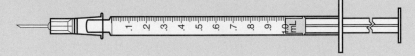

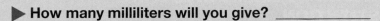

(Exercise continues on page 116)

5. Order: Cimetidine HCl 10 mg/kg PO qid for prophylaxis of duodenal ulcer. The dose on hand is 300 mg/5 mL. The child weighs 70 lb.

▶ **How many milliliters will you give?** _____

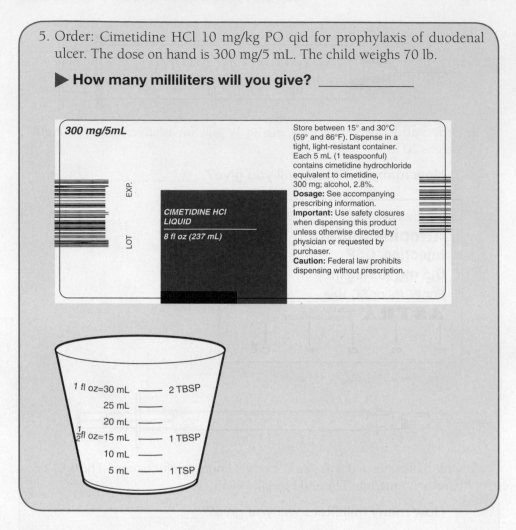

300 mg/5mL

CIMETIDINE HCl
LIQUID

8 fl oz (237 mL)

Store between 15° and 30°C (59° and 86°F). Dispense in a tight, light-resistant container. Each 5 mL (1 teaspoonful) contains cimetidine hydrochloride equivalent to cimetidine, 300 mg; alcohol, 2.8%.
Dosage: See accompanying prescribing information.
Important: Use safety closures when dispensing this product unless otherwise directed by physician or requested by purchaser.
Caution: Federal law prohibits dispensing without prescription.

1 fl oz=30 mL ——— 2 TBSP
25 mL ———
20 mL ———
$\frac{1}{2}$fl oz=15 mL ——— 1 TBSP
10 mL ———
5 mL ——— 1 TSP

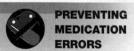

PREVENTING MEDICATION ERRORS

When reconstituting medication, always check a nursing drug reference to obtain information regarding the correct diluents and the correct amount of the diluents to be used to prevent **medication errors**.

MEDICATION PROBLEMS INVOLVING RECONSTITUTION

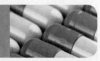

Some medications in vials are in a powder form and need reconstitution before administration. **Reconstitution** involves adding a specific amount of sterile solution (also called **diluent**) to the vial to change the powder to a liquid form. Information on how much diluent to add to the vial and what dosage of medication per milliliter will result after reconstitution (also called **yield** or **concentration**) can be obtained from a nursing drug reference, label, or package insert.

EXAMPLE 5.2

The physician orders Vancomycin 10 mg/kg IVPB every 6 hours for antibiotic-induced diarrhea. The child weighs 50 lb. The pharmacy sends a vial of medication labeled Vancomycin 500 mg. The nursing drug reference provides information to reconstitute 500 mg with 10 mL of sterile water for injection.

❋ **How many milliliters will you draw from the vial?**_____

Given quantity   = 10 mg/kg
Wanted quantity = mL
Dose on hand   = 500 mg/10 mL
Weight   = 50 lb

Unit Path

Given Quantity				Conversion Computation	Wanted Quantity

$$\frac{10 \text{ mg}}{\text{kg}} \left| \frac{1 \text{ kg}}{2.2 \text{ lb}} \right| \frac{50 \text{ lb}}{} \left| \frac{10 \text{ (mL)}}{500 \text{ mg}} \right| \frac{10 \times 1 \times 5 \times 1}{2.2 \times 5} \left| \frac{50}{11} \right. = 4.54 \text{ mL or } 4.5 \text{ mL}$$

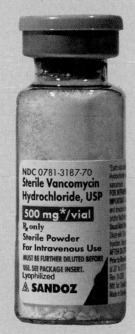

NDC 0781-3187-70
Sterile Vancomycin Hydrochloride, USP
500 mg*/vial
R, only
Sterile Powder
For Intravenous Use
MUST BE FURTHER DILUTED BEFORE USE. SEE PACKAGE INSERT.
Lyophilized
⚠ **SANDOZ**

© First Databank, Inc.

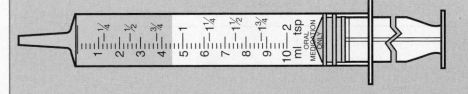

⬤ *4.5 mL is the wanted quantity and the answer to the problem.*

PREVENTING MEDICATION ERRORS

When adding reconstituted medications to an IV solution, always check a nursing drug reference for compatibility of the solutions. To prevent precipitation and/or to avoid extravasations, certain medications must be mixed in certain fluids and then further diluted.

Example: **Dilantin®** (phenytoin) must be reconstituted with normal saline (0.9% NaCl) and never administered into an IV line of dextrose in water (D_5W). Dilantin may only be further diluted with normal saline (0.9% NaCl).

Example: **Erythromycin** must be reconstituted with sterile water and may be further diluted in normal saline (0.9% NaCl) or dextrose in water (D_5W).

Example: **Acyclovir** must be reconstituted with sterile water and further diluted in varying strengths and combinations of normal saline (0.9% NaCl) and dextrose in water (D_5W).

EXAMPLE 5.3

Order: Solu-Medrol 40 mg IV every 4 hours for inflammation.

✿ **How many milliliters will you draw from the vial?** _____

Solu-Medrol®

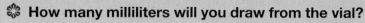

Upjohn

brand of methylprednisolone sodium succinate sterile powder
(methylprednisolone sodium succinate for injection, USP)

For Intravenous or Intramuscular Administration

125 mg Act-O-Vial System (Single-Dose Vial)—Each 2 mL (when mixed) contains methylprednisolone sodium succinate equivalent to 125 mg methylprednisolone; also 1.6 mg monobasic sodium phosphate anhydrous; 17.4 mg dibasic sodium phosphate dried; 17.6 mg benzyl alcohol added as preservative

DOSAGE AND ADMINISTRATION

When high dose therapy is desired, the recommended dose of SOLU-MEDROL Sterile Powder is 30 mg/kg administered intravenously over at least 30 minutes. This dose may be repeated every 4 to 6 hours for 48 hours.

In general, high dose corticosteroid therapy should be continued only until the patient's condition has stabilized; usually not beyond 48 to 72 hours.

Although adverse effects associated with high dose short-term corticoid therapy are uncommon, peptic ulceration may occur. Prophylactic antacid therapy may be indicated.

In other indications initial dosage will vary from 10 to 40 mg of methylprednisolone depending on the clinical problem being treated. The larger doses may be required for short-term management of severe, acute conditions. The initial dose usually should be given intravenously over a period of several minutes. Subsequent doses may be given intravenously or intramuscularly at intervals dictated by the patient's response and clinical condition. Corticoid therapy is an adjunct to, and not replacement for conventional therapy.

Dosage may be reduced for infants and children but should be governed more by the severity of the condition and response of the patient than by age or size. It should not be less than 0.5 mg per kg every 24 hours.

Dosage must be decreased or discontinued gradually when the drug has been administered for more than a few days. If a period of spontaneous remission occurs in a chronic condition, treatment should be discontinued. Routine laboratory studies, such as urinalysis, two-hour postprandial blood sugar, determination of blood pressure and body weight, and a chest X-ray should be made at regular intervals during prolonged therapy. Upper GI X-rays are desirable in patients with an ulcer history or significant dyspepsia.

SOLU-MEDROL may be administered by intravenous or intramuscular injection or by intravenous infusion, the preferred method for initial emergency use being intravenous injection. To administer by intravenous (or intramuscular) injection, prepare solution as directed. The desired dose may be administered intravenously over a period of several minutes. If desired, the medication may be administered in diluted solutions by adding Water for Injection or other suitable diluent (see below) to the **Act-O-Vial** and withdrawing the indicated dose.

To prepare solutions for intravenous infusion, first prepare the solution for injection as directed. This solution may then be added to indicated amounts of 5% dextrose in water, isotonic saline solution or 5% dextrose in isotonic saline solution.

Multiple Sclerosis

In treatment of acute exacerbations of multiple sclerosis, daily doses of 200 mg of prednisolone for a week followed by 80 mg every other day for 1 month have been shown to be effective (4 mg of methylprednisolone is equivalent to 5 mg of prednisolone).

DIRECTIONS FOR USING THE ACT-O-VIAL SYSTEM

1. Press down on plastic activator to force diluent into the lower compartment.
2. Gently agitate to effect solution.
3. Remove plastic tab covering center of stopper.
4. Sterilize top of stopper with a suitable germicide.
5. Insert needle **squarely through center** of stopper until tip is just visible. Invert vial and withdraw dose.

STORAGE CONDITIONS

Store unreconstituted product at controlled room temperature 15° to 30° C (59° to 86° F). Store solution at controlled room temperature 15° to 30° C (59° to 86° F). Use solution within 48 hours after mixing.

HOW SUPPLIED

SOLU-MEDROL Sterile Powder is available in the following packages:

40 mg Act-O-Vial System (Single-Dose Vial)	**500 mg** Vial NDC 0009-0758-01
1 mL NDC 0009-0113-12	**500 mg** Vial with Diluent NDC 0009-0887-01
25—1 mL NDC 0009-0113-13	**500 mg Act-O-Vial System (Single-Dose Vial)**
25—1 mL NDC 0009-0113-19	4 mL NDC 0009-0765-02
125 mg Act-O-Vial System (Single-Dose Vial)	**1 gram** Vial NDC 0009-0698-01
2 mL NDC 0009-0190-09	**1 gram Act-O-Vial System (Single-Dose Vial)**
25—2 mL NDC 0009-0190-10	8 mL NDC 0009-3389-01
25—2 mL NDC 0009-0190-16	**2 gram** Vial NDC 0009-0988-01
	2 gram Vial with Diluent NDC 0009-0796-01

Courtesy of the Upjohn Company.

Given quantity = 40 mg
Wanted quantity = mL
Dose on hand   = 125 mg/2 mL (yield from 2 mL Act-O-Vial)

Sequential method:

$$\frac{40\text{ mg}}{} \Bigg| \frac{2\ \text{(mL)}}{125\text{ mg}} \Bigg| \frac{40 \times 2}{125} \Bigg| \frac{80}{125} = 0.64\text{ mL or } 0.6\text{ mL}$$

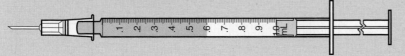

● **0.6 mL is the wanted quantity and the answer to the problem.**

EXAMPLE 5.4

Order: Claforan 50 mg/kg IV every 8 hours for infection. The infant weighs 12 kg.

✤ **How many milliliters will you draw from the vial after reconstitution?** _____

719000-2/95

Claforan®

Sterile (sterile cefotaxime sodium)
and
Injection (cefotaxime sodium injection)

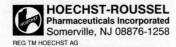

HOECHST-ROUSSEL
Pharmaceuticals Incorporated
Somerville, NJ 08876-1258
REG TM HOECHST AG

Neonates, Infants, and Children
The following dosage schedule is recommended:

    Neonates (birth to 1 month):
        0-1 week of age   50 mg/kg per dose every 12 hours IV
        1-4 weeks of age   50 mg/kg per dose every 8 hours IV
    It is not necessary to differentiate between premature and normal-gestational age infants.
    Infants and Children (1 month to 12 years): For body weights less than 50 kg, the recommended daily dose is 50 to 180 mg/kg IM or IV body weight divided into four to six equal doses. The higher dosages should be used for more severe or serious infections, including meningitis. For body weights 50 kg or more, the usual adult dosage should be used; the maximum daily dosage should not exceed 12 grams.

Courtesy of Hoechst-Roussel Pharmaceuticals.

Supply: Claforan 1 g/10 mL
The package insert states: Reconstitute vials with at least 10 mL of sterile water for injection.
Given quantity   = 50 mg/kg
Wanted quantity = mL
Dose on hand   = 1 g/10 mL
Weight   = 12 kg

(Example continues on page 120)

Random method:

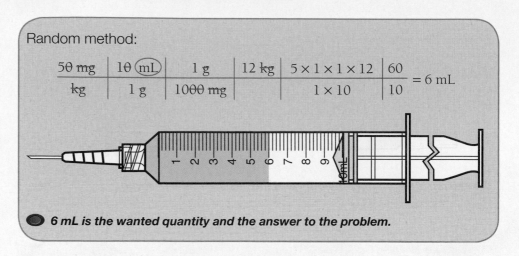

$$\frac{50 \text{ mg}}{\text{kg}} \quad \frac{10 \text{ (mL)}}{1 \text{ g}} \quad \frac{1 \text{ g}}{1000 \text{ mg}} \quad \frac{12 \text{ kg}}{} \quad \frac{5 \times 1 \times 1 \times 12}{1 \times 10} \quad \frac{60}{10} = 6 \text{ mL}$$

6 mL is the wanted quantity and the answer to the problem.

Exercise 5.2   **Medication Problems Involving Reconstitution**

(See pages 145 for answers)

1. Order: cefazolin 500 mg IV every 8 hours for infection.

   ▶ **How many milliliters will you draw out of the vial after reconstitution?** _____

   (Cefazolin is reconstituted using 50 mL sodium chloride.)

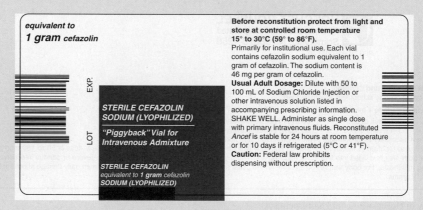

equivalent to **1 gram** cefazolin	Before reconstitution protect from light and store at controlled room temperature **15° to 30°C (59° to 86°F).** Primarily for institutional use. Each vial contains cefazolin sodium equivalent to 1 gram of cefazolin. The sodium content is 46 mg per gram of cefazolin.
STERILE CEFAZOLIN SODIUM (LYOPHILIZED) "Piggyback" Vial for Intravenous Admixture STERILE CEFAZOLIN equivalent to **1 gram** cefazolin SODIUM (LYOPHILIZED)	**Usual Adult Dosage:** Dilute with 50 to 100 mL of Sodium Chloride Injection or other intravenous solution listed in accompanying prescribing information. SHAKE WELL. Administer as single dose with primary intravenous fluids. Reconstituted *Ancef* is stable for 24 hours at room temperature or for 10 days if refrigerated (5°C or 41°F). **Caution:** Federal law prohibits dispensing without prescription.

2. Order: Primaxin 250 mg IV every 6 hours for infection.

   Supply: Primaxin vial labeled 500 mg. Reconstitute with 10 mL of compatible diluent and shake well.

   ▶ **How many milliliters will you draw from the vial after reconstitution?** _____

3. Order: Unasyn (ampicillin) 50 mg/kg IV every 4 hours for infection.

   Supply: Unasyn 1.5-g vial

   Nursing drug reference: Reconstitute each Unasyn 1.5-g vial with 4 mL of sterile water to yield 375 mg/mL.

   The child weighs 40 kg.

   ▶ **How many milliliters will you draw from the vial after reconstitution?** _____

4. Order: erythromycin 750 mg IV every 6 hours for infection.

   Supply: erythromycin 1-g vial labeled: Reconstitute with 20 mL of sterile water for injection.

   ▶ **How many milliliters will you draw from the vial after reconstitution?** _____

5. Order: Fortaz 30 mg/kg IV every 8 hours for infection

   Supply: Fortaz 500-mg vial labeled: Reconstitute with 5 mL of sterile water for injection.

   The child weighs 65 lb.

   ▶ **How many milliliters will you draw from the vial after reconstitution?** _____

MEDICATION PROBLEMS INVOLVING INTRAVENOUS PUMPS

Intravenous (IV) medications are administered by drawing a specific amount of medication from a vial or ampule and inserting that medication into an existing IV line. All IV medications must be given with specific thought to exactly how much *time* it should take to administer the medication. Information regarding time may be obtained from a nursing drug reference, label, or package insert, or may be specifically ordered by the physician.

Although IV medications can be administered IV push, the time involved often requires the use of an IV pump. All IV pumps deliver milliliters per hour (mL/hr) but may vary in operational capacity or size.

Below is an example of the dimensional analysis problem-solving method with basic terms applied to a medication problem involving an IV pump.

Unit Path

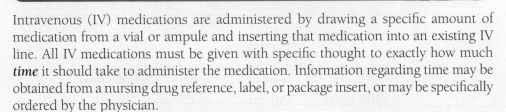

	Conversion Factor for Given Quantity (Numerator)	Conversion Computation	Wanted Quantity
Given Quantity			
$\dfrac{1500 \text{ Units}}{\text{hr}}$	$\dfrac{250 \text{ mL}}{25{,}000 \text{ Units}}$	$\dfrac{15}{\text{hr}}$	$= 15 \text{ mL}$

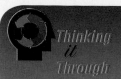

The two-factor–given quantity (the physician's order) contains a **numerator** (the dosage of medication) and a **denominator** (time). The wanted quantity (the answer to the problem) also contains a numerator (mL) and a denominator (time). This is called a two-factor–given quantity to a two-factor–wanted quantity medication problem. The denominator of the given quantity (hr) corresponds with the denominator of the wanted quantity (hr); therefore, only the numerator of the given quantity (units) needs to be canceled from the problem.

After factoring in the dose on hand, the unwanted unit (units) is canceled from the problem and the wanted unit (mL) remains in the numerator to correspond with the wanted quantity. The same number values are canceled from the numerator and denominator, leaving 15 mL/hr.

EXAMPLE 5.5

The physician orders heparin 1500 units/hr IV. The pharmacy sends an IV bag labeled: Heparin 25,000 units in 250 mL of D5W.

❋ **Calculate the IV pump setting for milliliters per hour.**

Given quantity   = 1500 units/hr
Wanted quantity = mL/hr
Dose on hand   = 25,000 units/250 mL

Sequential method:

Step 1 **Begin by identifying the given quantity. Establish the unit path to the wanted quantity.**

Unit Path

Given Quantity	Conversion Factor for Given Quantity (Numerator)	Conversion Computation	Wanted Quantity
$\dfrac{1500\ \text{Units}}{\text{hr}}$			$= \dfrac{\text{mL}}{\text{hr}}$

Step 2

Unit Path

Given Quantity	Conversion Factor for Given Quantity (Numerator)	Conversion Computation	Wanted Quantity
$\dfrac{1500\ \cancel{\text{Units}}}{\cancel{\text{hr}}}$	$\dfrac{250\ \text{mL}}{25,000\ \cancel{\text{Units}}}$		$= \dfrac{\text{mL}}{\text{hr}}$

Step 3

Unit Path

Given Quantity	Conversion Factor for Given Quantity (Numerator)	Conversion Computation	Wanted Quantity
$\dfrac{1500\ \cancel{\text{Units}}}{\cancel{\text{hr}}}$	$\dfrac{250\ \text{mL}}{25,000\ \cancel{\text{Units}}}$	15	$= \dfrac{15\ \text{mL}}{\text{hr}}$

⬤ ***15 mL/hr is the wanted quantity and the answer to the problem.***

EXAMPLE 5.6

The physician orders 500 mL of 0.45% NS with 20 mEq of KCl to infuse over 8 hours.

❀ **Calculate the number of milliliters per hour to set the IV pump.**

Given quantity   = 500 mL/8 hr
Wanted quantity = mL/hr

Sequential method:

$$\frac{500 \enclose{circle}{\text{mL}}}{8 \enclose{circle}{\text{hr}}} \quad \frac{500}{8} = \frac{62.5 \text{ mL}}{} \text{ or } \frac{63 \text{ mL}}{\text{hr}}$$

⬤ **63 mL/hr is the wanted quantity and the answer to the problem.**

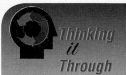

Thinking it Through

In this problem, the needed two factors are already identified in the given quantity and, therefore, require no additional conversions. The 20 mEq of KCl added to the IV bag is included as part of the 500 mL and is additional information for the nurse, but not part of the calculation.

EXAMPLE 5.7

The physician orders aminophylline 44 mg/hr IV. The pharmacy sends an IV bag labeled: Aminophylline 1 g/250 mL NS.

❀ **Calculate the milliliters per hour to set the IV pump.**

Given quantity   = 44 mg/hr
Wanted quantity = mL/hr
Dose on hand   = 1 g/250 mL

Random method:

$$\frac{44 \text{ mg}}{\enclose{circle}{\text{hr}}} \quad \frac{250 \enclose{circle}{\text{mL}}}{1 \text{ g}} \quad \frac{1 \text{ g}}{1000 \text{ mg}} \quad \frac{44 \times 25}{100} \quad \frac{1100}{100} = \frac{11 \text{ mL}}{\text{hr}}$$

⬤ **11 mL/hr is the wanted quantity and the answer to the problem.**

Thinking it Through

The given quantity has been identified as what the physician orders, but also can be information that the nurse has obtained. The nurse may know that the IV pump is set to deliver 11 mL/hr, but wants to know if the dosage of medication the patient is receiving is within a safe dosage range.

EXAMPLE 5.8

The nurse checks the IV pump and documents that the pump is set at and delivering 11 mL/hr and that the IV bag hanging is labeled: Aminophylline 1 g/250 mL.

❀ **How many milligrams per hour is the patient receiving?**

Given quantity   = 11 mL/hr
Wanted quantity = mg/hr
Dose on hand   = 1 g/250 mL

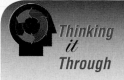

Thinking it Through

The dose on hand is factored in and allows the unwanted unit (mL) to be canceled.

(Example continues on page 124)

Sequential method:

Step 1

$$\frac{11 \text{ mL}}{\text{hr}} \Bigg| = \frac{\text{mg}}{\text{hr}}$$

Step 2

$$\frac{11 \text{ mL}}{\text{hr}} \left| \frac{1 \text{ g}}{250 \text{ mL}} \right. = \frac{\text{mg}}{\text{hr}}$$

Step 3

$$\frac{11 \text{ mL}}{\text{hr}} \left| \frac{1 \text{ g}}{250 \text{ mL}} \right| \frac{1000 \text{ mg}}{1 \text{ g}} \left| \frac{11 \times 100}{25} \right| \frac{1100}{25} = \frac{44 \text{ mg}}{\text{hr}}$$

⬤ *44 mg/hr is the wanted quantity and the answer to the problem.*

Exercise 5.3   **Medication Problems Involving Intravenous Pumps**

(See pages 145–146 for answers)

1. Order: heparin 1800 units/hr IV

   Supply: heparin 25,000 units/250 mL D5W

   ▶ **Calculate the milliliters per hour to set the IV pump.** _____

2. Order: aminophylline 35 mg/hr IV

   Supply: aminophylline 1 g/250 mL NS

   ▶ **Calculate the milliliters per hour to set the IV pump.** _____

3. Information obtained by the nurse: heparin 25,000 units in 250 mL D5W is infusing at 30 mL/hr.

   ▶ **How many units per hour is the patient receiving?** _____

4. Information obtained by the nurse: aminophylline 1 g/250 mL NS is infusing at 15 mL/hr.

   ▶ **How many milligrams per hour is the patient receiving?** _____

5. Order: heparin 900 units/hr IV

Supply: heparin 25,000 units/500 mL D5W

▶ **Calculate the milliliters per hour to set the IV pump.** _____

MEDICATION PROBLEMS INVOLVING DROP FACTORS

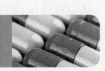

Although IV pumps are used whenever possible, there are situations (no IV pumps available) and circumstances (outpatient or home care) that arise when IV pumps are not available and IV fluids or medications might be administered using gravity flow. **Gravity flow** involves calculating the drops per minute (gtt/min) required to infuse IV fluids or medications. When IV fluids or medications are administered using gravity flow, it is important to know the drop factor for the IV tubing that is being used. **Drop factor** is the drops per milliliter (gtt/mL) that the IV tubing will produce..Two types of IV tubing are available for gravity flow. *Macrotubing* delivers a large drop and is available in 10 gtt/mL, 15 gtt/mL, and 20 gtt/mL (Table 5.1); and *microtubing* delivers a small drop and is available in 60 gtt/mL.

Regardless of the IV tubing used, the problem can be solved by dimensional analysis. Below is an example of a medication problem involving drop factors using the dimensional analysis method.

Unit Path

Given Quantity	Conversion Factor for Given Quantity (Numerator)	Conversion Computation		Wanted Quantity

$$\frac{250 \text{ mL}}{30 \text{ min}} \mid \frac{10 \text{ gtt}}{\text{mL}} \mid \frac{250 \times 1}{3} \mid \frac{250}{3} = \frac{83.3 \text{ gtt}}{\text{min}} \text{ or } \frac{83 \text{ gtt}}{\text{min}}$$

TABLE 5.1	**Examples of Different Macrodrip Factors**

Manufacturer	Drops per milliliter (gtt/mL)
Travenol	10
Abbott	15
McGaw	15
Cutter	20

PREVENTING MEDICATION ERRORS

When IV fluids are administered by gravity (without the use of an IV pump), it is the responsibility of the nurse to investigate the history of each patient to ensure safe delivery of IV fluids.

IV fluids that flow by gravity need to be monitored closely because the flow of the fluids can change with the position of the hand or arm. Some patients with a history of congestive heart failure do not tolerate large volumes of IV fluids.

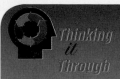

Thinking
it
Through

The given quantity and the wanted quantity both include two factors; therefore, this is a two-factor–given quantity to a two-factor–wanted quantity medication problem.

The denominators are the same (min). The numerator in the given quantity (mL) is an unwanted unit and needs to be canceled.

When the drop factor is factored in, the unwanted unit (mL) is canceled, and the wanted unit (gtt) is placed in the numerator to correspond with the wanted quantity.

After you cancel the unwanted units from the problem, multiply the numerators, multiply the denominators, and divide the product of the numerators by the product of the denominators to provide the wanted quantity.

EXAMPLE 5.9

The physician orders 250 mL of normal saline to infuse in 30 minutes. The drop factor listed on the IV tubing box is 10 gtt/mL.

❃ **Calculate the number of drops per minute required to infuse the IV bolus.**

Given quantity   = 250 mL/30 min
Wanted quantity = gtt/min
Drop factor   = 10 gtt/mL

Sequential method:

Step 1 **Begin by identifying the given quantity and establishing a unit path to the wanted quantity.**

Unit Path

Given Quantity	Conversion Factor for Given Quantity (Numerator)	Conversion Computation	Wanted Quantity
$\dfrac{250 \text{ mL}}{30 \text{ min}}$			$= \dfrac{\text{gtt}}{\text{min}}$

Step 2

Unit Path

Given Quantity	Conversion Factor for Given Quantity (Numerator)	Conversion Computation	Wanted Quantity
$\dfrac{250 \text{ mL}}{30 \text{ min}}$	$\dfrac{10 \text{ gtt}}{\text{mL}}$		$= \dfrac{\text{gtt}}{\text{min}}$

Step 3

Unit Path

Given Quantity	Conversion Factor for Given Quantity (Numerator)	Conversion Computation		Wanted Quantity
$\dfrac{250 \text{ mL}}{30 \text{ min}}$	$\dfrac{10 \text{ gtt}}{\text{mL}}$	$\dfrac{250 \times 1}{3}$	$\dfrac{250}{3}$	$= \dfrac{83.3 \text{ gtt}}{\text{min}}$ or $\dfrac{83 \text{ gtt}}{\text{min}}$

⬤ *83 gtt/min is the wanted quantity and the answer to the problem.*

EXAMPLE 5.10

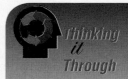

In some situations (home care), it may be important for the nurse to know exactly how long a specific amount of IV fluid will take to infuse. The physician may order a limited amount of IV fluid to infuse at a specific number of drops per minute (gtt/min).

The physician orders 1000 mL of D5W and 0.45% NS to infuse over 8 hours. The drop factor is 20 gtt/mL.

❋ **Calculate the number of drops per minute required to infuse the IV volume.**

Given quantity = 1000 mL/8 hr
Wanted quantity = gtt/min
Drop factor = 20 gtt/mL

Sequential method:

Step 1
_____

$$\frac{1000 \text{ mL}}{8 \text{ hr}} \left| \frac{20 \text{ gtt}}{\text{mL}} \right. = \frac{\text{gtt}}{\text{min}}$$

Step 2
_____

$$\frac{1000 \text{ mL}}{8 \text{ hr}} \left| \frac{20 \text{ gtt}}{\text{mL}} \right| \frac{1 \text{ hr}}{60 \text{ min}} = \frac{\text{gtt}}{\text{min}}$$

Step 3
_____

$$\frac{1000 \text{ mL}}{8 \text{ hr}} \left| \frac{20 \text{ gtt}}{\text{mL}} \right| \frac{1 \text{ hr}}{60 \text{ min}} \left| \frac{1000 \times 2 \times 1}{8 \times 6} \right| \frac{2000}{48} = \frac{41.66 \text{ gtt}}{\text{min}}$$

$$\frac{41.66 \text{ gtt}}{\text{min}} \quad \text{or} \quad \frac{42 \text{ gtt}}{\text{min}}$$

⬤ *42 gtt/min is the wanted quantity and the answer to the problem.*

Thinking it Through

The unwanted unit (mL) is canceled, and the wanted unit (gtt) is placed in the numerator. Another unwanted unit (hr) needs to be canceled from the unit path.

The conversion factor (1 hr = 60 min) has been factored in to allow the unwanted unit (hr) to be canceled and the wanted unit (min) is placed in the denominator.

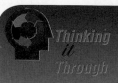

Thinking it Through

The given quantity and the wanted quantity have been identified and are both in the numerator; therefore, this is a one-factor–given quantity to a one-factor–wanted quantity medication problem.

The drop factor (10 gtt/mL) has been factored in using the sequential method to cancel the unwanted unit (mL).

The infusing rate of 21 gtt/min has now been factored in to cancel the unwanted unit (gtt).

The conversion factor (1 hr = 60 min) has been factored in to cancel the unwanted unit (min). The wanted unit (hr) remains in the numerator, which corresponds to the wanted quantity.

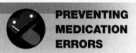

PREVENTING MEDICATION ERRORS

It is the responsibility of the nurse to ensure that an IV does not run dry and endanger the patient due to air in the IV line.

Check an IV bag infusing by gravity every 1 to 2 hours and/or instruct the patient to report when the IV has only a small amount (100 mL) left in the IV bag.

EXAMPLE 5.11

It is safe nursing practice to monitor an infusing IV every 2 hours to make sure it is infusing without difficulty and on time. It may be necessary to hang the next IV after $7\frac{1}{2}$ hours (before the estimated completion time) to keep the IV from running dry.

The physician orders 1000 mL of D5W. The drop factor is 10 gtt/mL. The infusion is dripping at 21 gtt/min.

❀ **How many hours will it take for the IV to infuse?**

Given quantity   = 1000 mL
Wanted quantity = hr
Drop factor   = 10 gtt/mL

Step 1

$$\frac{1000\ \text{mL}}{} = \text{hr}$$

Step 2

$$\frac{1000\ \text{mL}}{}\ \frac{10\ \text{gtt}}{\text{mL}} = \text{hr}$$

Step 3

$$\frac{1000\ \cancel{\text{mL}}}{}\ \frac{10\ \text{gtt}}{\cancel{\text{mL}}}\ \frac{\text{min}}{21\ \text{gtt}} = \text{hr}$$

Step 4

$$\frac{1000\ \cancel{\text{mL}}}{}\ \frac{10\ \text{gtt}}{\cancel{\text{mL}}}\ \frac{\cancel{\text{min}}}{21\ \cancel{\text{gtt}}}\ \frac{1\ \text{hr}}{60\ \cancel{\text{min}}} = \text{hr}$$

Step 5

$$\frac{1000\ \cancel{\text{mL}}}{}\ \frac{10\ \cancel{\text{gtt}}}{\cancel{\text{mL}}}\ \frac{\cancel{\text{min}}}{21\ \cancel{\text{gtt}}}\ \frac{1\ \text{hr}}{60\ \cancel{\text{min}}}\ \frac{1000 \times 1 \times 1}{21 \times 6}\ \frac{1000}{126} = 7.93\ \text{hr or } 7.9\ \text{hr}$$

⬤ *8 hours is the wanted quantity and the answer to the problem.*

Exercise 5.4	**Medication Problems Involving Drop Factors**

(See page 146 for answers)

1. Order: 800 mL D5W to infuse in 8 hours

   Drop factor: 15 gtt/mL

   ▶ **Calculate the number of drops per minute.** _____

2. Order: Infuse 250 mL NS

   Drop factor: 15 gtt/mL

   Infusion rate: 60 gtt/min

   ▶ **Calculate the hours to infuse.** _____

3. Order: 150 mL over 60 minutes

   Drop factor: 10 gtt/mL

   ▶ **Calculate the number of drops per minute.** _____

4. Order: 1000 mL D5W/0.9% NS

   Drop factor: 15 gtt/mL

   Infusion rate: 50 gtt/min

   ▶ **Calculate the number of hours to infuse.** _____

5. Order: 500 mL over 4 hours

   Drop factor: 15 gtt/mL

   ▶ **Calculate the number of drops per minute.** _____

MEDICATION PROBLEMS INVOLVING INTERMITTENT INFUSION

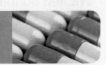

Intravenous medications can be delivered over a specific amount of time by *intermittent infusion*. These medications require the use of an **infusion pump**. Some must be reconstituted and further diluted in a specific type and amount of IV fluid and delivered over a limited time. Others do not need to be reconstituted, but must be further diluted in a specific type and amount of IV fluid and delivered over a limited time.

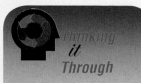

This order contains two problems. The first involves how many milliliters to draw from the vial after reconstitution, and the second involves how many milliliters per hour to set the IV pump.

EXAMPLE 5.12

The physician ordered erythromycin 500 mg IV every 6 hours for infection. The pharmacy sends a vial labeled: Erythromycin 1 g. The nursing drug reference provides information to reconstitute 1 g of erythromycin with 20 mL of sterile water and further dilute in 250 mL of 0.9% NS and to infuse over 1 hour.

❀ **How many milliliters will you draw from the vial after reconstitution?**

❀ **Calculate the milliliters per hour to set the IV pump.**

Step 1

❀ **How many milliliters will you draw from the vial after reconstitution?**

Given quantity = 500 mg
Wanted quantity = mL
Dose on hand   = 1 g/20 mL

Random method:

$$\frac{500 \text{ mg}}{} \cdot \frac{20 \text{ mL}}{1 \text{ g}} \cdot \frac{1 \text{ g}}{1000 \text{ mg}} \cdot \frac{5 \times 2}{1} \cdot \frac{10}{1} = 10 \text{ mL}$$

⬤ *The wanted quantity is 10 mL, and is the amount that will need to be drawn from the vial and added to the 100 mL of 0.9% NS. After adding the 10 mL to the IV bag, the IV bag will now contain 110 mL.*

Step 2

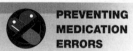

PREVENTING MEDICATION ERRORS

When adding reconstituted solutions to an IV bag, the general rule is to include the volume in the total amount to be calculated for IV administration if the reconstituted solution is 10% or more of the total IV solution (Example: 10% of 100 mL = 10 mL = 110 mL or 10% of 50 mL = 5 mL or 55 mL).

❀ **Calculate the milliliters per hour to set the IV pump.**

Given quantity = 110 mL/1 hr
Wanted quantity = mL/hr

Sequential method:

$$\frac{110 \text{ mL}}{1 \text{ hr}} \cdot \frac{110}{1} = \frac{110 \text{ mL}}{\text{hr}}$$

⬤ *The IV pump is set at 110 mL/hr to infuse the 500 mg of erythromycin ordered by the physician.*

Step 2 (alternative): If an IV pump was unavailable, the infusion could be delivered by gravity using IV tubing with a drop factor of 10 gtt/mL.

❀ **Calculate the drops per minute required to infuse the IV volume.**

Given quantity = 110 mL/1 hr
Wanted quantity = gtt/min
Drop factor   = 10 gtt/mL

Sequential method:

$$\frac{110 \text{ mL}}{1 \text{ hr}} \cdot \frac{10 \text{ gtt}}{\text{mL}} \cdot \frac{1 \text{ hr}}{60 \text{ min}} \cdot \frac{110 \times 1 \times 1}{1 \times 6} \cdot \frac{110}{6} = \frac{18.33 \text{ or } 18 \text{ gtt}}{\text{min}}$$

Exercise 5.5	**Medication Problems Involving Intermittent Infusion**

(See pages 146–147 for answers)

1. Order: ampicillin 250 mg IV every 4 hours for infection

   Supply: ampicillin 1-g vial

   Nursing drug reference: Reconstitute with 10 mL of 0.9% NS and further dilute in 50 mL NS. Infuse over 15 min.

   ▶ **How many milliliters will you draw from the vial after reconstitution?** _____

   ▶ **Calculate the milliliters per hour to set the IV pump.** _____

   ▶ **Calculate the drops per minute with a drop factor of 10 gtt/mL.** _____

2. Order: Clindamycin 0.3 g IV every 6 hours for infection

   Supply: Clindamycin 600 mg/4-mL vial

   Nursing drug reference: Dilute with 50 mL 0.9% NS and infuse over 15 min.

   ▶ **How many milliliters will you draw from the vial?** _____

   ▶ **Calculate the milliliters per hour to set the IV pump.** _____

   ▶ **Calculate the drops per minute with a drop factor of 15 gtt/mL.** _____

3. Order: Vancomycin 1 g IVPB every 12 hours for methicillin-resistant staphylococci

   Supply: Vancomycin 1-g vial

   Nursing drug reference: Reconstitute each 1-g vial with 20 mL of sterile water and further dilute in 100 mL of 0.9% NS to infuse over 60 minutes.

   ▶ **How many milliliters will you draw from the vial after reconstitution?** _____

   ▶ **Calculate the milliliters per hour to set the IV pump.** _____

(Exercise continues on page 132)

▶ **Calculate the drops per minute with a drop factor of 20 gtt/mL.** _____

4. Order: Unasyn 1000 mg IV every 6 hours for infection

   Supply: Unasyn 1.5-g vial

   Nursing drug reference: Reconstitute with 4 mL of 0.9% NS and further dilute with 100 mL NS to infuse over 1 hr.

   ▶ **How many milliliters will you draw from the vial after reconstitution?** _____

   ▶ **Calculate the milliliters per hour to set the IV pump.** _____

   ▶ **Calculate the drops per minute with a drop factor of 20 gtt/mL.** _____

5. Order: Zantac 50 mg IV every 6 hours for ulcers

   Supply: Zantac 25-mg/mL vial

   Nursing drug reference: Dilute with 50 mL 0.9% NS to infuse over 30 min.

   ▶ **How many milliliters will you draw from the vial?** _____

   ▶ **Calculate the milliliters per hour to set the IV pump.** _____

   ▶ **Calculate the drops per minute with a drop factor of 10 gtt/mL.** _____

Summary

This chapter has taught you to calculate two-factor medication problems involving the weight of the patient, reconstitution of medications, and the amount of time over which medications and intravenous fluids can be safely administered. To demonstrate your ability to calculate medication problems accurately, complete the following practice problems.

Practice Problems for Chapter 5

Two-Factor Medication Problems

(See pages 147–148 for answers)

1. Order: verapamil 0.2 mg/kg IV for arrhythmia

   Supply: verapamil (Isoptin) 5 mg/2 mL

   Child's weight: 10 lb

   ❋ **How many milliliters will you give?** _____

2. Order: Tylenol Elixir 10 mg/kg every 4 hours prn for fever

   Supply: Tylenol Elixir 160 mg/5 mL

   Child's weight: 8 kg

   ❋ **How many milliliters will you give?** _____

3. Order: Fortaz 1.25 g IV every 8 hours for infection

   Supply: Fortaz 2-g vial

   Nursing drug reference: Dilute each 2 g with 10 mL sterile water for injection.

   ❋ **How many milliliters will you draw from the vial after reconstitution?** _____

4. Order: Unasyn 750 mg IV every 8 hours for infection

   Supply: Unasyn 1.5-g vial

   Nursing drug reference: Reconstitute with 4 mL of sterile water for injection.

   ❋ **How many milliliters will you draw from the vial after reconstitution?** _____

5. Order: heparin 700 units/hr for anticoagulation

   Supply: heparin 25,000 units/250 mL NS

   ❋ **At how many milliliters per hour will you set the IV pump?** _____

6. Information obtained by the nurse: Zantac 150 mg in 250 mL NS is infusing at 11 mL/hr.

   ❋ **How many milligrams per hour is the patient receiving?** _____

(Practice Problems continue on page 134)

7. Order: 1000 mL D5W/0.9% NS to infuse over 8 hours

   Drop factor: 20 gtt/mL

   ❋ **Calculate the number of drops per minute.** _____

8. Order: Infuse 750 mL NS

   Drop factor: 15 gtt/mL

   Infusion rate: 18 gtt/min

   ❋ **Calculate the number of hours to infuse.** _____

9. Order: vancomycin 10 mg/kg IV every 8 hours for infection

   Supply: vancomycin 500-mg vial

   Infant's weight: 20 lb

   Nursing drug reference: Dilute each 500-mg vial with 10 mL of sterile water for injection and further dilute in 100 mL of 0.9% NS to infuse over 1 hr.

   ❋ **How many milliliters will you draw from the vial after reconstitution?** _____

   ❋ **Calculate the milliliters per hour to set the IV pump.** _____

   ❋ **Calculate the drops per minute with a drop factor of 10 gtt/mL.** _____

10. Order: acyclovir 355 mg IV every 8 hours for herpes

    Supply: acyclovir 500-mg vial

    Nursing drug reference: Reconstitute each 500 mg with 10 mL of sterile water for injection and further dilute in 100 mL NS to infuse over 1 hour.

    ❋ **How many milliliters will you draw from the vial after reconstitution?** _____

    ❋ **Calculate the milliliters per hour to set the IV pump.** _____

    ❋ **Calculate the drops per minute with a drop factor of 20 gtt/mL.** _____

11. Order: Diltiazem hydrochloride (Cardizem) 0.25 mg/kg IV push over 2 minutes for atrial fibrillation.

    Supply: Cardizem vial labeled 5 mg/mL

    Nursing drug reference: May be administered by direct IV over 2 minutes or as an infusion.

    Patient's weight: 80 kg

    ❋ **How many milliliters will you give via IV push over 2 minutes?** _____

12. Order: Pantoprazole sodium (Protonix) 40 mg IV every 12 hours to infuse over 15 minutes for treatment of ulcerated GERD

    Supply: Protonix 40 mg powder

    Nursing drug reference: Reconstitute 40 mg powder with 10 mL 0.9% NS and further dilute in 100 mL 0.9% NS or D5W to yield 0.4 mg/mL.

    ✳ **Calculate the milliliters per hour to set the IV pump to administer the infusion over 15 minutes.** _____

13. Order: Diltiazem hydrochloride (Cardizem) 10 mg/hr continuous IV infusion for atrial fibrillation

    Supply: Cardiazem 125 mg/25 mL syringe

    Nursing drug reference: May be administered by direct IV over 2 minutes or as an infusion. For IV infusion, add Cardizem to 100 mL of 0.9% NS or D5W (100 mL + 25 mL = 125 mL) to yield 1 mg/mL.

    ✳ **Calculate the milliliters per hour to set the IV pump.** _____

14. Order: Benazepril hydrochloride (Lotensin) 0.2 mg/kg PO as monotherapy for hypertension

    Supply: Lotensin suspension 150 mL yields 2 mg/mL

    Child's weight: 40 kg

    ✳ **How many milliliters will you give?** _____

15. Order: Lithium carbonate (Lithium) 1.2 g/day in three divided doses PO for manic-depressive disorder

    Supply: Lithium 300 mg/5 mL syrup

    ✳ **How many milliliters per dose will you give?** _____

16. Order: Levofloxacin (Levaquin) 250 mg IV over 90 minutes for gonococcal infection

    Supply: Levaquin premixed 500 mg/100 mL D5W (yields 5 mg/mL)

    ✳ **How many milliliters per hour will you set the IV pump?** _____

17. Order: Heparin 1200 units/hr continuous IV infusion

    Supply: Heparin 25,000 units/250 mL of D5W

    ✳ **How many milliliters per hour will you set the IV pump?** _____

(Practice Problems continue on page 136)

18. The nurse checks the IV pump and documents that the pump is set at and delivering 18 mL/hr of heparin. The IV bag hanging is labeled: Heparin 25,000 units/250 mL.

    ✳ **How many units per hour is the patient receiving?** _____

19. Order: 1000 mL 0.9% NS/D5W to infuse over 8 hours

    Drop factor: 10 gtt/mL

    ✳ **Calculate the number of drops per minute.** _____

20. Order: 1000 mL D5W/0.9% NS

    Drop factor: 10 gtt/mL

    Infusion rate: 15 gtt/min

    ✳ **Calculate the number of hours to infuse.** _____

21. Order: Caldolor (Ibuprofen) 400 mg IV every 6 hours prn for severe pain

    Supply: Caldolor 400 mg/4-mL vial

    Nursing drug reference: Further dilute in 100 mL D5W or 0.9% NS and infuse over 30 minutes.

    ✳ **How many mL will you draw from the vial?** _____

    ✳ **How many milliliters per hour will you set the IV pump?** _____

22. Order: Banzel (Rufinamide) 10 mg/kg PO every other day for seizures associated with Lennox-Gastaut syndrome

    Supply: Banzel 40 mg/mL oral suspension

    Child's weight: 60 lb

    ✳ **How many milliliters will you give?** _____

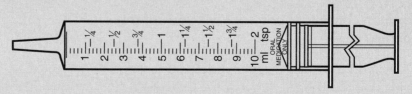

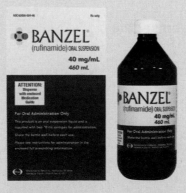

23. Order: Rimantadine (Flumadine) 5 mg/kg PO every day for prevention of influenza A in high-risk children

    Supply: Rimantadine 100-mg tablets

    Child's weight: 50 lb

    ❋ **How many tablets will you give?** _____

24. Order: Carbinoxamine (Karbinal ER) 0.4 mg/kg PO every 12 hours for relief of seasonal allergies

    Supply: Carbinoxamine 4 mg/5 mL oral suspension in strawberry banana

    Child's weight: 35 lb

    ❋ **How many milliliters will you give?**

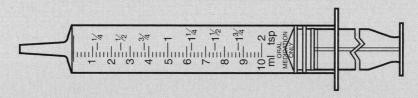

25. Order: Cefazolin 1 g IV every 12 hours for urinary tract infection

    Supply: The pharmacy sends an IV bag labeled Cefazolin 1 g/50 mL to infuse over 30 minutes

    ❋ **How many milliliters per hour will you set the IV pump?** _____

Chapter 5 Post-Test

Two-Factor Medication Problems

Name _____   Date _____

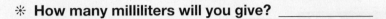

1. Order: Furosemide 2 mg/kg PO every 8 hours for congestive heart failure
   The child weighs 10 kg.

   ❋ **How many milliliters will you give?** _____

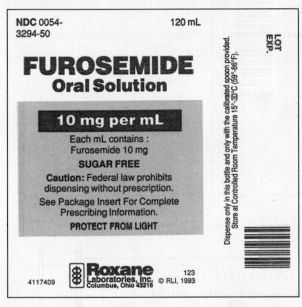

NDC 0054-
3294-50   120 mL

LOT
EXP.

FUROSEMIDE
Oral Solution

10 mg per mL

Each mL contains :
Furosemide 10 mg

SUGAR FREE

Caution: Federal law prohibits
dispensing without prescription.

See Package Insert For Complete
Prescribing Information.

PROTECT FROM LIGHT

Dispense only in this bottle and only with the calibrated spoon provided.
Store at Controlled Room Temperature 15°-30°C (59°-86°F).

4117409   ⚕ **Roxane**   123
          Laboratories, Inc.   © RLI, 1993
          Columbus, Ohio 43216

Courtesy of Roxane Laboratories.

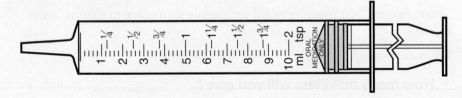

(Post-Test continues on page 140)

2. Order: meperidine 1.5 mg/kg PO every 4 hours for pain

The child weighs 22 lb.

✳ **How many milliliters will you give?** _____

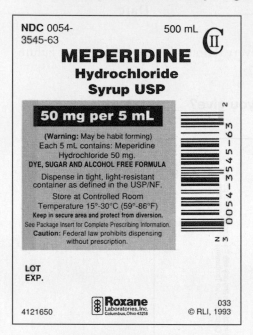

NDC 0054-
3545-63   500 mL

MEPERIDINE

**Hydrochloride
Syrup USP**

50 mg per 5 mL

(Warning: May be habit forming)
Each 5 mL contains: Meperidine
Hydrochloride 50 mg.
DYE, SUGAR AND ALCOHOL FREE FORMULA

Dispense in tight, light-resistant
container as defined in the USP/NF.

Store at Controlled Room
Temperature 15°-30°C (59°-86°F)
Keep in secure area and protect from diversion.
See Package Insert for Complete Prescribing Information.
Caution: Federal law prohibits dispensing
without prescription.

LOT
EXP.

Roxane
Laboratories, Inc.
Columbus, Ohio 43216

4121650   033
                                       © RLI, 1993

Courtesy of Roxane Laboratories.

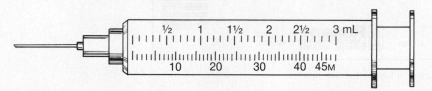

3. Order: Epogen 100 units/kg IV tid for anemia secondary to chronic renal failure

The patient weighs 160 lb.

✳ **How many milliliters will you give?** _____

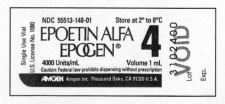

Single Use Vial
U.S. License No. 1080
NDC 55513-148-01   Store at 2° to 8°C

**EPOETIN ALFA
EPOGEN®**   **4**

4000 Units/mL   Volume 1 mL
Caution: Federal law prohibits dispensing without prescription
AMGEN Amgen Inc. Thousand Oaks, CA 91320 U.S.A.

Courtesy of Amgen, Inc.

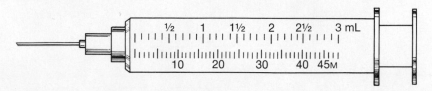

4. Order: amoxicillin/clavulanate potassium 10 mg/kg PO every 8 hours for otitis media

   Nursing drug reference: Dilute with 1 teaspoon (5 mL) of tap water and shake vigorously to yield 125 mg per 5 mL.

   The child weighs 25 kg.

   ❋ **How many milliliters will you give after reconstitution?** _____

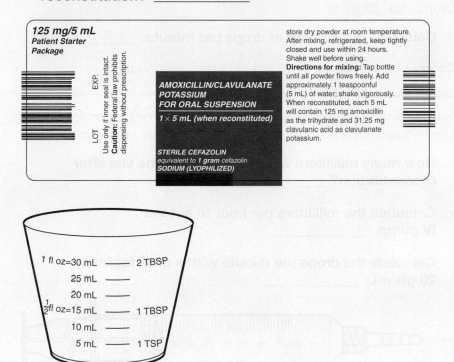

5. The physician orders heparin to infuse at 1300 units/hr continuous IV infusion.

   The pharmacy sends an IV bag labeled heparin 25,000 units in 250 mL.

   ❋ **Calculate the milliliters per hour to set the IV pump.** _____

6. A patient is receiving heparin 25,000 units in 250 mL infused at 25 mL/hr.

   ❋ **How many units per hour is the patient receiving?** _____

(Post-Test continues on page 142)

7. The physician orders morphine sulfate 2 mg/hr continuous IV for intractable pain related to end-stage lung cancer.

   The pharmacy sends an IV bag labeled morphine sulfate 100 mg in 250 mL.

   ❋ **Calculate the milliliters per hour to set the IV pump.** _____

8. Order: 1000 mL D5W/1/2 NS with 20 mEq of KCl to infuse in 12 hours

   Drop factor: 20 gtt/mL.

   ❋ **Calculate the number of drops per minute.** _____

9. Order: Azactam 500 mg IV every 12 hours for septicemia

   Supply: Azactam 1-g vials

   Nursing drug reference: Dilute each 1-g vial with 10 mL of sterile water for injection and further dilute in 100 mL of NS to infuse over 60 minutes.

   ❋ **How many milliliters will you draw from the vial after reconstitution?** _____

   ❋ **Calculate the milliliters per hour to set the IV pump.** _____

   ❋ **Calculate the drops per minute with a drop factor of 20 gtt/mL.** _____

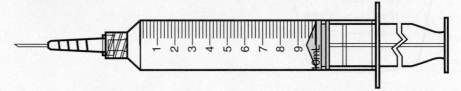

10. Order: Cefazolin 6.25 mg/kg IV every 6 hours for pneumonia

    The child weighs 38.2 kg.

    Nursing drug reference: Dilute each 1-g vial with 10 mL of sterile water for injection and further dilute 50 mL of NS to infuse over 30 minutes.

    ❋ **How many milliliters will you draw from the vial after reconstitution?** _____

    ❋ **Calculate the milliliters per hour to set the IV pump.** _____

    ❋ **Calculate the drops per minute with a drop factor of 10 gtt/mL.** _____

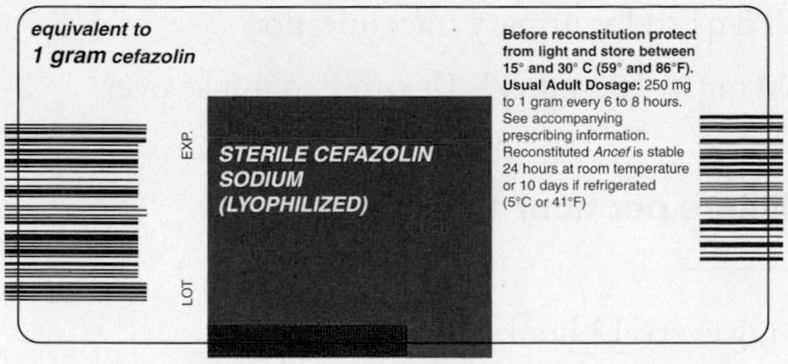

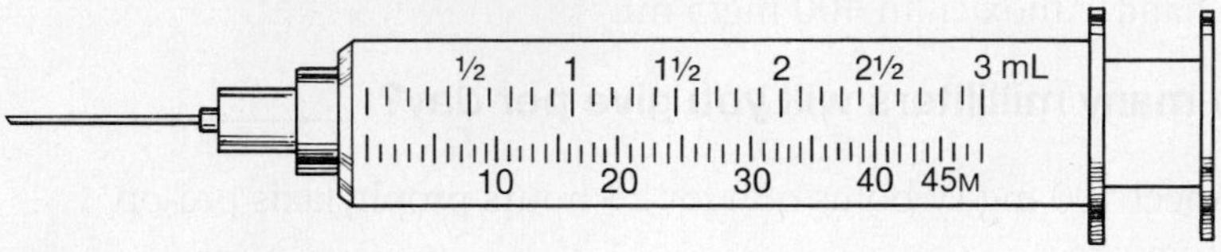

11. Order: 1000 mL D5W 0.45% NS over 8 hours

    Drop factor: 15 gtt/mL

    ✻ **Calculate the number of drops per minute.** ____________

12. Order: Procrit 50 units/kg three times weekly for anemia

    Client's weight: 140 lb

    Dose on hand: Procrit 3000 units per mL

    ✻ **How many milliliters will you give?** ____________

13. Order: 1 liter 0.9% NS to infuse over 12 hours

    Drop factor: 10 gtt/mL

    ✻ **Calculate the number of drops per minute.** ____________

14. Order: Tagamet 400 mg in 50 mL D5W for a duodenal ulcer to infuse over 1 hour

    Drop factor: 15 gtt/mL

    ✻ **Calculate the number of drops per minute.** ____________

15. Order: Lasix 40 mg PO in three divided doses for CHF

    Dose on hand: Lasix 20-mg tablets

    ✻ **How many tablets will you give each day?** ____________

16. Order: Heparin 10,000 units in 1 L 0.9% NS over 12 hours status post-hip replacement

    ✻ **How many units per hour is the patient receiving?** ____________

17. Order: 2 mg of a medication in 1000 mL D5W at 5 mcg/minute

    Drop factor: 10 gtt/mL

    ✻ **Calculate the number of drops per minute.** ____________

(Post-Test continues on page 144)

18. Order: Cipro 200 mg IVPB q12h for urinary tract infection

    Dose on hand: Cipro 200 mg in 100 mL 5% Dextrose to infuse over 60 minutes

    ✳ **Calculate the milliliters per hour to set the IV pump.** _____

19. Order: Amoxicillin 400 mg every 12 hours for ear infection

    Dose on hand: Amoxicillin 400 mg/5 mL

    ✳ **How many milliliters will you give per day?** _____

20. Order: Ancef 500 mg IV bolus q8h for 24 hours prophylaxis pre-op hysterectomy

    Nursing drug reference: Dilute each 1-g vial with 10 mL sterile water and administer IV over 3–5 minutes.

    ✳ **How many milliliters will you give per day?** _____

ANSWER KEY FOR CHAPTER 5: TWO-FACTOR MEDICATION PROBLEMS

Exercise 5.1	**Pediatric Medication Problems Involving Weight**

1

Sequential method:

$$\frac{1 \text{ mg}}{\text{kg}} \left| \frac{\text{mL}}{10 \text{ mg}} \right| \frac{1 \text{ kg}}{2.2 \text{ lb}} \left| 45 \text{ lb} \right| \frac{1 \times 1 \times 45}{10 \times 2.2} \left| \frac{45}{22} \right| = \frac{2.04 \text{ or}}{2 \text{ mL}}$$

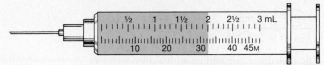

2

Sequential method:

$$\frac{0.01 \text{ mg}}{\text{kg}} \left| \frac{\text{mL}}{0.1 \text{ mg}} \right| \frac{1 \text{ kg}}{2.2 \text{ lb}} \left| 20 \text{ lb} \right| \frac{0.01 \times 1 \times 20}{0.1 \times 2.2} \left| \frac{0.2}{0.22} \right| = 0.9 \text{ mL}$$

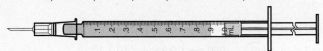

3

Sequential method:

$$\frac{0.5 \text{ mg}}{\text{kg}} \left| \frac{\text{mL}}{25 \text{ mg}} \right| \frac{1 \text{ kg}}{2.2 \text{ lb}} \left| 45 \text{ lb} \right| \frac{0.5 \times 1 \times 45}{25 \times 2.2} \left| \frac{22.5}{55} \right| = 0.4 \text{ mL}$$

4

Random method:

$$\frac{50 \text{ mcg}}{\text{kg}} \left| \frac{\text{mL}}{8 \text{ mg}} \right| \frac{1 \text{ mg}}{1000 \text{ mcg}} \left| \frac{1 \text{ kg}}{2.2 \text{ lb}} \right| 75 \text{ lb} \left| \frac{5 \times 1 \times 1 \times 75}{8 \times 100 \times 2.2} \right| \frac{375}{1760} = 0.2 \text{ mL}$$

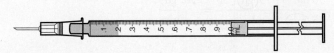

5

Random method:

$$\frac{10 \text{ mg}}{\text{kg}} \left| \frac{1 \text{ kg}}{2.2 \text{ lb}} \right| 70 \text{ lb} \left| \frac{5 \text{ mL}}{300 \text{ mg}} \right| \frac{10 \times 1 \times 7 \times 5}{2.2 \times 30} \left| \frac{350}{66} \right| = 5.3 \text{ or } 5 \text{ mL}$$

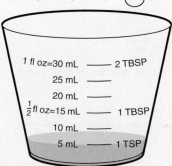

Exercise 5.2	**Medication Problems Involving Reconstitution**

1

Random method:

$$\frac{500 \text{ mg}}{1 \text{ g}} \left| \frac{50 \text{ mL}}{1000 \text{ mg}} \right| \frac{1}{2} \text{ g} \left| \frac{5 \times 5}{1} \right| \frac{25}{1} = 25 \text{ mL}$$

2

Sequential method:

$$\frac{250 \text{ mg}}{500 \text{ mg}} \left| \frac{10 \text{ mL}}{} \right| \frac{25 \times 1}{5} \left| \frac{25}{5} \right| = 5 \text{ mL}$$

3

Random method:

$$\frac{50 \text{ mg}}{\text{kg}} \left| \frac{4 \text{ mL}}{1.5 \text{ g}} \right| \frac{1 \text{ g}}{1000 \text{ mg}} \left| 40 \text{ kg} \right| \frac{5 \times 4 \times 1 \times 4}{1.5 \times 10} \left| \frac{80}{15} \right| = \frac{5.33 \text{ or}}{5 \text{ mL}}$$

Random method using yield:

$$\frac{50 \text{ mg}}{\text{kg}} \left| \frac{1 \text{ mL}}{375 \text{ mg}} \right| 40 \text{ kg} \left| \frac{50 \times 1 \times 40}{375} \right| \frac{2000}{375} = \frac{5.33 \text{ or}}{5 \text{ mL}}$$

4

Random method:

$$\frac{750 \text{ mg}}{1 \text{ g}} \left| \frac{20 \text{ mL}}{1000 \text{ mg}} \right| 1 \text{ g} \left| \frac{75 \times 2 \times 1}{1 \times 10} \right| \frac{150}{10} = 15 \text{ mL}$$

5

Sequential method:

$$\frac{30 \text{ mg}}{\text{kg}} \left| \frac{5 \text{ mL}}{500 \text{ mg}} \right| \frac{1 \text{ kg}}{2.2 \text{ lb}} \left| 65 \text{ lb} \right| \frac{3 \times 5 \times 1 \times 65}{50 \times 2.2} \left| \frac{975}{110} \right| = \frac{8.86 \text{ or}}{8.9 \text{ mL}}$$

Exercise 5.3	**Medication Problems Involving Intravenous Pumps**

1

Sequential method:

$$\frac{1800 \text{ units}}{\text{hr}} \left| \frac{250 \text{ mL}}{25,000 \text{ units}} \right| \frac{18}{} = \frac{18 \text{ mL}}{\text{hr}}$$

2

Random method:

$$\frac{35 \text{ mg}}{\text{hr}} \left| \frac{250 \text{ mL}}{1 \text{ g}} \right| \frac{1}{2} \text{ g} \left| \frac{1000 \text{ mg}}{} \right| \frac{35 \times 25}{100} \left| \frac{875}{100} \right| = \frac{8.75 \text{ or } 9 \text{ mL}}{\text{hr}}$$

3

Sequential method:

$$\frac{30 \text{ mL}}{\text{hr}} \bigg| \frac{25,000 \text{ units}}{250 \text{ mL}} \bigg| \frac{30 \times 2500}{25} \bigg| \frac{75,000}{25} = \frac{3000 \text{ units}}{\text{hr}}$$

4

Sequential method:

$$\frac{15 \text{ mL}}{\text{hr}} \bigg| \frac{1 \text{ g}}{250 \text{ mL}} \bigg| \frac{1000 \text{ mg}}{1 \text{ g}} \bigg| \frac{15 \times 100}{25} \bigg| \frac{1500}{25} = \frac{60 \text{ mg}}{\text{hr}}$$

5

Sequential method:

$$\frac{900 \text{ units}}{\text{hr}} \bigg| \frac{500 \text{ mL}}{25,000 \text{ units}} \bigg| \frac{90 \times 5}{25} \bigg| \frac{450}{25} = \frac{18 \text{ mL}}{\text{hr}}$$

Exercise 5.4   **Medication Problems Involving Drop Factors**

1

Sequential method:

$$\frac{800 \text{ mL}}{8 \text{ hr}} \bigg| \frac{15 \text{ gtt}}{\text{mL}} \bigg| \frac{1 \text{ hr}}{60 \text{ min}} \bigg| \frac{80 \times 15 \times 1}{8 \times 6} \bigg| \frac{1200}{48} = \frac{25 \text{ gtt}}{\text{min}}$$

2

Sequential method:

$$\frac{250 \text{ mL}}{\text{mL}} \bigg| \frac{15 \text{ gtt}}{60 \text{ gtt}} \bigg| \frac{\text{min}}{60 \text{ min}} \bigg| \frac{1 \text{ hr}}{60 \times 60} \bigg| \frac{250 \times 15 \times 1}{3600} \bigg| \frac{3750}{3600} = \frac{1.04 \text{ or}}{1 \text{ hr}}$$

3

Sequential method:

$$\frac{150 \text{ mL}}{60 \text{ min}} \bigg| \frac{10 \text{ gtt}}{\text{mL}} \bigg| \frac{150 \times 1}{6} \bigg| \frac{150}{6} = \frac{25 \text{ gtt}}{\text{min}}$$

4

Sequential method:

$$\frac{1000 \text{ mL}}{\text{mL}} \bigg| \frac{15 \text{ gtt}}{50 \text{ gtt}} \bigg| \frac{\text{min}}{60 \text{ min}} \bigg| \frac{1 \text{ hr}}{5 \times 6} \bigg| \frac{10 \times 15 \times 1}{30} \bigg| \frac{150}{30} = 5 \text{ hr}$$

5

Sequential method:

$$\frac{500 \text{ mL}}{4 \text{ hr}} \bigg| \frac{15 \text{ gtt}}{\text{mL}} \bigg| \frac{1 \text{ hr}}{60 \text{ min}} \bigg| \frac{50 \times 15 \times 1}{4 \times 6} \bigg| \frac{750}{24} = \frac{31.25 \text{ or } 31 \text{ gtt}}{\text{min}}$$

Exercise 5.5   **Medication Problems Involving Intermittent Infusion**

1

Random method:

$$\frac{250 \text{ mg}}{\text{mL}} \bigg| \frac{10 \text{ mL}}{1 \text{ g}} \bigg| \frac{1 \text{ g}}{1000 \text{ mg}} \bigg| \frac{25 \times 1}{10} \bigg| \frac{25}{10} = 2.5 \text{ mL}$$

Calculate milliliters per hour to set the IV pump.

Sequential method:

$$\frac{50 \text{ mL}}{15 \text{ min}} \bigg| \frac{60 \text{ min}}{1 \text{ hr}} \bigg| \frac{50 \times 60}{15 \times 1} \bigg| \frac{3000}{15} = \frac{200 \text{ mL}}{\text{hr}}$$

Calculate drops per minute with a drop factor of 10 gtt/mL.

Sequential method:

$$\frac{50 \text{ mL}}{15 \text{ min}} \bigg| \frac{10 \text{ gtt}}{\text{mL}} \bigg| \frac{50 \times 10}{15} \bigg| \frac{500}{15} = \frac{33.33 \text{ or } 33 \text{ gtt}}{\text{min}}$$

2

Random method:

$$\frac{0.3 \text{ g}}{\text{mL}} \bigg| \frac{4 \text{ mL}}{600 \text{ mg}} \bigg| \frac{1000 \text{ mg}}{1 \text{ g}} \bigg| \frac{0.3 \times 4 \times 10}{6 \times 1} \bigg| \frac{12}{6} = 2 \text{ mL}$$

Calculate milliliters per hour to set the IV pump.

Sequential method:

$$\frac{50 \text{ mL}}{15 \text{ min}} \bigg| \frac{60 \text{ min}}{1 \text{ hr}} \bigg| \frac{50 \times 60}{15 \times 1} \bigg| \frac{3000}{15} = \frac{200 \text{ mL}}{\text{hr}}$$

Calculate drops per minute with a drop factor of 15 gtt/mL.

Sequential method:

$$\frac{50 \text{ mL}}{15 \text{ min}} \bigg| \frac{15 \text{ gtt}}{\text{mL}} \bigg| \frac{50}{1} = \frac{50 \text{ gtt}}{\text{min}}$$

3

Sequential method:

$$\frac{1 \text{ g}}{1 \text{ g}} \bigg| \frac{20 \text{ mL}}{1 \text{ g}} \bigg| \frac{20}{1} = 20 \text{ mL}$$

Calculate the milliliters per hour to set the IV pump.

Sequential method:

$$\frac{120 \text{ mL}}{60 \text{ min}} \bigg| \frac{60 \text{ min}}{1 \text{ hr}} \bigg| \frac{120}{1} = \frac{120 \text{ mL}}{\text{hr}}$$

Calculate the drops per minute with a drop factor of 20 gtt/mL.

Sequential method:

$$\frac{120 \text{ mL}}{1 \text{ hr}} \bigg| \frac{20 \text{ gtt}}{\text{mL}} \bigg| \frac{1 \text{ hr}}{60 \text{ min}} \bigg| \frac{120 \times 2}{6} \bigg| \frac{240}{6} = \frac{40 \text{ gtt}}{\text{min}}$$

4

Random method:

$$\frac{1000 \text{ mg}}{} \cdot \frac{4 \text{ mL}}{1.5 \text{ g}} \cdot \frac{1 \text{ g}}{1000 \text{ mg}} \cdot \frac{4 \times 1}{1.5} \cdot \frac{4}{1.5} = 2.66 \text{ or } 2.7 \text{ mL}$$

Calculate milliliters per hour to set the IV pump.

Sequential method:

$$\frac{100 \text{ mL}}{1 \text{ hr}} \cdot \frac{100}{1} = \frac{100 \text{ mL}}{\text{hr}}$$

Calculate drops per minute with a drop factor of 20 gtt/mL.

Sequential method:

$$\frac{100 \text{ mL}}{1 \text{ hr}} \cdot \frac{20 \text{ gtt}}{\text{mL}} \cdot \frac{1 \text{ hr}}{60 \text{ min}} \cdot \frac{100 \times 2}{6} \cdot \frac{200}{6} = 33.33 \text{ or } 33 \frac{\text{gtt}}{\text{min}}$$

5

Sequential method:

$$\frac{50 \text{ mg}}{} \cdot \frac{\text{mL}}{25 \text{ mg}} \cdot \frac{50}{25} = 2 \text{ mL}$$

Calculate milliliters per hour to set the IV pump.

Random method:

$$\frac{50 \text{ mL}}{30 \text{ min}} \cdot \frac{60 \text{ min}}{1 \text{ hr}} \cdot \frac{50 \times 6}{3 \times 1} \cdot \frac{300}{3} = \frac{100 \text{ mL}}{\text{hr}}$$

Calculate drops per minute with a drop factor of 10 gtt/mL.

Sequential method:

$$\frac{50 \text{ mL}}{30 \text{ min}} \cdot \frac{10 \text{ gtt}}{\text{mL}} \cdot \frac{50 \times 1}{3} \cdot \frac{50}{3} = 16.66 \text{ or } 17 \frac{\text{gtt}}{\text{min}}$$

Practice Problems

1

Sequential method:

$$\frac{0.2 \text{ mg}}{\text{kg}} \cdot \frac{2 \text{ mL}}{5 \text{ mg}} \cdot \frac{1 \text{ kg}}{2.2 \text{ lb}} \cdot \frac{10 \text{ lb}}{} \cdot \frac{0.2 \times 2 \times 1 \times 10}{5 \times 2.2} \cdot \frac{4}{11} = 0.36 \text{ or } 0.4 \text{ mL}$$

2

Sequential method:

$$\frac{10 \text{ mg}}{\text{kg}} \cdot \frac{5 \text{ mL}}{160 \text{ mg}} \cdot \frac{8 \text{ kg}}{} \cdot \frac{1 \times 5 \times 8}{16} \cdot \frac{40}{16} = 2.5 \text{ mL}$$

3

Sequential method:

$$\frac{1.25 \text{ g}}{} \cdot \frac{10 \text{ mL}}{2 \text{ g}} \cdot \frac{1.25 \times 10}{2} \cdot \frac{12.5}{2} = 6.25 \text{ or } 6.3 \text{ mL}$$

4

Random method:

$$\frac{750 \text{ mg}}{1.5 \text{ g}} \cdot \frac{4 \text{ mL}}{1000 \text{ mg}} \cdot \frac{1 \text{ g}}{1.5 \times 100} \cdot \frac{75 \times 4 \times 1}{150} \cdot \frac{300}{150} = 2 \text{ mL}$$

5

Sequential method:

$$\frac{700 \text{ units}}{\text{hr}} \cdot \frac{250 \text{ mL}}{25{,}000 \text{ units}} \cdot \frac{7}{} = 7 \frac{\text{mL}}{\text{hr}}$$

6

Sequential method:

$$\frac{11 \text{ mL}}{\text{hr}} \cdot \frac{150 \text{ mg}}{250 \text{ mL}} \cdot \frac{11 \times 15}{25} \cdot \frac{165}{25} = 6.6 \frac{\text{mg}}{\text{hr}}$$

7

Sequential method:

$$\frac{1000 \text{ mL}}{8 \text{ hr}} \cdot \frac{20 \text{ gtt}}{\text{mL}} \cdot \frac{1 \text{ hr}}{60 \text{ min}} \cdot \frac{1000 \times 2 \times 1}{8 \times 6} \cdot \frac{2000}{48} = 41.66 \text{ or } 42 \frac{\text{gtt}}{\text{min}}$$

8

Sequential method:

$$\frac{750 \text{ mL}}{} \cdot \frac{15 \text{ gtt}}{\text{mL}} \cdot \frac{\text{min}}{18 \text{ gtt}} \cdot \frac{1 \text{ hr}}{60 \text{ min}} \cdot \frac{75 \times 15 \times 1}{18 \times 6} \cdot \frac{1125}{108} = 10.41 \text{ or } 10 \text{ hr}$$

9

Sequential method:

$$\frac{10 \text{ mg}}{\text{kg}} \cdot \frac{10 \text{ mL}}{500 \text{ mg}} \cdot \frac{1 \text{ kg}}{2.2 \text{ lb}} \cdot \frac{20 \text{ lb}}{} \cdot \frac{1 \times 1 \times 1 \times 20}{5 \times 2.2} \cdot \frac{20}{11} = 1.8 \text{ mL}$$

Sequential method:

$$\frac{100 \text{ mL}}{1 \text{ hr}} \cdot \frac{100}{1} = \frac{100 \text{ mL}}{\text{hr}}$$

Sequential method:

$$\frac{100 \text{ mL}}{1 \text{ hr}} \cdot \frac{10 \text{ gtt}}{\text{mL}} \cdot \frac{1 \text{ hr}}{60 \text{ min}} \cdot \frac{100 \times 1}{6} \cdot \frac{100}{6} = 16.666 \text{ or } 17 \frac{\text{gtt}}{\text{min}}$$

10

Sequential method:

$$\frac{355 \text{ mg}}{} \cdot \frac{10 \text{ mL}}{500 \text{ mg}} \cdot \frac{355 \times 1}{50} \cdot \frac{355}{50} = 7.1 \text{ or } 7 \text{ mL}$$

Calculate mL per hour to set the IV pump.

$$\frac{100 \text{ mL}}{1 \text{ hr}} \cdot \frac{100}{1} = \frac{100 \text{ mL}}{\text{hr}}$$

Calculate drops per minute with a drop factor of 20 gtt/mL.

Sequential method:

$$\frac{100 \text{ mL}}{1 \text{ hr}} \cdot \frac{20 \text{ gtt}}{\text{mL}} \cdot \frac{1 \text{ hr}}{60 \text{ min}} \cdot \frac{100 \times 2}{6} \cdot \frac{200}{6} = 33.33 \text{ or } 33 \frac{\text{gtt}}{\text{min}}$$

11

$$\frac{0.25 \text{ mg}}{\text{kg}} \left| \frac{\text{mL}}{5 \text{ mg}} \right| \frac{80 \text{ kg}}{} \left| \frac{0.25 \times 80}{5} \right| \frac{20}{5} = \begin{array}{l} 4 \text{ mL IV push} \\ \text{over 2 minutes} \end{array}$$

12

$$\frac{40 \text{ mg}}{15 \text{ min}} \left| \frac{\text{mL}}{0.4 \text{ mg}} \right| \frac{60 \text{ min}}{1 \text{ hr}} \left| \frac{40 \times 60}{15 \times 0.4 \times 1} \right| \frac{2400}{6} = 400 \; \frac{\text{mL}}{\text{hr}}$$

13

$$\frac{10 \text{ mg}}{\text{hr}} \left| \frac{125 \text{ mL}}{125 \text{ mg}} \right| \frac{10}{} = 10 \; \frac{\text{mL}}{\text{hr}}$$

OR

$$\frac{10 \text{ mg}}{\text{hr}} \left| \frac{1 \text{ mL}}{1 \text{ mg}} \right| \frac{10}{} = 10 \; \frac{\text{mL}}{\text{hr}}$$

14

$$\frac{0.2 \text{ mg}}{\text{kg}} \left| \frac{\text{mL}}{2 \text{ mg}} \right| \frac{40 \text{ kg}}{} \left| \frac{0.2 \times 40}{2} \right| \frac{8}{2} = 4 \text{ mL}$$

15

$$\frac{1.2 \text{ g}}{\text{day}} \left| \frac{5 \text{ mL}}{3 \text{ dose}} \right| \frac{1000 \text{ mg}}{300 \text{ mg}} \left| \frac{1.2 \times 5 \times 10}{3 \times 3 \times 1} \right| \frac{60}{9} = \begin{array}{l} 6.66 \text{ or} \\ 7 \text{ mL dose} \end{array}$$

16

$$\frac{250 \text{ mg}}{90 \text{ min}} \left| \frac{100 \text{ mL}}{500 \text{ mg}} \right| \frac{60 \text{ min}}{1 \text{ hr}} \left| \frac{250 \times 1 \times 6}{9 \times 5 \times 1} \right| \frac{1500}{45} = 33.3 \text{ or } 33 \; \frac{\text{mL}}{\text{hr}}$$

OR

$$\frac{250 \text{ mg}}{90 \text{ min}} \left| \frac{\text{mL}}{5 \text{ mg}} \right| \frac{60 \text{ min}}{1 \text{ hr}} \left| \frac{250 \times 6}{9 \times 5 \times 1} \right| \frac{1500}{45} = 33.3 \text{ or } 33 \; \frac{\text{mL}}{\text{hr}}$$

17

$$\frac{1200 \text{ units}}{\text{hr}} \left| \frac{250 \text{ mL}}{25,000 \text{ units}} \right| \frac{12}{} = 12 \; \frac{\text{mL}}{\text{hr}}$$

18

$$\frac{18 \text{ mL}}{\text{hr}} \left| \frac{25,000 \text{ units}}{250 \text{ mL}} \right| \frac{18 \times 2500}{25} \left| \frac{45,000}{25} \right| = 1800 \; \frac{\text{units}}{\text{hr}}$$

19

$$\frac{1000 \text{ mL}}{8 \text{ hr}} \left| \frac{10 \text{ gtt}}{\text{mL}} \right| \frac{1 \text{ hr}}{60 \text{ min}} \left| \frac{1000 \times 1 \times 1}{8 \times 6} \right| \frac{1000}{48} = 20.83 \text{ or } 21 \; \frac{\text{gtt}}{\text{min}}$$

20

$$\frac{1000 \text{ mL}}{\text{mL}} \left| \frac{10 \text{ gtt}}{15 \text{ gtt}} \right| \frac{\text{min}}{60 \text{ min}} \left| \frac{1 \text{ hr}}{} \right| \frac{1000 \times 1 \times 1}{15 \times 6} \left| \frac{1000}{90} \right| = 11.11 \text{ or } 11 \text{ hr}$$

21

Sequential method:

$$\frac{400 \text{ mg}}{} \left| \frac{4 \text{ mL}}{400 \text{ mg}} \right| \frac{4}{} = 4 \text{ mL}$$

Calculate how many milliliters per hour you will set the IV pump.

$$\frac{100 \text{ mL}}{30 \text{ min}} \left| \frac{60 \text{ min}}{1 \text{ hr}} \right| \frac{100 \times 6}{3 \times 1} \left| \frac{600}{3} \right| = 200 \; \frac{\text{mL}}{\text{hr}}$$

22

Sequential method:

$$\frac{10 \text{ mg}}{\text{kg}} \left| \frac{1 \text{ kg}}{2.2 \text{ lb}} \right| \frac{60 \text{ lb}}{} \left| \frac{\text{mL}}{40 \text{ mg}} \right| \frac{10 \times 1 \times 6}{2.2 \times 4} \left| \frac{60}{8.8} \right| = 6.8 \text{ mL}$$

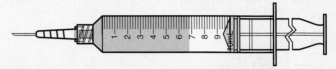

23

Sequential method:

$$\frac{5 \text{ mg}}{\text{kg}} \left| \frac{1 \text{ kg}}{2.2 \text{ lb}} \right| \frac{50 \text{ lb}}{} \left| \frac{\text{tablet}}{100 \text{ mg}} \right| \frac{5 \times 1 \times 5}{2.2 \times 10} \left| \frac{25}{22} \right| = 1.13 \text{ or } 1 \text{ tablet}$$

24

Sequential method:

$$\frac{0.4 \text{ mg}}{\text{kg}} \left| \frac{1 \text{ kg}}{2.2 \text{ lb}} \right| \frac{35 \text{ lb}}{4 \text{ mg}} \left| \frac{5 \text{ mL}}{} \right| \frac{0.4 \times 1 \times 35 \times 5}{2.2 \times 4} \left| \frac{70}{8.8} \right| = 7.95 \text{ or } 8 \text{ mL}$$

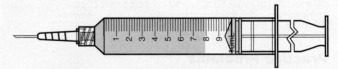

25

Sequential method:

$$\frac{50 \text{ mL}}{30 \text{ min}} \left| \frac{60 \text{ min}}{1 \text{ hr}} \right| \frac{50 \times 6}{3 \times 1} \left| \frac{300}{3} \right| = 100 \; \frac{\text{mL}}{\text{hr}}$$

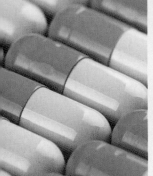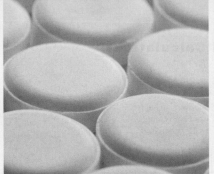

Three-Factor Medication Problems

Objectives

After completing this chapter, you will successfully be able to:

1. Calculate three-factor–given quantity to one-factor–, two-factor–, or three-factor–wanted quantity medication problems involving a specific amount of medication or intravenous (IV) fluid based on the weight of the patient and the time required for safe administration.

2. Calculate problems requiring reconstitution or preparation of medications using information from a nursing drug reference, label, or package insert.

When medications are ordered for infants and children, the dosage of medication (g, mg, mcg, gr) based on the **weight** of the child must be considered as well as how much medication the child can receive per **dose** or **day**.

Although the **physician or nurse practitioner** orders the medications, the nurse must be aware of the safe dosage range for administration of medications. It is the responsibility of the nurse to check a nursing drug reference for the **right dosage** before administering a medication to a child to prevent **medication errors**.

When physicians or nurse practitioners order medications for critically ill patients, the patients must be closely monitored by the nurse for effectiveness of the medications. Often, the medications or intravenous (IV) fluids must be *titrated* for effectiveness, with an increase or decrease in the dosage based on the patient's response.

Factors involved in the safe administration of medications or IV fluids for the critically ill patient include the **dosage** of medication based on the **weight** of the patient and the **time** required for administration. The medication may need reconstitution or preparation by the nurse for immediate administration in a critical situation. The weight of the patient also may need to be obtained daily to ensure accurate correlation with the dosage of medication ordered. A nursing drug reference provides the nurse with information related to **dosage**, **weight**, and **time** for safe administration of medication.

To be able to calculate three-factor–given quantity to one-factor–, two-factor–, or three-factor–wanted quantity medication problems, it is necessary to understand all of the components of the medication order and to be able to calculate medication problems in a critical situation. This chapter will teach you to calculate medication problems involving the dosage of medication based on the weight of the patient and the time required for safe administration using dimensional analysis.

Three-factor–given quantity medication problems can be solved implementing the sequential method or the random method of dimensional analysis. The *given quantity* or the physician's order now contains three parts, including a **numerator** (the *dosage* of medication ordered) and two **denominators** (the *weight* of the patient and the *time* required for safe administration).

Example 6.1 demonstrates the problem-solving method showing placement of basic dimensional analysis terms applied to a three-factor medication problem.

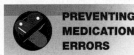
PREVENTING MEDICATION ERRORS

When caring for critically ill patients, the nurse is responsible for titrating medication for the desired effectiveness (decrease in chest pain, increase in urine output, or increase in blood pressure).

The weight of a patient is extremely important when administering medications to a critically ill patient because a change in weight (either increased or decreased) can change the effectiveness of the medication. To prevent **medication errors**, a daily weight is obtained on every critically ill patient.

Unit Path

Given Quantity	Conversion Factor for Given Quantity (Numerator)	Conversion Factor for Given Quantity (Denominator)	Conversion Computation		Wanted Quantity
$\dfrac{30 \text{ mg}}{\text{kg/day}}$	$\dfrac{5 \text{ mL}}{300 \text{ mg}}$	22 kg	$\dfrac{30 \times 5 \times 22}{300}$	$\dfrac{3300}{300} =$	$\dfrac{11 \text{ mL}}{\text{day}}$

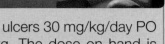

EXAMPLE 6.1

The physician orders Tagamet for gastrointestinal ulcers 30 mg/kg/day PO in four divided doses for a child weighing 22 kg. The dose on hand is Tagamet 300 mg/5 mL.

❖ How many milliliters per day will the child receive?

Given quantity	= 30 mg/kg/day
Wanted quantity	= mL/day
Dose on hand	= 300 mg/5 mL
Weight	= 22 kg

Step 1 Identify the three-factor–given quantity (the physician's order), which contains three parts: a *numerator* (30 mg) and two denominators (kg/day). Establish the unit path from the given *quantity* (30 mg/kg/day) to the *two-factor–wanted quantity* (mL/day) using the sequential method of dimensional analysis and the necessary conversion factors.

Sequential method:

$$\frac{30 \text{ mg}}{\text{kg/day}} \bigg| = \frac{\text{mL}}{\text{day}}$$

Step 2

Unit Path

Given Quantity	Conversion Factor for Given Quantity (Numerator)	Conversion Factor for Given Quantity (Denominator)	Conversion Computation		Wanted Quantity
$\dfrac{30 \text{ mg}}{\text{kg/day}}$	$\dfrac{5 \text{ mL}}{300 \text{ mg}}$				$\dfrac{\text{mL}}{\text{day}}$

Step 3

Unit Path

Given Quantity	Conversion Factor for Given Quantity (Numerator)	Conversion Factor for Given Quantity (Denominator)	Conversion Computation		Wanted Quantity
$\dfrac{30 \text{ mg}}{\text{kg/day}}$	$\dfrac{5 \text{ mL}}{300 \text{ mg}}$	22 kg			$\dfrac{\text{mL}}{\text{day}}$

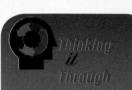

Thinking it Through

The three-factor–given quantity has been set up with a numerator (30 mg) and two denominators (kg/day) leading across the unit path to a two-factor–wanted quantity, with a numerator (mL) and a denominator (day). The conversion factors can now be factored into the unit path to allow cancellation of unwanted units.

The *dose on hand* (300 mg/5 mL) has been factored in and placed so that the wanted unit (mL) correlates with the *wanted quantity* (mL) and the unwanted unit (mg) is canceled.

The child's weight (22 kg) has been factored in and set up to allow the unwanted unit (kg) to be canceled.

All the unwanted units have been canceled, and the wanted units are placed to correlate with the two-factor–wanted quantity (mL/day). Multiply numerators, multiply denominators, and divide the product of the numerators by the product of the denominators to provide the numerical answer. The wanted quantity is 11 mL/day.

Step 4

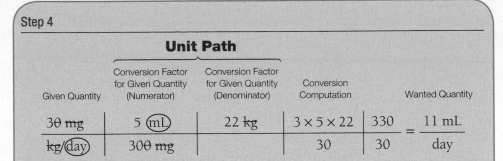

Unit Path

Given Quantity	Conversion Factor for Given Quantity (Numerator)	Conversion Factor for Given Quantity (Denominator)	Conversion Computation		Wanted Quantity
$\dfrac{30 \text{ mg}}{\text{kg/day}}$	$\dfrac{5 \text{ mL}}{300 \text{ mg}}$	22 kg	$\dfrac{3 \times 5 \times 22}{30}$	$\dfrac{330}{30}$	$= \dfrac{11 \text{ mL}}{\text{day}}$

The child is to receive 11 mL/day in four divided doses; therefore, the *conversion factor* involves how many doses are in a day (4 divided doses = day).

Step 5 **Using dimensional analysis, calculate how many milliliters per dose the child should receive.**

Given quantity   = 11 mL/day
Wanted quantity = mL/dose

$$\frac{11 \text{ mL}}{\text{day}} \left| \quad \right. = \frac{\text{mL}}{\text{dose}}$$

Step 6

$$\frac{11 \text{ mL}}{\text{day}} \left| \frac{\text{day}}{4 \text{ doses}} \right| \frac{11}{4} = 2.75 \text{ or } \frac{2.8 \text{ mL}}{\text{dose}}$$

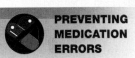 *The wanted quantity is 2.8 mL/dose, and the child will receive this orally (PO) four times a day (qid).*

The problem could have been set up to find the wanted quantity of milliliters per dose.

Step 6 (alternative).

Given quantity   = 30 mg/kg/day
Wanted quantity = mL/dose
Dose on hand   = 300 mg/5 mL
Weight   = 22 kg

Sequential method:

$$\frac{30 \text{ mg}}{\text{kg/day}} \left| \frac{5 \text{ mL}}{300 \text{ mg}} \right| 22 \text{ kg} \left| \frac{\text{day}}{4 \text{ doses}} \right| \frac{3 \times 5 \times 22}{30 \times 4} \left| \frac{330}{120} \right. = 2.75 \text{ or } \frac{2.8 \text{ mL}}{\text{dose}}$$

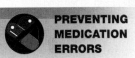 *The wanted quantity is 2.8 mL/dose, and the child will receive this orally (PO) four times a day (qid).*

PREVENTING MEDICATION ERRORS

Every new medication order for a child should be carefully reviewed for errors related to **dosage, route,** and **frequency**. Many **medication** errors can be eliminated if a double-check system is in place for all new medication orders.

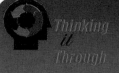

Thinking it Through

The **two-factor–given quantity** (2.8 mL/dose) has been factored in with a *numerator* (2.8 mL) and a *denominator* (dose). The **three-factor–wanted quantity** (mg/kg/day) also has been factored in with a *numerator* (mg) and two *denominators* (kg/day).

The **conversion factors** have been added, and all unwanted units have been canceled from the problem. The wanted unit (mg) is placed in the numerator to correlate with the **wanted quantity** (mg) also in the numerator. The wanted units (kg and day) are in the denominator to correlate with the wanted quantity (kg and day) in the denominator.

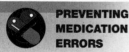

PREVENTING MEDICATION ERRORS

Knowing the **Six Rights** of medication administration can help to eliminate **medication errors** but another important consideration is being aware of the safe dosage range for each medication being administered.

A Nursing Drug Reference lists the safe dosage range for adults, children, and infants. It is the responsibility of the nurse to be familiar with safe dosage ranges to prevent **medication errors**.

EXAMPLE 6.2

As a prudent nurse, you are concerned that the child may be receiving an unsafe dosage of Tagamet; therefore, you want to identify how many milligrams per kilogram per day (mg/kg/day) the child weighing 22 kg is receiving. The dosage of medication being given four times a day is 2.8 mL/dose. The dosage on hand is 300 mg/5 mL.

❧ **How many milligrams per kilogram per day is the child receiving?**

Given quantity   = 2.8 mL/dose
Wanted quantity = mg/kg/dose
Dose on hand   = 300 mg/5 mL
Child's weight   = 22 kg

Sequential method:

Step 1

$$\frac{2.8 \text{ mL}}{\text{dose}} \bigg| \hspace{5cm} = \frac{\text{mg}}{\text{kg/day}}$$

Step 2

$$\frac{2.8 \text{ mL}}{\text{dose}} \bigg| \frac{300 \text{ mg}}{5 \text{ mL}} \bigg| \frac{4 \text{ doses}}{\text{day}} \bigg| \frac{}{22 \text{ kg}} = \frac{\text{mg}}{\text{kg/day}}$$

Step 3

$$\frac{2.8 \text{ mL}}{\text{dose}} \bigg| \frac{300 \text{ mg}}{5 \text{ mL}} \bigg| \frac{4 \text{ doses}}{\text{day}} \bigg| \frac{}{22 \text{ kg}} \bigg| \frac{2.8 \times 300 \times 4}{5 \times 22} \bigg| \frac{3360}{110} = \frac{30.54 \text{ or } 30.5 \text{ mg}}{\text{kg/day}}$$

⬤ *The three-factor–wanted quantity is 30.5 mg/kg/day. The nursing drug reference identifies that 20 to 40 mg/kg/day in four divided doses is a safe dosage of Tagamet for children. Therefore, the nurse is assured that the child is receiving a correct dosage. Dimensional analysis assists you to critically think through any type of medication problem.*

EXAMPLE 6.3

The physician orders dobutamine 5 mcg/kg/min IV for cardiac failure. The pharmacy sends an IV bag labeled: dobutamine 250 mg/50 mL D5W/0.45% NS. The patient weighs 165 lb.

❧ **Calculate the milliliters per hour at which to set the IV pump.**

Given quantity   = 5 mcg/kg/min
Wanted quantity = mL/hr
Dose on hand   = 250 mg/50 mL
Weight   = 165 lb

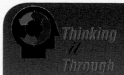

Step 1   Identify the *three-factor–given quantity* (the physician's order) containing three parts, including the *numerator* (5 mg) and two *denominators* (kg/min). Establish the unit path from the three-factor–given quantity to the two-factor–wanted quantity (mL/hr).

Random method:

$$\frac{5 \text{ mcg}}{\text{kg/min}} \left|\rule{0pt}{20pt}\right. = \frac{\text{mL}}{\text{hr}}$$

Step 2

$$\frac{5 \text{ mcg}}{\text{kg/\cancel{min}}} \left|\frac{60 \text{ \cancel{min}}}{1 \text{ hr}}\right. = \frac{\text{mL}}{\text{hr}}$$

Step 3

$$\frac{5 \text{ mcg}}{\text{kg/\cancel{min}}} \left|\frac{60 \text{ \cancel{min}}}{1 \text{ \textcircled{hr}}}\right|\frac{50 \text{ \textcircled{mL}}}{250 \text{ mg}} = \frac{\text{mL}}{\text{hr}}$$

Step 4

$$\frac{5 \text{ \cancel{mcg}}}{\text{kg/\cancel{min}}} \left|\frac{60 \text{ \cancel{min}}}{1 \text{ \textcircled{hr}}}\right|\frac{50 \text{ \textcircled{mL}}}{250 \text{ mg}}\left|\frac{1 \text{ mg}}{1000 \text{ \cancel{mcg}}}\right. = \frac{\text{mL}}{\text{hr}}$$

Step 5

$$\frac{5 \text{ \cancel{mcg}}}{\text{\cancel{kg}/\cancel{min}}} \left|\frac{60 \text{ \cancel{min}}}{1 \text{ \textcircled{hr}}}\right|\frac{50 \text{ \textcircled{mL}}}{250 \text{ mg}}\left|\frac{1 \text{ mg}}{1000 \text{ \cancel{mcg}}}\right|\frac{1 \text{ kg}}{2.2 \text{ \cancel{lb}}}\left|\frac{165 \text{ \cancel{lb}}}{} \right. = \frac{\text{mL}}{\text{hr}}$$

Step 6

$$\frac{5 \text{ \cancel{mcg}}}{\text{\cancel{kg}/\cancel{min}}} \left|\frac{6\cancel{0} \text{ \cancel{min}}}{\cancel{1} \text{ \textcircled{hr}}}\right|\frac{5\cancel{0} \text{ \textcircled{mL}}}{25\cancel{0} \text{ \cancel{mg}}}\left|\frac{\cancel{1} \text{ \cancel{mg}}}{100\cancel{0} \text{ \cancel{mcg}}}\right|\frac{1 \text{ \cancel{kg}}}{2.2 \text{ \cancel{lb}}}\left|\frac{165 \text{ \cancel{lb}}}{} \right. = \frac{\text{mL}}{\text{hr}}$$

$$\frac{5 \times 6 \times 5 \times 1 \times 165}{25 \times 100 \times 2.2} \left|\frac{24{,}750}{5500}\right. = \frac{4.5 \text{ mL}}{\text{hr}}$$

⬤ ***The 4.5 mL/hr is the wanted quantity and is the answer to the problem. Intravenous pumps used in critical care can be set to deliver amounts including decimal points so it is not necessary to round up the answer.***

Thinking it Through

The three-factor–given quantity has been set up with a **numerator** (5 mg) and **two denominators** (kg/min) leading across the unit path to a two-factor–wanted quantity with a *numerator* (mL) and a **denominator** (hr). By using the random method of dimensional analysis, the **conversion factors** are factored to cancel out unwanted units.

The unwanted unit (min) has been canceled by factoring the **conversion factor** (1 hr = 60 min), and the wanted unit corresponds with the **wanted quantity denominator** (hr).

The **dose on hand** (250 mg/50 mL) has been factored in and placed so that the *wanted unit* (mL) corresponds with the wanted quantity numerator (mL).

The *conversion factor* (1 mg = 1000 mcg) has been factored in to cancel the unwanted units (mg and mcg).

The final **conversion factors** (1 kg = 2.2 lb) and the *weight* of the patient have been factored in to cancel the remaining unwanted units (kg and lb). All the unwanted units have been canceled, and the wanted units (mL and hr) remain in position to correlate with the **two-factor–wanted quantity** (mL/hr). Multiply the numerators, multiply the denominators, and divide the product of the numerators by the product of the denominators to provide the numerical value for the two-factor–wanted quantity.

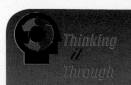

The **two-factor–given quantity** is identified as the information that the nurse obtained from the IV pump, and the **three-factor–wanted quantity** is the information that the physician has requested.

The *dose on hand* (the IV fluid that is presently infusing) has been factored in to cancel the unwanted unit (mL).

The *conversion factor* (1 mg = 1000 mcg) has been factored in to cancel the unwanted unit (mg). The wanted unit (mcg) remains and corresponds with the wanted quantity in the *numerator*.

The *conversion factor* (1 hr = 60 min) has been factored in to cancel the unwanted unit (hr). The wanted unit (min) remains placed in the *denominator*.

The *conversion factor* (1 kg = 2.2 lb) has been factored in to correspond with the *wanted quantity denominator* (kg). The *weight* of the patient also is factored in to cancel the unwanted unit (lb). After all unwanted units have been canceled and the wanted units have been identified, multiply the numerators, multiply the denominators, and divide the product of the numerators by the product of the denominators to provide the numerical value for the *wanted quantity*.

EXAMPLE 6.4

The nurse has been monitoring the hemodynamic readings of a patient weighing 165 lb receiving dobutamine, 250 mg in 50 mL of D5W/0.45% NS, and has received additional orders from the physician to *titrate* for effectiveness.

❋ **The IV pump is now set at 9 mL/hr, and the physician wants to know how many micrograms per kilogram per minute the patient is now receiving.**

Given quantity   = 9 mL/hr
Wanted quantity = mcg/kg/min
Dose on hand   = 250 mg/50 mL
Weight   = 165 lb

Step 1

$$\frac{9 \text{ mL}}{\text{hr}} = \frac{\text{mcg}}{\text{kg/min}}$$

Step 2

Sequential method:

$$\frac{9 \text{ mL}}{\text{hr}} \,\Big|\, \frac{250 \text{ mg}}{50 \text{ mL}} = \frac{\text{mcg}}{\text{kg/min}}$$

Step 3

$$\frac{9 \text{ mL}}{\text{hr}} \,\Big|\, \frac{250 \text{ mg}}{50 \text{ mL}} \,\Big|\, \frac{1000 \text{ (mcg)}}{1 \text{ mg}} = \frac{\text{mcg}}{\text{kg/min}}$$

Step 4

$$\frac{9 \text{ mL}}{\text{hr}} \,\Big|\, \frac{250 \text{ mg}}{50 \text{ mL}} \,\Big|\, \frac{1000 \text{ (mcg)}}{1 \text{ mg}} \,\Big|\, \frac{1 \text{ hr}}{60 \text{ (min)}} = \frac{\text{mcg}}{\text{kg/min}}$$

Step 5

$$\frac{9 \text{ mL}}{\text{hr}} \,\Big|\, \frac{250 \text{ mg}}{50 \text{ mL}} \,\Big|\, \frac{1000 \text{ (mcg)}}{1 \text{ mg}} \,\Big|\, \frac{1 \text{ hr}}{60 \text{ (min)}} \,\Big|\, \frac{2.2 \text{ lb}}{1 \text{ (kg)} \,\Big|\, 165 \text{ lb}} = \frac{\text{mcg}}{\text{kg/min}}$$

Step 6

$$\frac{9 \text{ mL}}{\text{hr}} \,\Big|\, \frac{250 \text{ mg}}{50 \text{ mL}} \,\Big|\, \frac{1000 \text{ (mcg)}}{1 \text{ mg}} \,\Big|\, \frac{1 \text{ hr}}{60 \text{ (min)}} \,\Big|\, \frac{2.2 \text{ lb}}{1 \text{ (kg)} \,\Big|\, 165 \text{ lb}} = \frac{\text{mcg}}{\text{kg/min}}$$

$$\frac{9 \times 25 \times 100 \times 2.2}{5 \times 6 \times 1 \times 165} \,\Big|\, \frac{49{,}500}{4950} = \frac{10 \text{ mcg}}{\text{kg/min}}$$

⬤ *The nurse can inform the physician that the patient is now receiving 10 mcg/kg/min infusing at 9 mL/hr.*

Dimensional analysis is a problem-solving method that uses critical thinking. When implementing the *sequential method* or the *random method* of dimensional analysis, the medication problem can be set up in a number of different ways, with a focus on the correct placement of *conversion factors* to allow unwanted units to be canceled from the unit path.

Dimensional analysis is a problem-solving method that nurses can use to calculate a variety of medication problems in the hospital, outpatient, or home care environment. The medication problems may involve one-factor–, two-factor–, or three-factor–given quantity medication orders, resulting in one-factor–, two-factor–, or three-factor–wanted quantity answers.

With advanced nursing and home care nursing resulting in increased autonomy, it is more important than ever that nurses be able to accurately calculate medication problems. Dimensional analysis provides the opportunity to use one problem-solving method for any type of medication problem, thereby increasing consistency and decreasing confusion when calculating medication problems.

Exercise 6.1	**Medication Problems Involving Dosage, Weight, and Time**

(See pages 171–172 for answers)

1. Order: Furosemide 2 mg/kg/day PO in two divided doses for congestive heart failure

   Supply: Furosemide 40 mg/5 mL

   Child's weight: 20 kg

▶ **How many milliliters per dose will you give?** _____

NDC 0054-8298

DELIVERS 5 mL

FUROSEMIDE
40 mg per 5 mL

Oral Solution
SUGAR FREE
Caution: Federal law prohibits
dispensing without prescription.
See Package Insert

⑧ **Roxane**
Laboratories, Inc.
Columbus, Ohio 43216

PEEL
086

Courtesy of Roxane Laboratories.

(Exercise continues on page 156)

2. Order: Cefazolin 40 mg/kg/day in divided doses every 8 hours for infection

Supply: Cefazolin 1 g

Child's weight: 30 lb

Nursing drug reference: Reconstitute with 10 mL of sterile water for injection.

▶ **How many milliliters per dose will you draw from the vial after reconstitution?** _____

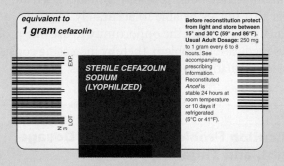

3. Order: Dilantin 6 mg/kg/day in divided doses every 12 hours for seizures

Supply: Dilantin 125 mg/5 mL

Child's weight: 45 lb

▶ **How many milliliters per dose will you give?** _____

4. Order: prednisolone 1.5 mg/kg/day in four divided doses for inflammation

Supply: prednisolone 6.7 mg/5 mL

Child's weight: 20 kg

▶ **How many milliliters per dose will you give?** _____

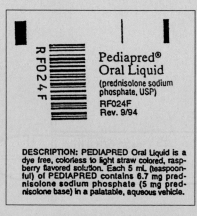

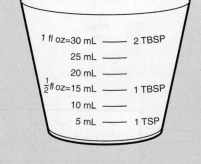

Courtesy of Fisons Pharmaceuticals.

5. Order: Cleocin 10 mg/kg/day IV in divided doses every 8 hours for infection

   Supply: Cleocin 300 mg/2 mL

   Child's weight: 50 lb

   ▶ **How many milliliters per dose will you give?** _____

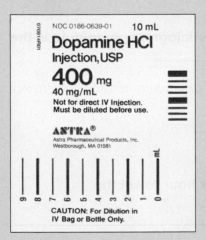

Upjohn

Cleocin Phosphate®
brand of clindamycin phosphate sterile solution
and clindamycin phosphate IV solution
(clindamycin phosphate injection, USP and
clindamycin phosphate injection in 5% dextrose)
Sterile Solution is for Intramuscular and Intravenous Use
CLEOCIN PHOSPHATE in the ADD-Vantage™ Vial is For
Intravenous Use Only

DESCRIPTION
   CLEOCIN PHOSPHATE Sterile Solution in vials contains
clindamycin phosphate, a water soluble ester of clindamycin
and phosphoric acid. Each mL contains the equivalent of 150
mg clindamycin, 0.5 mg disodium edetate and 9.45 mg benzyl
alcohol added as preservative in each mL. Clindamycin is a
semisynthetic antibiotic produced by a 7(S)-chloro-substitu-
tion of the 7(R)-hydroxyl group of the parent compound
lincomycin.

Courtesy of Upjohn Company.

6. Order: dopamine 5 mcg/kg/min IV to increase blood pressure

   Supply: dopamine 400-mg vial

   Supply: 250 cc D5W

   Patient's weight: 200 lb

   ▶ **How many milliliters will you draw from the vial**
     to equal 400 mg? _____

   ▶ **Calculate the milliliters per hour to set the**
     IV pump. _____

NDC 0186-0639-01   10 mL

Dopamine HCl
Injection, USP

400 mg
40 mg/mL
Not for direct IV Injection.
Must be diluted before use.

ASTRA®
Astra Pharmaceutical Products, Inc.
Westborough, MA 01581

mL

9 8 7 6 5 4 3 2 1 0

CAUTION: For Dilution in
IV Bag or Bottle Only.

Courtesy of Astra Pharmaceutical Products.

(Exercise continues on page 158)

Dopamine Hydrochloride Injection, USP

DOSAGE AND ADMINISTRATION
WARNING: <u>This is a potent drug. It must be diluted before administration to patient.</u>
Suggested Dilution
Transfer contents of one or more additive syringes of dopamine hydrochloride by aseptic technique to either a 250 mL, or 500 mL container of one of the following sterile intravenous solutions:

1. Sodium Chloride Injection, USP
2. Dextrose 5% Injection, USP
3. Dextrose (5%) and Sodium Chloride (0.9%) Injection, USP
4. Dextrose (5%) and Sodium Chloride (0.45%) Injection, USP
5. Dextrose (5%) in Lactated Ringer's Injection
6. Sodium Lactate (1/6 Molar) Injection, USP
7. Lactated Ringer's Injection, USP

Dopamine HCl has been found to be stable for a minimum of 24 hours after dilution in the sterile intravenous solutions listed above. However, as with all intravenous admixtures, dilution should be made just prior to administration.
Do NOT add dopamine HCl to 5% Sodium Bicarbonate or other alkaline intravenous solution, since the drug is inactivated in alkaline solution.

Rate of Administration
Dopamine HCl, after dilution, is administered intravenously through a suitable intravenous catheter or needle. An IV drip chamber or other suitable metering device is essential for controlling the rate of flow in drops/minute. Each patient must be individually titrated to the desired hemodynamic and/or renal response with dopamine HCl. In titrating to the desired increase in systolic blood pressure, the optimum dosage rate for renal response may be exceeded, thus necessitating a reduction in rate after the hemodynamic condition is stabilized.
Administration at rates greater than 50 mcg/kg/minute have safely been used in advanced circulatory decompensation states. If unnecessary fluid expansion is of concern, adjustment of drug concentration may be preferred over increasing the flow rate of a less concentrated dilution.

Suggested Regimen
1. When appropriate, increase blood volume with whole blood or plasma until central venous pressure is 10 to 15 cm H_2O or pulmonary wedge pressure is 14 to 18 mm Hg.
2. Begin administration of diluted solution at doses of 2–5 mcg/kg/minute dopamine HCl in patients who are likely to respond to modest increments of heart force and renal perfusion.
   In more seriously ill patients, begin administration of diluted solution at doses of 5 mcg/kg/minute dopamine HCl and increase gradually using 5–10 mcg/kg/minute increments up to 20–50 mcg/kg/minute as needed. If doses of dopamine HCl in excess of 50 mcg/kg/minute are required, it is suggested that urine output be checked frequently. Should urine flow begin to decrease in the absence of hypotension, reduction of dopamine HCl dosage should be considered. Multiclinic trials have shown that more than 50% of the patients were satisfactorily maintained on doses of dopamine HCl of less than 20 mcg/kg/minute. In patients who do not respond to these doses with adequate arterial pressures or urine flow, additional increments of dopamine HCl may be employed in an effort to produce an appropriate arterial pressure and central perfusion.
3. Treatment of all patients requires constant evaluation of therapy in terms of the blood volume, augmentation of myocardial contractility, and distribution of peripheral perfusion. Dosage of dopamine HCl should be adjusted according to the patient's response, with particular attention to diminution of established urine flow rate, increasing tachycardia or development of new dysrhythmias as indices for decreasing or temporarily suspending the dosage.
4. As with all potent administered drugs, care should be taken to control the rate of administration to avoid inadvertent administration of a bolus of drug.
Parenteral drug products should be inspected visually for particulate matter and discoloration prior to administration, whenever solution and container permit.

HOW SUPPLIED
Dopamine HCl 200 mg is supplied in the following form:
Additive Syringe   5 mL (40 mg/mL)   NDC 0186-0638-01

Dopamine HCl 800 mg is supplied in the following form:
Additive Syringe   5 mL (160 mg/mL)   NDC 0186-0642-01

Dopamine HCl 400 mg is supplied in the following forms:
Additive Syringe   5 mL (80 mg/mL)   NDC 0186-0641-01
                   10 mL (40 mg/mL)   NDC 0186-0639-01

Packages are color coded according to the total dosage content; 200 mg coded blue/white, 400 mg coded green/white and 800 mg coded yellow/white.
Store at controlled room temperature 15°–30°C (59°–86°F). Protect from light.
Avoid contact with alkalies (including sodium bicarbonate), oxidizing agents, or iron salts.
NOTE: Do not use the Injection if it is darker than slightly yellow or discolored in any way.

ASTRA® | Astra Pharmaceutical Products, Inc.
         | Westborough, MA 01581   021861R07   3/92 (7)

Courtesy of Astra Pharmaceutical Products.

7. Information obtained by the nurse: Nipride 50 mg/250 mL D5W is infusing at 22 mL/hr.

   Patient's weight: 160 lb

   ▶ **How many micrograms per kilogram per minute is the patient receiving?** _____

8. Order: Milrinone 0.5 mcg/kg/min continuous infusion for congestive heart failure

   Supply: Milrinone 20 mg/100 mL of D5W

   Patient's weight: 180 lb

   ▶ **Calculate the milliliters per hour to set the IV pump.** _____

9. Information obtained by the nurse: Nipride 50 mg/250 mL D5W is infusing at 46 mL/hr.

   Patient's weight: 160 lb

   ▶ **How many micrograms per kilogram per minute is the patient receiving?** _____

10. Order: Procainamide 4 mg/min maintenance infusion for life-threatening arrhythmia (2–6 mg/min safe dosage range)

    Supply: Procainamide 1 g/50 mL D5W

    ▶ **Calculate the milliliters per hour to set the IV pump.** _____

    Information obtain by the nurse: Procainamide 1 g/50 mL D5W is infusing at 15 mL/hr.

    ▶ **How many milliliters per minute is the patient now receiving? Is this dosage within the safe dosage range?** _____

Summary

This chapter has taught you to calculate three-factor medication problems involving the **dosage** of medication, the **weight** of the patient, and the amount of **time** over which medications or IV fluids can be safely administered. Using the sequential method or the random method of dimensional analysis, demonstrate your ability to calculate medication problems accurately by completing the following practice problems.

Practice Problems for Chapter 6

Three-Factor Medication Problems

(See pages 172–173 for answers)

1. Order: amrinone 8 mcg/kg/min IV for congestive heart failure

   Supply: amrinone 100 mg/100 mL of 0.9% NS

   Patient's weight: 198 lb

   ✳ **Calculate the milliliters per hour to set the IV pump.** _____

2. Order: Tagamet 40 mg/kg/day PO in four divided doses for gastrointestinal ulcers

   Supply: Tagamet 300 mg/5 mL

   Child's weight: 80 lb

   ✳ **How many milliliters per dose will you give?** _____

3. Information obtained by the nurse: Dopamine 200 mg in 500 mL D5W is infusing at 45 mL/hr for a patient weighing 60 kg.

   ✳ **How many micrograms per kilogram per minute is the patient receiving?** _____

4. Order: Dopamine 2 mcg/kg/min IV for decreased cardiac output

   Supply: Dopamine 400 mg/500 mL

   Patient's weight: 176 lb

   ✳ **Calculate the milliliters per hour to set the IV pump.** _____

5. Order: Neupogen 5 mcg/kg/day SQ for 2 weeks for neutropenia

   Supply: Neupogen 300 mcg/mL

   Patient's weight: 130 lb

   ✳ **How many micrograms per day will you give?** _____

6. Order: aminophylline 0.5 mg/kg/hr IV loading dose for bronchodilation

   Supply: aminophylline 250 mg/250 mL D5W

   Patient's weight: 132 lb

   ❋ **Calculate the milliliters per hour to set the IV pump.** _____

7. Order: furosemide 2 mg/kg/day PO for congestive heart failure

   Supply: furosemide 10 mg/mL

   Child's weight: 40 kg

   ❋ **How many milliliters per day will you give?** _____

8. Information obtained by the nurse: Nipride 200 mg in 1000 mL D5W is infusing at 15 mL/hr for a patient weighing 100 kg.

   ❋ **How many micrograms per kilogram per minute is the patient receiving?** _____

9. Information obtained by the nurse: A child weighing 65 lb is receiving 10 mL of Tagamet PO qid from a stock bottle labeled: Tagamet 300 mg/5 mL.

   ❋ **How many milligrams per kilogram per day is the child receiving?** _____

10. Information obtained by the nurse: Aminophylline 250 mg/250 mL 0.9% NS is infusing at 25 mL/hr for a patient weighing 50 kg.

    ❋ **How many milligrams per kilogram per hour is the patient receiving?** _____

11. Order: Gabapentin (Neurontin) 10 mg/kg/day PO in three divided doses for seizures

    Supply: Neurontin 250 mg/5 mL solution

    Child's weight: 60 lb

    ❋ **How many milliliters per dose will the child receive?** _____

12. Information obtained by the nurse: A 10-year-old child weighing 60 lb is receiving 2 mL/dose PO three times a day of gabapentin (Neurontin) for seizures from a stock bottle labeled 250 mg/5 mL.

    Nursing drug reference: Children ages 3–12 years should be receiving 10–15 mg/kg/day in three divided doses.

    ❋ **How many mg/kg/day is the child receiving?** _____

(Practice Problems continue on page 162)

13. Order: Tobramycin sulfate 3 mg/kg/day IV in three doses every 8 hours for infection

    Patient's weight: 60 kg

    Supply: Tobramycin 60 mg in 100 mL D5W

    Nursing drug reference: Mix 60 mg/mL in 100 mL D5W and infuse over 60 minutes.

    ✳ **How many milligrams per dose should the patient receive?** _____

    ✳ **Calculate the milliliters per hour to set the IV pump.** _____

14. Order: Amiodarone hydrochloride (Cordarone) 7 mcg/kg/min IV for unstable ventricular tachycardia

    Supply: Amiodarone 500 mg/250 mL 0.9% NS

    Patient's weight: 80 kg

    ✳ **Calculate the milliliters per hour to set the IV pump.** _____

15. Information obtained by the nurse: A patient who weighs 80 kg is receiving 15 mL/hr of Amiodarone hydrochloride (Cordarone) for unstable ventricular tachycardia from an IV bag labeled 500 mg/250 mL 0.9% NS.

    ✳ **How many mcg/kg/min is the patient receiving?** _____

16. Order: Pentamidine isethionate (Pentam 300) 4 mg/kg/day IV for 14 days for pneumonia secondary to Pneumocystis carinii

    Supply: Pentamidine 300 mg/250 mL D5W

    Nursing drug reference: Infuse slowly over 60 minutes

    Patient's weight: 80 kg

    ✳ **Calculate the milliliters per hour to set the IV pump.** _____

17. Order: Dopamine hydrochloride (Dopamine) 20 mcg/kg/min IV for cardiogenic shock

    Supply: Dopamine 400 mg/250 mL 0.9% NS

    Patient's weight: 180 lb

    ✳ **Calculate the milliliters per hour to set the IV pump.** _____

18. Information obtained by the nurse: Dopamine hydrochloride (Dopamine) 400 mg in 250 mL 0.9% NS is infusing at 30 mL/hr.

    Patient's weight: 180 lb

    ✳ **How many micrograms per kilogram per minute is the patient receiving?** _____

19. Order: Nitroprusside sodium (Nitropress) 5 mcg/kg/min IV for hypertensive crisis

    Supply: Nitropress 50 mg/250 mL D5W

    Patient's weight: 80 kg

    ✳ **Calculate the milliliters per hour to set the IV pump.** _____

20. Information obtained by the nurse: Nitroprusside sodium (Nitropress) 50 mg in 250 mL D5W is infusing at 80 mL/hr

    Patient's weight: 80 kg

    ✳ **How many micrograms per kilogram per minute is the patient receiving?** _____

21. Order: Nitroprusside sodium (Nipride) 0.25 mcg/kg/min IV for hypertensive crisis

    Supply: Nitroprusside 50 mg/250 mL D5W

    Patient's weight: 195 lb

    ✳ **Calculate the milliliters per hour to set the IV pump.** _____

22. Order: Esmolol (Brevibloc) 0.1 mg/kg/min IV for supraventricular tachycardia

    Supply: Esmolol 2500 mg/250 mL D5W

    Patient's weight: 80 kg

    ✳ **Calculate the milliliters per hour to set the IV pump.** _____

23. Information obtained by the nurse: Nitroprusside sodium (Nipride) 50 mg/250 mL D5W is infusing at 8 mL/hr.

    Patient's weight: 195 lb

    ✳ **How many micrograms per kilogram per minute is the patient receiving?** _____

24. Order: Dobutamine 0.5 mcg/kg/min IV initially for decreased cardiac output

    Supply: Dobutamine 250 mg/250 mL D5W

    Patient's weight: 250 lb

    ✳ **Calculate the milliliters per hour to set the IV pump.** _____

25. Information obtained by the nurse: Dobutamine 250 mg/250 mL D5W is infusing at 5 mL/hr.

    Patient's weight: 250 lb

    ✳ **How many micrograms per kilogram per minute is the patient receiving?** _____

Chapter 6 Post-Test

Three-Factor Medication Problems

Name _____   Date _____

1. Order: morphine sulfate 0.3 mg/kg/dose PO every 4 hours for pain

   Supply: morphine sulfate 10 mg/5 mL

   Child's weight: 20 lb

※ **How many milliliters per dose will you give?** _____

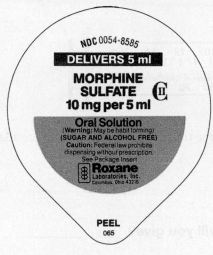

NDC 0054-8585

DELIVERS 5 ml

MORPHINE SULFATE Ⅽᴵᴵ
10 mg per 5 ml

Oral Solution
(Warning: May be habit forming)
(SUGAR AND ALCOHOL FREE)
Caution: Federal law prohibits
dispensing without prescription.
See Package Insert
Roxane
Laboratories, Inc.
Columbus, Ohio 43216

PEEL
065

Courtesy of Roxane Laboratories, Inc.

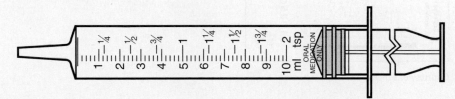

(Post-Test continues on page 166)

2. Order: filgrastim 5 mcg/kg/day for myelosuppression secondary to chemotherapy administration

   Supply: filgrastim 480 mcg/1.6 mL

   Patient's weight: 100 lb

   ✳ **How many milliliters per day will you give?** _____

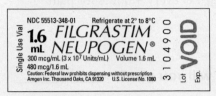

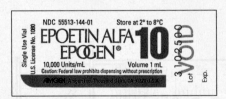

Courtesy of Amgen, Inc.

3. Order: Epogen 100 units/kg/day SQ three times weekly for anemia secondary to AZT administration

   Supply: Epogen 10,000 units/mL

   Patient's weight: 180 lb

   ✳ **How many milliliters per day will you give?** _____

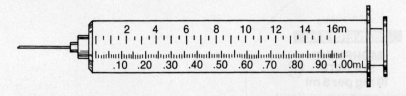

Courtesy of Amgen, Inc.

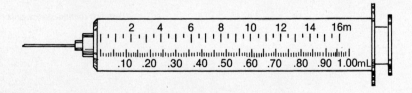

4. Order: digoxin 25 mcg/kg/day PO every 8 hours for congestive heart failure

   Supply: digoxin 0.25 mg/5 mL

   Child's weight: 25 lb

   ✳ **How many milliliters will you give per day?** _____

   ✳ **How many milliliters will you give per dose?** _____

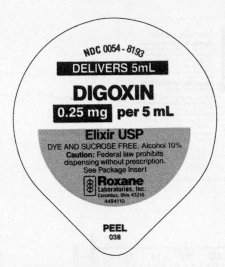

Courtesy of Roxane Laboratories, Inc.

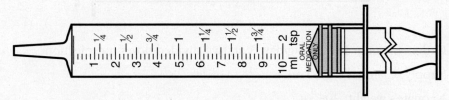

(Post-Test continues on page 168)

5. Order: clindamycin 10 mg/kg/day IV in three divided doses for respiratory tract infection

Supply: clindamycin 150 mg/mL

Child's weight: 10 kg

❋ **How many milliliters per dose will you draw from the vial?** _____

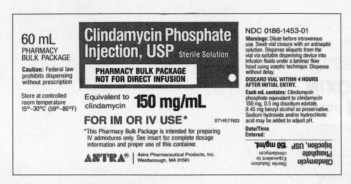

Courtesy of Astra Pharmaceutical Products.

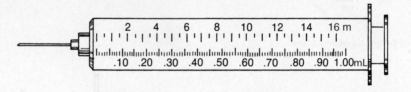

6. Order: Claforan 100 mg/kg/day IV in two divided doses for infection

Supply: Claforan 1 g/10 mL

Neonate's weight: 2045 g

❋ **How many milliliters per dose will you draw from the vial?** _____

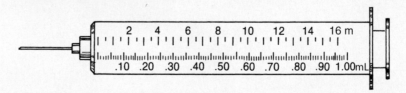

7. Order: gentamicin 2.5 mg/kg/dose IV every 12 hours for gram-negative bacillary infection

Supply: gentamicin 40 mg/mL

Neonate's weight: 1182 g

❋ **How many milligrams per dose will the neonate receive?** _____

8. Order: ampicillin 100 mg/kg/day IV in divided doses every 12 hours for respiratory tract infection

    Supply: ampicillin 125 mg/5 mL

    Neonate's weight: 1182 g

    ❋ **How many milligrams per dose will the neonate receive?** _____

    ❋ **How many milliliters per dose will you draw from the vial?** _____

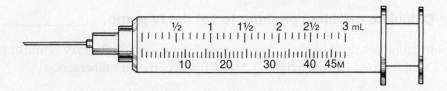

9. Order: Solu-Medrol 5.4 mg/kg/hr IV for acute spinal cord injury

    Supply: Solu-Medrol 125 mg/2 mL

    Patient's weight: 160 lb

    ❋ **How many milligrams per hour will the patient receive?** _____

10. Order: aminophylline 0.8 mg/kg/hr IV for respiratory distress

    Supply: aminophylline 250 mg/100 mL

    Child's weight: 65 lb

    ❋ **Calculate the milliliters per hour to set the IV pump.** _____

11. Order: Daptomycin 4 mg/kg IVPB over 30 minutes once daily for bacterial infection

    Supply: 500 mg vial

    Client's weight: 185 lb

    Nursing drug reference: Reconstitute with 10 mL of 0.9% sodium chloride and further dilute in 50 mL of 0.9% sodium chloride to yield 50 mg/mL.

    ❋ **Calculate the milliliters per hour to set the IV pump.** _____

12. Order: Intropin 10 mcg/kg/min for decreased cardiac output

    Supply: 200 mg/250 mL D5W

    Client's weight: 140 lb

    ❋ **Calculate the milliliters per hour to set the IV pump.** _____

(Post-Test continues on page 170)

13. Order: Cefazolin 25 mg/kg/30 min IVPB for severe otitis media

    Supply: 500 mg/50 mL 0.9% NS

    Drop factor: 10 gtt/mL

    Child's weight: 40 lb

    ❋ **Calculate the number of drops per minute.** _____

14. Order: Dopamine 5 mcg/kg/min IV for hypotension

    Supply: 400 mg/250 mL 0.9% NS

    Client's weight: 85 kg

    ❋ **Calculate milliliters per hour to set the IV pump.** _____

15. Information obtained by the nurse: Nipride 50 mg in 250 mL D5W is infusing at 15 mL/hr for a patient weighing 220 lb for hypertensive emergency.

    ❋ **How many micrograms per kilogram per minute is the patient receiving?** _____

16. Information obtained by the nurse: Aminophylline 250 mg in 250 mL D5W is infusing at 30 mL/hr for a patient weighing 132 lb for bronchodilation.

    ❋ **How many milligrams per kilogram per hour is the patient receiving?** _____

17. Order: Heparin 18 units/kg/hr IV for pulmonary embolism

    Supply: 25,000 units/250 mL D5W

    Client's weight: 82 kg

    ❋ **Calculate the milliliters per hour to set the IV pump.** _____

18. Order: Cordarone 6 mcg/kg/min for unstable ventricular tachycardia

    Supply: 500 mg/250 mL 0.9%

    Client's weight: 176 lb

    ❋ **Calculate the milliliters per hour to set the IV pump.** _____

19. Order: Intropin 1 mcg/kg/min for renal perfusion

    Instructions: Add 400 mg to 500 mL 0.9% NS

    Client's weight: 212 lb

    ❋ **Calculate the milliliters per hour to set the IV pump.** _____

20. Information obtained by the nurse: Dopamine 400 mg in 250 mL D5W is infusing at 10 mL/hr for a patient weighing 110 lb for decreased cardiac output.

    ❋ **How many micrograms per kilogram per minute is the patient receiving?** _____

ANSWER KEY FOR CHAPTER 6: THREE-FACTOR MEDICATION PROBLEMS

Exercise 6.1 Medication Problems Involving Dosage, Weight, and Time

1

Sequential method:

$$\frac{2\ \text{mg}}{\text{kg/day}} \left| \frac{5\ \text{mL}}{40\ \text{mg}} \right| \frac{20\ \text{kg}}{} \left| \frac{\text{day}}{2\ \text{doses}} \right| \frac{2 \times 5 \times 2}{4 \times 2} \left| \frac{20}{8} \right| = \frac{2.5\ \text{mL}}{\text{dose}}$$

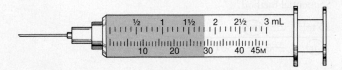

2

Random method:

$$\frac{40\ \text{mg}}{\text{kg/day}} \left| \frac{10\ \text{mL}}{\frac{1}{4}\ \text{g}} \right| \frac{\text{day}}{3\ \text{doses}} \left| \frac{\frac{1}{4}\ \text{kg}}{2.2\ \text{lb}} \right| \frac{30\ \text{lb}}{} \left| \frac{\frac{1}{4}\ \text{g}}{1000\ \text{mg}} \right| = \frac{\text{mL}}{\text{dose}}$$

$$\frac{4 \times 1 \times 3}{3 \times 2.2} \left| \frac{12}{6.6} \right| = 1.81\ \text{or}\ 1.8 \ \frac{\text{mL}}{\text{dose}}$$

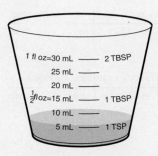

3

Sequential method:

$$\frac{6\ \text{mg}}{\text{kg/day}} \left| \frac{5\ \text{mL}}{125\ \text{mg}} \right| \frac{1\ \text{kg}}{2.2\ \text{lb}} \left| \frac{45\ \text{lb}}{} \right| \frac{\text{day}}{2\ \text{doses}} = \frac{\text{mL}}{\text{dose}}$$

$$\frac{6 \times 5 \times 1 \times 45}{125 \times 2.2 \times 2} \left| \frac{1350}{550} \right| = 2.45\ \text{or}\ 2.5 \ \frac{\text{mL}}{\text{dose}}$$

4

Sequential method:

$$\frac{1.5\ \text{mg}}{\text{kg/day}} \left| \frac{5\ \text{mL}}{6.7\ \text{mg}} \right| \frac{20\ \text{kg}}{} \left| \frac{\text{day}}{4\ \text{doses}} \right| \frac{1.5 \times 5 \times 20}{6.7 \times 4} = \frac{\text{mL}}{\text{dose}}$$

$$\frac{150}{26.8} = 5.59\ \text{or}\ 5.6 \ \frac{\text{mL}}{\text{dose}}$$

5

Sequential method:

$$\frac{10\ \text{mg}}{\text{kg/day}} \left| \frac{2\ \text{mL}}{300\ \text{mg}} \right| \frac{1\ \text{kg}}{2.2\ \text{lb}} \left| \frac{1\ \text{day}}{3\ \text{doses}} \right| \frac{50\ \text{lb}}{} \left| \frac{1 \times 2 \times 1 \times 1 \times 5}{3 \times 2.2 \times 3} \right| \frac{10}{19.8} = \frac{0.5\ \text{mL}}{\text{dose}}$$

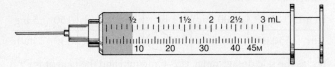

6

Random method:

$$\frac{400\ \text{mg}}{} \left| \frac{\text{mL}}{40\ \text{mg}} \right| \frac{40}{4} = 10\ \text{mL}$$

Random method:

$$\frac{5\ \text{mcg}}{\text{kg/min}} \left| \frac{60\ \text{min}}{\frac{1}{4}\ \text{hr}} \right| \frac{\frac{1}{4}\ \text{kg}}{2.2\ \text{lb}} \left| \frac{200\ \text{lb}}{} \right| \frac{250\ \text{mL}}{400\ \text{mg}} \left| \frac{1\ \text{mg}}{1000\ \text{mcg}} \right| = \frac{\text{mL}}{\text{hr}}$$

$$\frac{5 \times 6 \times 2 \times 25 \times 1}{2.2 \times 4 \times 10} \left| \frac{1500}{88} \right| = 17.04\ \text{or}\ 17 \ \frac{\text{mL}}{\text{hr}}$$

7

Sequential method:

$$\frac{22\ \text{mL}}{\text{hr}} \left| \frac{50\ \text{mg}}{250\ \text{mL}} \right| \frac{\frac{1}{4}\ \text{hr}}{60\ \text{min}} \left| \frac{1000\ \text{mcg}}{\frac{1}{4}\ \text{mg}} \right| \frac{2.2\ \text{lb}}{1\ \text{kg}} \left| \frac{}{160\ \text{lb}} \right| = \frac{\text{mcg}}{\text{kg/min}}$$

$$\frac{22 \times 5 \times 10 \times 2.2}{25 \times 6 \times 1 \times 16} \left| \frac{2420}{2400} \right| = 1.008\ \text{or}\ 1 \ \frac{\text{mcg}}{\text{kg/min}}$$

8

Sequential method:

$$\frac{0.5\ \text{mcg}}{\text{kg/min}} \left| \frac{60\ \text{min}}{1\ \text{hr}} \right| \frac{1\ \text{kg}}{2.2\ \text{lb}} \left| \frac{180\ \text{lb}}{} \right| \frac{\frac{1}{4}\ \text{mg}}{1000\ \text{mcg}} \left| \frac{100\ \text{mL}}{20\ \text{mg}} \right| \frac{0.5 \times 6 \times 1 \times 18}{2.2 \times 2} \left| \frac{54}{4.4} \right| =$$

$$12.27\ \text{or}\ 12.3 \ \frac{\text{mL}}{\text{hr}}$$

9

Sequential method:

$$\frac{46\ \text{mL}}{\text{hr}} \left| \frac{50\ \text{mg}}{250\ \text{mL}} \right| \frac{\frac{1}{4}\ \text{hr}}{60\ \text{min}} \left| \frac{1000\ \text{mcg}}{\frac{1}{4}\ \text{mg}} \right| \frac{2.2\ \text{lb}}{1\ \text{kg}} \left| \frac{}{160\ \text{lb}} \right| = \frac{\text{mcg}}{\text{kg/min}}$$

$$\frac{46 \times 5 \times 10 \times 2.2}{25 \times 6 \times 1 \times 16} \left| \frac{5060}{2400} \right| = 2.1\ \text{or}\ 2 \ \frac{\text{mcg}}{\text{kg/min}}$$

10

Sequential method:

$$\frac{4 \text{ mg}}{\text{min}} \cdot \frac{60 \text{ min}}{1 \text{ hr}} \cdot \frac{1 \text{ g}}{1000 \text{ mg}} \cdot \frac{50 \text{ mL}}{1 \text{ g}} \cdot \frac{4 \times 6 \times 5}{1 \times 10} \cdot \frac{120}{10} = \frac{12 \text{ mL}}{\text{hr}}$$

Information obtained by the nurse: Procainamide 1 g/50 mL D5W is infusing at 15 mL/hr.

Sequential method:

$$\frac{15 \text{ mL}}{\text{hr}} \cdot \frac{1 \text{ g}}{50 \text{ mL}} \cdot \frac{1000 \text{ mg}}{1 \text{ g}} \cdot \frac{1 \text{ hr}}{60 \text{ min}} \cdot \frac{15 \times 10 \times 1}{5 \times 6} \cdot \frac{150}{30} = \frac{5 \text{ mg}}{\text{min}}$$

Yes, as the safe dosage range is 2–6 mg/min and the patient is receiving 5 mg/min.

Practice Problems

1

Random method:

$$\frac{8 \text{ mcg}}{\text{kg/min}} \cdot \frac{100 \text{ mL}}{100 \text{ mg}} \cdot \frac{1 \text{ mg}}{1000 \text{ mcg}} \cdot \frac{1 \text{ kg}}{2.2 \text{ lb}} \cdot \frac{198 \text{ lb}}{} \cdot \frac{60 \text{ min}}{1 \text{ hr}} = \frac{\text{mL}}{\text{hr}}$$

$$\frac{8 \times 1 \times 198 \times 6}{100 \times 2.2} \cdot \frac{9504}{220} = \frac{43.2 \text{ mL}}{\text{hr}}$$

2

Sequential method:

$$\frac{40 \text{ mg}}{\text{kg/day}} \cdot \frac{5 \text{ mL}}{300 \text{ mg}} \cdot \frac{1 \text{ kg}}{2.2 \text{ lb}} \cdot \frac{80 \text{ lb}}{} \cdot \frac{\text{day}}{4 \text{ doses}} = \frac{\text{mL}}{\text{dose}}$$

$$\frac{4 \times 5 \times 1 \times 8}{3 \times 2.2 \times 4} \cdot \frac{160}{26.4} = \frac{6.06 \text{ or } 6 \text{ mL}}{\text{dose}}$$

3

Sequential method:

$$\frac{45 \text{ mL}}{\text{hr}} \cdot \frac{200 \text{ mg}}{500 \text{ mL}} \cdot \frac{1000 \text{ mcg}}{1 \text{ mg}} \cdot \frac{1 \text{ hr}}{60 \text{ min}} \cdot \frac{}{60 \text{ kg}} = \frac{\text{mcg}}{\text{kg/min}}$$

$$\frac{45 \times 2 \times 10}{5 \times 6 \times 6} \cdot \frac{900}{180} = \frac{5 \text{ mcg}}{\text{kg/min}}$$

4

Random method:

$$\frac{2 \text{ mcg}}{\text{kg/min}} \cdot \frac{500 \text{ mL}}{400 \text{ mg}} \cdot \frac{1 \text{ mg}}{1000 \text{ mcg}} \cdot \frac{60 \text{ min}}{1 \text{ hr}} \cdot \frac{1 \text{ kg}}{2.2 \text{ lb}} \cdot \frac{176 \text{ lb}}{} = \frac{\text{mL}}{\text{hr}}$$

$$\frac{2 \times 5 \times 6 \times 1 \times 176}{4 \times 100 \times 2.2} \cdot \frac{10,560}{880} = \frac{12 \text{ mL}}{\text{hr}}$$

5

Random method:

$$\frac{5 \text{ mcg}}{\text{kg/day}} \cdot \frac{1 \text{ kg}}{2.2 \text{ lb}} \cdot \frac{130 \text{ lb}}{} \cdot \frac{5 \times 1 \times 130}{2.2} \cdot \frac{650}{2.2} = \frac{295.45 \text{ or } 296 \text{ mcg}}{\text{day}}$$

6

Sequential method:

$$\frac{0.5 \text{ mg}}{\text{kg/hr}} \cdot \frac{250 \text{ mL}}{250 \text{ mg}} \cdot \frac{1 \text{ kg}}{2.2 \text{ lb}} \cdot \frac{132 \text{ lb}}{} \cdot \frac{0.5 \times 1 \times 132}{2.2} \cdot \frac{66}{2.2} = \frac{30 \text{ mL}}{\text{hr}}$$

7

Sequential method:

$$\frac{2 \text{ mg}}{\text{kg/day}} \cdot \frac{\text{mL}}{10 \text{ mg}} \cdot \frac{40 \text{ kg}}{} \cdot \frac{2 \times 4}{1} \cdot \frac{8}{1} = \frac{8 \text{ mL}}{\text{day}}$$

8

Sequential method:

$$\frac{15 \text{ mL}}{\text{hr}} \cdot \frac{200 \text{ mg}}{1000 \text{ mL}} \cdot \frac{1 \text{ hr}}{60 \text{ min}} \cdot \frac{1000 \text{ mcg}}{1 \text{ mg}} \cdot \frac{}{100 \text{ kg}} \cdot \frac{15 \times 2}{60 \times 1} \cdot \frac{30}{60} = \frac{0.5 \text{ mcg}}{\text{kg/min}}$$

9

Sequential method:

$$\frac{10 \text{ mL}}{\text{dose}} \cdot \frac{300 \text{ mg}}{5 \text{ mL}} \cdot \frac{4 \text{ doses}}{\text{day}} \cdot \frac{2.2 \text{ lb}}{1 \text{ kg}} \cdot \frac{}{65 \text{ lb}} = \frac{\text{mg}}{\text{kg/day}}$$

$$\frac{10 \times 300 \times 4 \times 2.2}{5 \times 1 \times 65} \cdot \frac{26,400}{325} = 81.23 \text{ or } 81 \, \frac{\text{mg}}{\text{kg/day}}$$

10

Sequential method:

$$\frac{25 \text{ mL}}{\text{hr}} \cdot \frac{250 \text{ mg}}{250 \text{ mL}} \cdot \frac{}{50 \text{ kg}} \cdot \frac{25}{50} = 0.5 \, \frac{\text{mg}}{\text{kg/hr}}$$

11

$$\frac{10 \text{ mg}}{\text{kg/day}} \cdot \frac{5 \text{ mL}}{250 \text{ mg}} \cdot \frac{1 \text{ kg}}{2.2 \text{ lb}} \cdot \frac{60 \text{ lb}}{} \cdot \frac{\text{day}}{3 \text{ doses}} \cdot \frac{10 \times 5 \times 1 \times 6}{25 \times 2.2 \times 3} \cdot \frac{300}{165} = 1.8 \, \frac{\text{mL}}{\text{dose}}$$

12

$$\frac{2 \text{ mL}}{\text{dose}} \cdot \frac{250 \text{ mg}}{5 \text{ mL}} \cdot \frac{3 \text{ doses}}{\text{day}} \cdot \frac{2.2 \text{ lb}}{1 \text{ kg}} \cdot \frac{}{60 \text{ lb}} \cdot \frac{2 \times 25 \times 3 \times 2.2}{5 \times 1 \times 6} \cdot \frac{330}{30} = 11 \, \frac{\text{mg}}{\text{kg/day}}$$

13

$$\frac{3 \text{ mg}}{\text{kg/day}} \cdot \frac{60 \text{ kg}}{} \cdot \frac{\text{day}}{3 \text{ doses}} \cdot \frac{3 \times 60}{3} \cdot \frac{180}{3} = 60 \, \frac{\text{mg}}{\text{dose}}$$

$$\frac{60 \text{ mg}}{60 \text{ min}} \cdot \frac{100 \text{ mL}}{60 \text{ mg}} \cdot \frac{60 \text{ min}}{1 \text{ hr}} \cdot \frac{100}{1} = \frac{100 \text{ mL}}{\text{hr}}$$

14

$$\frac{7 \text{ mcg}}{\text{kg/min}} \cdot \frac{250 \text{ mL}}{500 \text{ mg}} \cdot \frac{1 \text{ mg}}{1000 \text{ mcg}} \cdot \frac{80 \text{ kg}}{} \cdot \frac{60 \text{ min}}{1 \text{ hr}} \cdot \frac{7 \times 25 \times 1 \times 8 \times 6}{50 \times 10 \times 1} \cdot \frac{8400}{500} = 16.8 \text{ or } 17 \, \frac{\text{mL}}{\text{hr}}$$

15

$$\frac{15 \text{ mL}}{\text{hr}} \cdot \frac{500 \text{ mg}}{250 \text{ mL}} \cdot \frac{1 \text{ hr}}{60 \text{ min}} \cdot \frac{1000 \text{ mcg}}{1 \text{ mg}} \cdot \frac{}{80 \text{ kg}} \cdot \frac{15 \times 50 \times 1 \times 10}{25 \times 6 \times 1 \times 8} \cdot \frac{7500}{1200} = 6.25 \text{ or } 6 \, \frac{\text{mcg}}{\text{kg/min}}$$

16

$$\frac{4\ \text{mg}}{\text{kg/day}} \left| \frac{250\ \text{mL}}{300\ \text{mg}} \right| \frac{80\ \text{kg}}{} \left| \frac{\text{day}}{24\ \text{hr}} \right| \frac{4 \times 25 \times 8}{3 \times 24} \left| \frac{800}{72} \right. = 11.11\ \text{or}\ 11\ \frac{\text{mL}}{\text{hr}}$$

17

$$\frac{20\ \text{mcg}}{\text{kg/min}} \left| \frac{1\ \text{kg}}{2.2\ \text{lb}} \right| \frac{180\ \text{lb}}{} \left| \frac{1\ \text{mg}}{1000\ \text{mcg}} \right| \frac{250\ \text{mL}}{400\ \text{mg}} \left| \frac{60\ \text{min}}{1\ \text{hr}} \right| \frac{2 \times 1 \times 18 \times 1 \times 25 \times 6}{2.2 \times 10 \times 4 \times 1} \left| \frac{5400}{88} \right. =$$

$$61.36\ \text{or}\ 61\ \frac{\text{mL}}{\text{hr}}$$

18

$$\frac{30\ \text{mL}}{\text{hr}} \left| \frac{1\ \text{hr}}{60\ \text{min}} \right| \frac{400\ \text{mg}}{250\ \text{mL}} \left| \frac{1000\ \text{mcg}}{1\ \text{mg}} \right| \frac{2.2\ \text{lb}}{1\ \text{kg}} \left| \frac{}{180\ \text{lb}} \right| \frac{30 \times 1 \times 40 \times 10 \times 2.2}{6 \times 25 \times 1 \times 1 \times 18} \left| \frac{26400}{2700} \right. =$$

$$9.7\ \text{or}\ 10\ \frac{\text{mcg}}{\text{kg/min}}$$

19

$$\frac{5\ \text{mcg}}{\text{kg/min}} \left| \frac{80\ \text{kg}}{} \right| \frac{60\ \text{min}}{1\ \text{hr}} \left| \frac{1\ \text{mg}}{1000\ \text{mcg}} \right| \frac{250\ \text{mL}}{50\ \text{mg}} \left| \frac{5 \times 8 \times 6 \times 1 \times 25}{1 \times 10 \times 5} \right| \frac{6000}{50} = 120\ \frac{\text{mL}}{\text{hr}}$$

20

$$\frac{80\ \text{mL}}{\text{hr}} \left| \frac{50\ \text{mg}}{250\ \text{mL}} \right| \frac{1\ \text{hr}}{60\ \text{min}} \left| \frac{}{80\ \text{kg}} \right| \frac{1000\ \text{mcg}}{1\ \text{mg}} \left| \frac{5 \times 100}{25 \times 6} \right| \frac{500}{150} = 3.33\ \text{or}\ 3\ \frac{\text{mcg}}{\text{kg/min}}$$

21

Sequential method:

$$\frac{0.25\ \text{mcg}}{\text{kg/min}} \left| \frac{1\ \text{kg}}{2.2\ \text{lb}} \right| \frac{195\ \text{lb}}{} \left| \frac{60\ \text{min}}{1\ \text{hr}} \right| \frac{1\ \text{mg}}{1000\ \text{mcg}} \left| \frac{250\ \text{mL}}{50\ \text{mg}} \right| \frac{0.25 \times 195 \times 6 \times 1 \times 25}{2.2 \times 10 \times 50} \left| \frac{7312.5}{1100} \right. =$$

$$6.6\ \frac{\text{mL}}{\text{hr}}$$

22

Sequential method:

$$\frac{0.1\ \text{mg}}{\text{kg/min}} \left| \frac{80\ \text{kg}}{} \right| \frac{60\ \text{min}}{1\ \text{hr}} \left| \frac{250\ \text{mL}}{2500\ \text{mg}} \right| \frac{0.1 \times 80 \times 6}{1} \left| \frac{48}{1} \right. = 48\ \frac{\text{mL}}{\text{hr}}$$

23

Sequential method:

$$\frac{8\ \text{mL}}{\text{hr}} \left| \frac{50\ \text{mg}}{250\ \text{mL}} \right| \frac{1\ \text{hr}}{60\ \text{min}} \left| \frac{1000\ \text{mcg}}{1\ \text{mg}} \right| \frac{2.2\ \text{lb}}{1\ \text{kg}} \left| \frac{}{195\ \text{lb}} \right| \frac{8 \times 50 \times 10 \times 2.2}{25 \times 6 \times 1 \times 195} \left| \frac{8800}{29250} \right. =$$

$$0.3\ \frac{\text{mcg}}{\text{kg/min}}$$

24

Sequential method:

$$\frac{0.5\ \text{mcg}}{\text{kg/min}} \left| \frac{1\ \text{kg}}{2.2\ \text{lb}} \right| \frac{250\ \text{lb}}{} \left| \frac{60\ \text{min}}{1\ \text{hr}} \right| \frac{1\ \text{mg}}{1000\ \text{mcg}} \left| \frac{250\ \text{mL}}{250\ \text{mg}} \right| \frac{0.5 \times 25 \times 6}{2.2 \times 10} \left| \frac{75}{22} \right. = 3.4\ \frac{\text{mL}}{\text{hr}}$$

25

Sequential method:

$$\frac{5\ \text{mL}}{\text{hr}} \left| \frac{1\ \text{hr}}{60\ \text{min}} \right| \frac{250\ \text{mg}}{250\ \text{mL}} \left| \frac{1000\ \text{mcg}}{1\ \text{mg}} \right| \frac{2.2\ \text{lb}}{1\ \text{kg}} \left| \frac{}{250\ \text{lb}} \right| \frac{5 \times 10 \times 2.2}{6 \times 1 \times 25} \left| \frac{110}{150} \right. = 0.73\ \text{or}\ 0.7\ \frac{\text{mcg}}{\text{kg/min}}$$

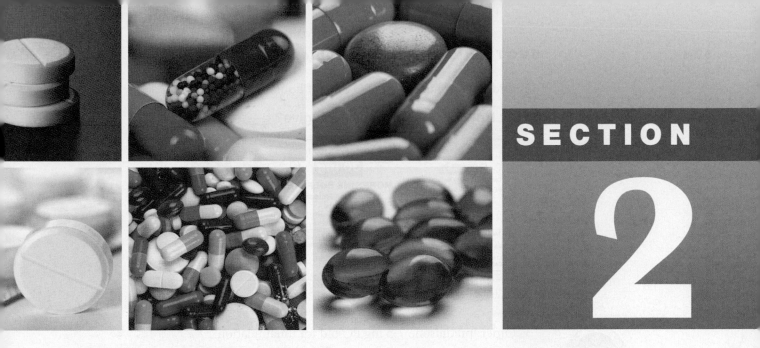

Practice Problems

Practice Problems

One-Factor Practice Problems

(See pages 209–211 for answers)

1. Order: trimethobenzamide HCl 200 mg qid IM for nausea and vomiting

   ✳ **How many milliliters will you give?** _____

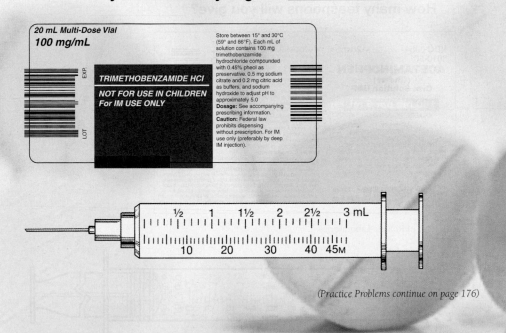

20 mL Multi-Dose Vial
100 mg/mL

EXP.

TRIMETHOBENZAMIDE HCI

NOT FOR USE IN CHILDREN
For IM USE ONLY

LOT

Store between 15° and 30°C
(59° and 86°F). Each mL of
solution contains 100 mg
trimethobenzamide
hydrochloride compounded
with 0.45% pheol as
preservative. 0.5 mg sodium
citrate and 0.2 mg citric acid
as buffers, and sodium
hydroxide to adjust pH to
approximately 5.0
Dosage: See accompanying
prescribing information.
Caution: Federal law
prohibits dispensing
without prescription. For IM
use only (preferably by deep
IM injection).

½ 1 1½ 2 2½ 3 mL

10   20   30   40 45м

(Practice Problems continue on page 176)

2. Order: morphine 30 mg PO every 4 hours for pain

✳ **How many tablets will you give?** _____

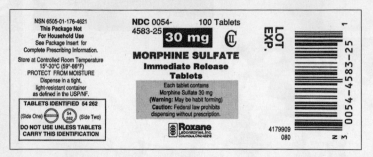

Courtesy of Roxane Laboratories.

3. Order: prednisone 7.5 mg PO bid for inflammation

✳ **How many tablets will you give?** _____

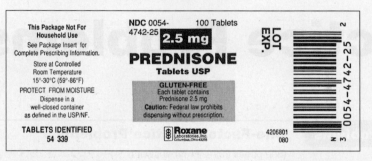

Courtesy of Roxane Laboratories.

4. Order: acetaminophen 160 mg PO every 4 hours for fever

✳ **How many teaspoons will you give?** _____

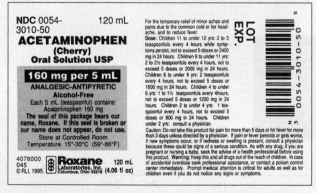

Courtesy of Roxane Laboratories.

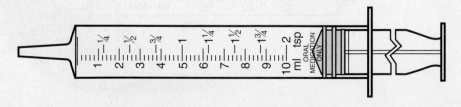

5. Order: Xanax 0.5 mg PO tid for anxiety

※ **How many tablets will you give?** _____

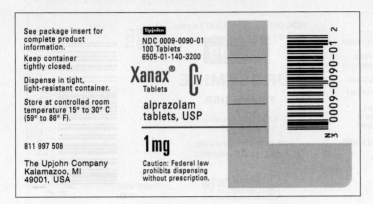

Courtesy of the Upjohn Company.

6. Order: Adalat 60 mg PO daily for hypertension

※ **How many tablets will you give?** _____

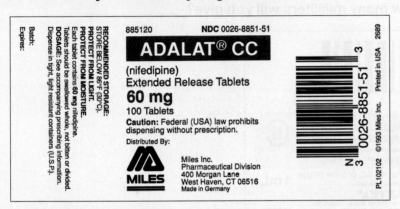

Courtesy of Miles Inc.

7. Order: Halcion 0.25 mg PO at hs for insomnia

※ **How many tablets will you give?** _____

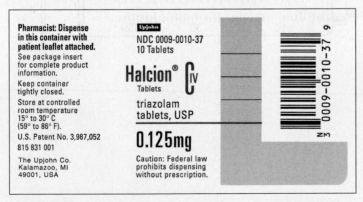

Courtesy of the Upjohn Company.

(Practice Problems continue on page 178)

8. Order: furosemide 80 mg PO daily for congestive heart failure

   ❋ **How many tablets will you give?** _____

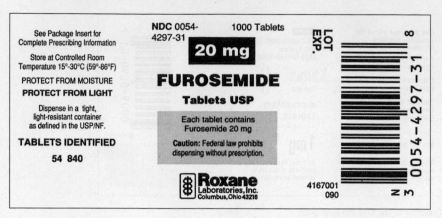

See Package Insert for
Complete Prescribing Information

Store at Controlled Room
Temperature 15°-30°C (59°-86°F)

PROTECT FROM MOISTURE

PROTECT FROM LIGHT

Dispense in a tight,
light-resistant container
as defined in the USP/NF.

TABLETS IDENTIFIED

54 840

NDC 0054-
4297-31   1000 Tablets

20 mg

FUROSEMIDE

Tablets USP

Each tablet contains
Furosemide 20 mg

Caution: Federal law prohibits
dispensing without prescription.

Roxane
Laboratories, Inc.
Columbus, Ohio 43216

LOT
EXP.

4167001
090

0054-4297-31

Courtesy of Roxane Laboratories.

9. Order: morphine sulfate 10 mg IM prn for pain

   ❋ **How many milliliters will you give?** _____

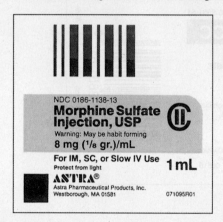

NDC 0186-1138-13

**Morphine Sulfate
Injection, USP**

Warning: May be habit forming

8 mg (¹/₈ gr.)/mL

For IM, SC, or Slow IV Use
Protect from light

ASTRA®
Astra Pharmaceutical Products, Inc.
Westborough, MA 01581

071095R01

1 mL

Courtesy of Astra Pharmaceutical Products.

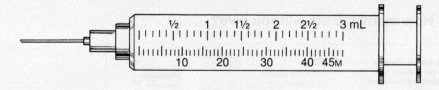

10. Order: naloxone HCl 100 mcg IVP prn for respiratory depression

❊ **How many milliliters will you give?** _____

Courtesy of Astra Pharmaceutical Products.

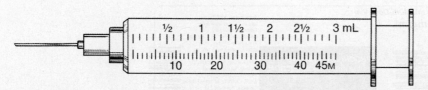

11. Order: Solu-Medrol 80 mg IVP every 4 hours for inflammation

❊ **How many milliliters will you give?** _____

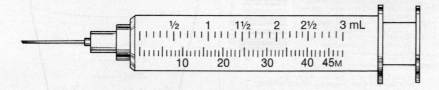

Courtesy of the Upjohn Company.

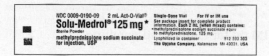

(Practice Problems continue on page 180)

12. Order: lactulose 20 g PO daily for constipation

❋ **How many milliliters will you give?** _____

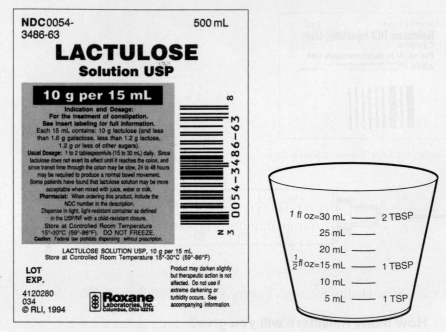

Courtesy of Roxane Laboratories.

13. Order: prochlorperazine 5 mg IM tid for nausea and vomiting

❋ **How many milliliters will you give?** _____

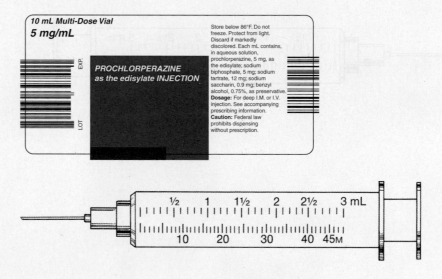

14. Order: amoxicillin/clavulanate potassium 250 mg PO every 8 hours for infection

    Supply: Amoxicillin 125 mg/5 mL

    ❋ **How many milliliters will you give?** _____

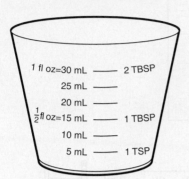

15. Order: trimethobenzamide HCl 200 mg PO tid for nausea and vomiting

    ❋ **How many capsules will you give?** _____

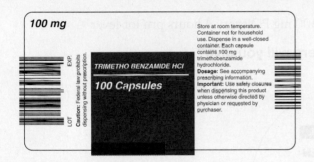

16. Order: prednisone 10 mg PO bid for adrenal insufficiency

    ❋ **How many tablets will you give?** _____

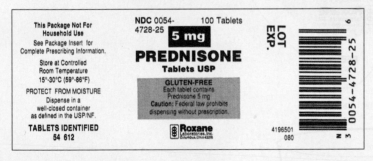

Courtesy of Roxane Laboratories.

(Practice Problems continue on page 182)

17. Order: hydromorphone 3 mg IM every 4 hours for pain

❋ **How many milliliters will you give?** _____

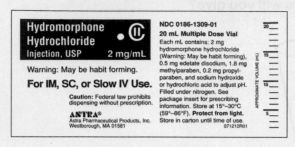

Courtesy of Astra Pharmaceutical Products.

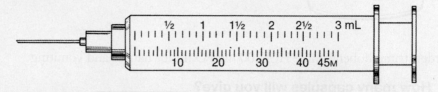

18. Order: acetaminophen 400 mg PO every 4 hours prn for fever

❋ **How many milliliters will you give?** _____

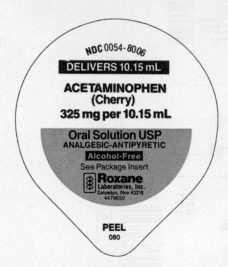

Courtesy of Roxane Laboratories.

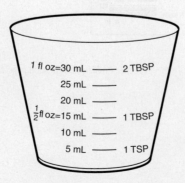

19. Order: magnesium sulfate 1000 mg IM times four doses for hypomagnesemia

   ✳ **How many milliliters will you give?** _____

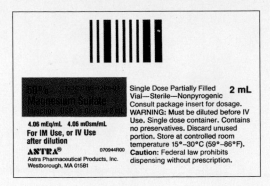

   Single Dose Partially Filled **2 mL**
   Vial—Sterile—Nonpyrogenic
   Consult package insert for dosage.
   **WARNING: Must be diluted before IV
   Use.** Single dose container. Contains
   no preservatives. Discard unused
   portion. Store at controlled room
   temperature 15°–30°C (59°–86°F).
   Caution: Federal law prohibits
   dispensing without prescription.

   50%
   Magnesium Sulfate
   Injection, USP 1 Gram in 2 mL
   4.06 mEq/mL 4.06 mOsm/mL
   **For IM Use, or IV Use
   after dilution**
   ASTRA® 070944R00
   Astra Pharmaceutical Products, Inc.
   Westborough, MA 01581

Courtesy of Astra Pharmaceutical Products.

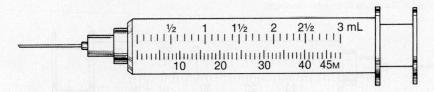

20. Order: prochlorperazine 10 mg PO qid prn for nausea and vomiting

   ✳ **How many teaspoons will you give?** _____

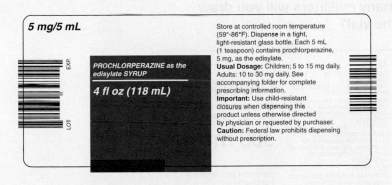

   5 mg/5 mL

   Store at controlled room temperature
   (59°-86°F). Dispense in a tight,
   light-resistant glass bottle. Each 5 mL
   (1 teaspoon) contains prochlorperazine,
   5 mg, as the edisylate.
   Usual Dosage: Children; 5 to 15 mg daily.
   Adults: 10 to 30 mg daily. See
   accompanying folder for complete
   prescribing information.
   Important: Use child-resistant
   closures when dispensing this
   product unless otherwise directed
   by physician or requested by purchaser.
   Caution: Federal law prohibits dispensing
   without prescription.

   **PROCHLORPERAZINE as the
   edisylate SYRUP**

   4 fl oz (118 mL)

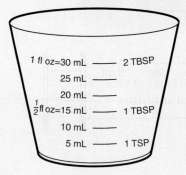

   1 fl oz=30 mL ——— 2 TBSP
       25 mL ———
       20 mL ———
   ½ fl oz=15 mL ——— 1 TBSP
       10 mL ———
       5 mL ——— 1 TSP

(Practice Problems continue on page 184)

21. Order: Hemabate 0.25 mg IM to control postpartum bleeding

    ✳ **How many milliliters will you give?** _____

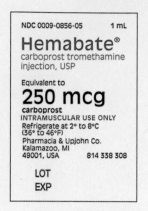

    NDC 0009-0856-05   1 mL

    Hemabate®
    carboprost tromethamine
    injection, USP

    Equivalent to
    250 mcg
    carboprost
    INTRAMUSCULAR USE ONLY
    Refrigerate at 2° to 8°C
    (36° to 46°F)
    Pharmacia & Upjohn Co.
    Kalamazoo, MI
    49001, USA   814 338 308

    LOT

    EXP

Courtesy of Pharmacia & Upjohn Company.

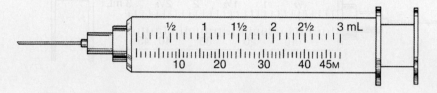

22. Order: Lincocin 500 mg every 8 hours IV for infection

    ✳ **How many milliliters will you draw**
    from the vial? _____

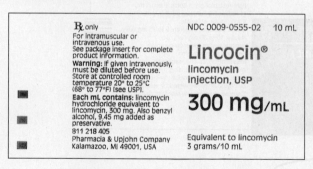

    ℞ only
    For intramuscular or
    intravenous use.
    See package insert for complete
    product information.
    Warning: If given intravenously,
    must be diluted before use.
    Store at controlled room
    temperature 20° to 25°C
    (68° to 77°F) (see USP).
    Each mL contains: lincomycin
    hydrochloride equivalent to
    lincomycin, 300 mg. Also benzyl
    alcohol, 9.45 mg added as
    preservative.
    811 218 405
    Pharmacia & Upjohn Company
    Kalamazoo, MI 49001, USA

    NDC 0009-0555-02   10 mL

    Lincocin®
    lincomycin
    injection, USP

    300 mg/mL

    Equivalent to lincomycin
    3 grams/10 mL

Courtesy of Pharmacia & Upjohn Company.

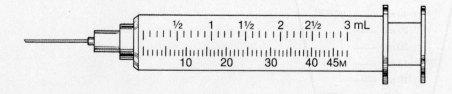

23. Order: Fragmin 2500 IU SQ daily for 10 days for thromboembolism prophylaxis

❋ **How many milliliters will you give?** _____

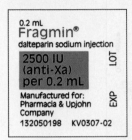

0.2 mL
Fragmin®
dalteparin sodium injection
2500 IU
(anti-Xa)
per 0.2 mL
LOT
Manufactured for:
Pharmacia & Upjohn
Company
132050198   KV0307-02
EXP

Courtesy of Pharmacia & Upjohn Company.

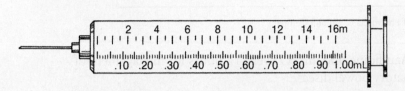

24. Order: Vantin 200 mg every 12 hours PO for infection

❋ **How many milliliters will you give?** _____

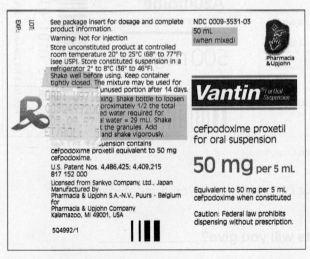

See package insert for dosage and complete product information.
Warning: Not for injection
Store unconstituted product at controlled room temperature 20° to 25°C (68° to 77°F) (see USP). Store constituted suspension in a refrigerator 2° to 8°C (36° to 46°F).
Shake well before using. Keep container tightly closed. The mixture may be used for ... unused portion after 14 days.
... xing: Shake bottle to loosen ... proximately 1/2 the total ... ed water required for ... al water = 29 mL). Shake ... t the granules. Add ... and shake vigorously.
...uspension contains cefpodoxime proxetil equivalent to 50 mg cefpodoxime.
U.S. Patent Nos. 4,486,425; 4,409,215 817 152 000
Licensed from Sankyo Company, Ltd., Japan
Manufactured by
Pharmacia & Upjohn S.A.-N.V., Puurs - Belgium
for
Pharmacia & Upjohn Company
Kalamazoo, MI 49001, USA
5Q4992/1

NDC 0009-3531-03
50 mL
(when mixed)

Pharmacia
&Upjohn

Vantin® For Oral Suspension

cefpodoxime proxetil
for oral suspension

50 mg per 5 mL

Equivalent to 50 mg per 5 mL
cefpodoxime when constituted

Caution: Federal law prohibits
dispensing without prescription.

Courtesy of Pharmacia & Upjohn Company.

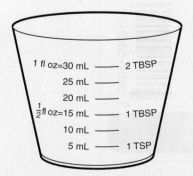

1 fl oz=30 mL —— 2 TBSP
25 mL ——
20 mL ——
½ fl oz=15 mL —— 1 TBSP
10 mL ——
5 mL —— 1 TSP

(Practice Problems continue on page 186)

25. Order: Cleocin 300 mg PO daily for *P. carinii* pneumonia

❋ **How many capsules will you give?** _____

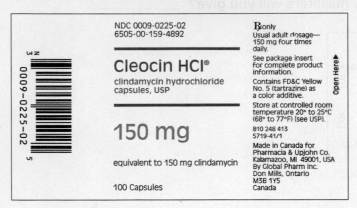

Courtesy of Pharmacia & Upjohn Company.

26. Order: Azulfidine 500 mg PO every 12 hours for management of inflammatory bowel disease

❋ **How many tablets will you give?** _____

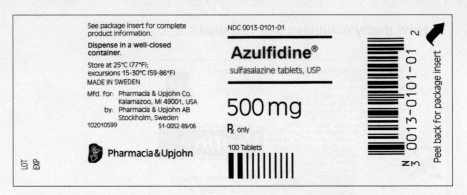

Courtesy of Pharmacia & Upjohn Company.

27. Order: Mirapex 0.25 mg PO tid for signs/symptoms of idiopathic Parkinson's disease

❋ **How many tablets will you give?** _____

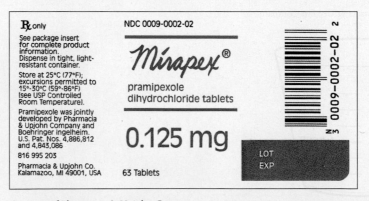

Courtesy of Pharmacia & Upjohn Company.

28. Order: Glyset 25 mg PO tid at the start of each meal for management of type 2 diabetes mellitus

   ❊ **How many tablets will you give?** _____

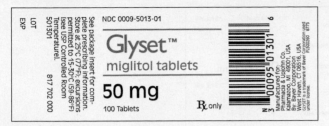

   Courtesy of Pharmacia & Upjohn Company.

29. Order: Micronase 5 mg PO daily for control of blood sugars associated with non–insulin-dependent diabetes mellitus

   ❊ **How many tablets will you give?** _____

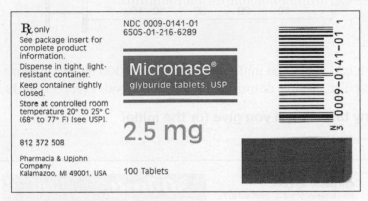

   Courtesy of Pharmacia & Upjohn Company.

30. Order: Xanax 0.5 mg PO tid for panic attacks

   ❊ **How many tablets will you give?** _____

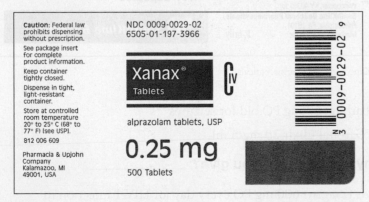

   Courtesy of Pharmacia & Upjohn Company.

(*Practice Problems continue on page 188*)

31. Order: Depo-Provera 150 mg IM within the first 5 days of menses for contraception

    ✳ **How many milliliters will you give?** _____

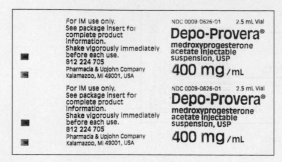

For IM use only.
See package insert for complete product information.
Shake vigorously immediately before each use.
812 224 705
Pharmacia & Upjohn Company
Kalamazoo, MI 49001, USA
NDC 0009-0626-01   2.5 mL Vial
Depo-Provera®
medroxyprogesterone acetate Injectable suspension, USP
400 mg /mL

For IM use only.
See package insert for complete product information.
Shake vigorously immediately before each use.
812 224 705
Pharmacia & Upjohn Company
Kalamazoo, MI 49001, USA
NDC 0009-0626-01   2.5 mL Vial
Depo-Provera®
medroxyprogesterone acetate Injectable suspension, USP
400 mg /mL

Courtesy of Pharmacia & Upjohn Company.

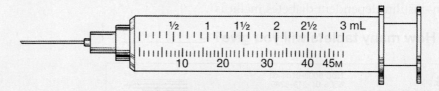

32. Order: Eskalith 600 mg PO tid initial dose followed by 300 mg PO qid for treatment of bipolar affective disorder. Check lithium levels every 3 months.

    ✳ **How many tablets will you give for the initial dose?** _____

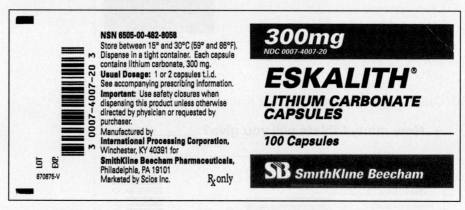

NSN 6505-00-482-8058
Store between 15° and 30°C (59° and 86°F). Dispense in a tight container. Each capsule contains lithium carbonate, 300 mg.
Usual Dosage: 1 or 2 capsules t.i.d. See accompanying prescribing information.
Important: Use safety closures when dispensing this product unless otherwise directed by physician or requested by purchaser.
Manufactured by
International Processing Corporation, Winchester, KY 40391 for
SmithKline Beecham Pharmaceuticals, Philadelphia, PA 19101
Marketed by Scios Inc.   ℞ only

300mg
NDC 0007-4007-20
ESKALITH®
LITHIUM CARBONATE CAPSULES
100 Capsules
SB SmithKline Beecham

Courtesy of SmithKline Beecham Pharmaceuticals.

33. Order: Phenobarbital 60 mg PO bid for seizures

    Supply: Phenobarbital Elixir 20 mg/5 mL

    ✳ **How many milliliters will you give?** _____

34. Order: Abacavir (Ziagen) 600 mg PO every day for HIV-1 infection in combination with Zidovudine

    Supply: Ziagen 300 mg/tablets

    ✳ **How many tablets will you give?** _____

35. Order: Zidovudine 100 mg PO every four hours for symptomatic HIV infection (600 mg/daily total)

Supply: Zidovudine 10 mg/mL syrup

✳ **How many milliliters will you give?** _____

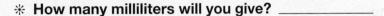

Practice Problems	**Two-Factor Practice Problems**
	(See pages 212–214 for answers)

1. Order: digoxin elixir 25 mcg/kg for congestive heart failure

Child's weight: 25 lb

✳ **How many milliliters will you give?** _____

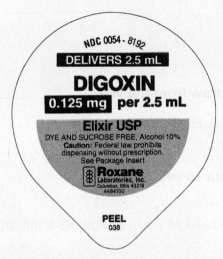

DELIVERS 2.5 mL

DIGOXIN

0.125 mg per 2.5 mL

Elixir USP
DYE AND SUCROSE FREE, Alcohol 10%
Caution: Federal law prohibits
dispensing without prescription.
See Package Insert

Roxane
Laboratories, Inc.
Columbus, Ohio 43216
4484100

PEEL
038

NDC 0054-8192

Courtesy of Roxane Laboratories.

2. Order: atropine sulfate 0.02 mg/kg IV every 4 hours for bradycardia

Child's weight: 35 lb

✳ **How many milliliters will you give?** _____

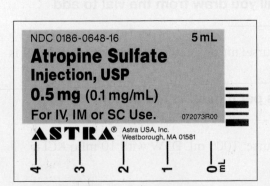

NDC 0186-0648-16   5 mL

Atropine Sulfate
Injection, USP

0.5 mg (0.1 mg/mL)

For IV, IM or SC Use.   072073R00

ASTRA® Astra USA, Inc.
Westborough, MA 01581

4   3   2   1   0
                    mL

Courtesy of Astra Pharmaceutical Products.

(Practice Problems continue on page 190)

3. Order: lidocaine 2 mg/min IV for arrhythmia

    Supply: lidocaine 2 g/500 mL D5W

    ❋ **Calculate the milliliters per hour to set the IV pump.** _____

4. Order: nafcillin 500 mg IVPB every 6 hours for respiratory infection

    Supply: nafcillin 1-g vial

    Nursing drug reference: Reconstitute each 1-g vial with 3.4 mL sterile water and further dilute in 50 mL 0.9% NS to infuse over 30 minutes.

    ❋ **How many milliliters will you draw from the vial after reconstitution?** _____

    ❋ **Calculate the milliliters per hour to set the IV pump.** _____

5. Order: gentamicin 1 mg/kg IV every 8 hours for infection

    Supply: gentamicin 40 mg/mL

    Child's weight: 94 lb

    ❋ **How many milliliters will you draw from the vial?** _____

6. Order: morphine 15 mg/hr IV for intractable pain

    Supply: morphine 300 mg/500 mL NS

    ❋ **Calculate the milliliters per hour to set the IV pump.** _____

7. Information obtained by the nurse: Dilaudid 50 mg in 250 mL NS is infusing at 25 mL/hr.

    ❋ **How many milligrams per hour is the patient receiving?** _____

8. Order: add 10 mEq KCl to 1000 mL D5W

    Supply: KCl 20 mEq/20 mL

    ❋ **How many milliliters will you draw from the vial to add to the IV bag?** _____

9. Information obtained by the nurse: nitroglycerin 50 mg in 500 mL D5W is infusing at 3 mL/hr.

    ❋ **How many micrograms per minute is the patient receiving?** _____

10. Information obtained by the nurse: 1000 mL D5W with 10 mEq KCl is infusing at 100 mL/hr.

    ❋ **How many milliequivalents of KCl is the patient receiving per hour?** _____

11. Order: infuse 1000 mL D5W at 250 mL/hr

    Drop factor: 20 gtt/mL

    ❋ **Calculate the number of drops per minute.** _____

12. Order: infuse 750 mL NS over 5 hours

    Drop factor: 10 gtt/mL

    ❋ **Calculate the number of drops per minute.** _____

13. Order: infuse 500 mL D5W over 8 hours

    Drop factor: 60 gtt/mL

    ❋ **Calculate the number of drops per minute.** _____

14. Order: infuse 750 mL D5W

    Drop factor: 15 gtt/mL

    Infusion rate: 18 gtt/min

    ❋ **Calculate the number of hours to infuse.** _____

15. Order: infuse 250 mL NS

    Drop factor: 15 gtt/mL

    Infusion rate: 50 gtt/min

    ❋ **Calculate the number of hours to infuse.** _____

16. Order: infuse 1000 mL D5W/0.45% NS

    Drop factor: 15 gtt/mL

    Infusion rate: 25 gtt/min

    ❋ **Calculate the number of hours to infuse.** _____

17. Order: fortaz 1.25 g IV every 12 hours for urinary tract infection

    Supply: fortaz 2-g vial

    Nursing drug reference: Dilute each 1 g with 10 mL of sterile water and further
    dilute in 100 mL 0.9% NS to infuse over 1 hour.

    ❋ **How many milliliters will you draw from the vial
    after reconstitution?** _____

    ❋ **Calculate the milliliters per hour
    to set the IV pump.** _____

    ❋ **Calculate the drops per minute with a drop factor
    of 10 gtt/mL.** _____

(Practice Problems continue on page 192)

18. Order: vancomycin 275 mg IV every 8 hours for infection

    Supply: vancomycin 500-mg vial

    Nursing drug reference: Reconstitute each 500-mg vial with 10 mL NS and further dilute with 250 mL NS to infuse over 1 hour.

    ✳ **How many milliliters will you draw from the vial after reconstitution?** _____

    ✳ **Calculate the milliliters per hour to set the IV pump.** _____

    ✳ **Calculate the drops per minute with a drop factor of 10 gtt/mL.** _____

19. Order: Nafcillin 1 g every 4 hours IVPB for severe respiratory infection

    Supply: Nafcillin 1-g vial

    Nursing drug reference: Reconstitute each 1-g vial with 3.4 mL sterile water and further dilute in 100 mL 0.9% NS to infuse over 60 minutes.

    ✳ **How many milliliters will you draw from the vial after reconstitution?** _____

    ✳ **Calculate the milliliters per hour to set the IV pump.** _____

    ✳ **Calculate the drops per minute with a drop factor of 20 gtt/mL.** _____

20. Order: gentamicin 23 mg IV every 8 hours for infection

    Supply: gentamicin 40 mg/mL

    Nursing drug reference: Dilute with 100 mL NS and infuse over 1 hour.

    ✳ **How many milliliters will you draw from the vial after reconstitution?** _____

    ✳ **Calculate the milliliters per hour to set the IV pump.** _____

    ✳ **Calculate the drops per minute with a drop factor of 15 gtt/mL.** _____

21. Order: Cortef 0.56 mg/kg PO daily for adrenal insufficiency

✷ **How many milliliters will you give a child weighing 18 kg?** _____

NDC 0009-0142-01
4 Fl Oz

Cortef®

hydrocortisone cypionate
oral suspension

10 mg/5 mL*

℞ only

810 322 608

**Pharmacia
&Upjohn**

NDC 0009-0142-01   4 Fl Oz
See package insert for complete product information.
Warning—This potent drug must be used only under the direct supervision of a physician.
Shake well before each use, until all visible sediment is resuspended.
Dispense in tight, light-resistant container. Store bottle inside carton. Keep container tightly closed. Store at controlled room temperature 20° to 25° C (68° to 77° F) [see USP].
Each 5 mL (teaspoonful) contains
*Hydrocortisone . . . . 10 mg
(as 13.4 mg hydrocortisone cypionate)
Contains FD&C Yellow No. 6 as a color additive.
810 330 507
Pharmacia & Upjohn Company
Kalamazoo, MI 49001, USA

Courtesy of Pharmacia & Upjohn Company.

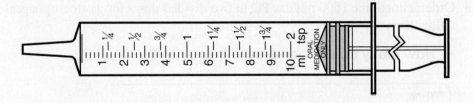

22. Order: Colestid 30 g/day PO in four divided doses for hypercholesterolemia or management of cholesterol

✷ **How many packets/dose will you give?** _____

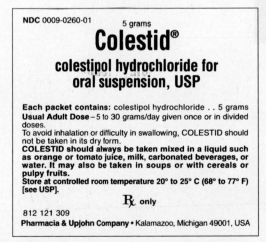

NDC 0009-0260-01   5 grams

Colestid®

colestipol hydrochloride for oral suspension, USP

Each packet contains: colestipol hydrochloride . . 5 grams
Usual Adult Dose – 5 to 30 grams/day given once or in divided doses.
To avoid inhalation or difficulty in swallowing, COLESTID should not be taken in its dry form.
COLESTID should always be taken mixed in a liquid such as orange or tomato juice, milk, carbonated beverages, or water. It may also be taken in soups or with cereals or pulpy fruits.
Store at controlled room temperature 20° to 25° C (68° to 77° F) [see USP].

℞ only

812 121 309
Pharmacia & Upjohn Company • Kalamazoo, Michigan 49001, USA

Courtesy of Pharmacia & Upjohn Company.

(Practice Problems continue on page 194)

23. Order: vincristine 10 mcg/kg IV weekly for treatment of Hodgkin's lymphoma

    ✳ **How many milliliters will you give a patient weighing 50 kg?** _____

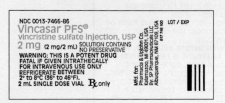

NDC 0013-7466-86
Vincasar PFS®
vincristine sulfate injection, USP
2 mg (2 mg/2 mL) SOLUTION CONTAINS NO PRESERVATIVE
WARNING: THIS IS A POTENT DRUG
FATAL IF GIVEN INTRATHECALLY
FOR INTRAVENOUS USE ONLY
REFRIGERATE BETWEEN
2° to 8°C (36° to 46°F).
2 mL SINGLE DOSE VIAL   ℞ only
LOT / EXP
Mfd for:
Pharmacia & Upjohn Co.
Kalamazoo, MI 49001, USA
By SP Pharmaceuticals LLC
Albuquerque, NM 87109, USA

Courtesy of Pharmacia & Upjohn Company.

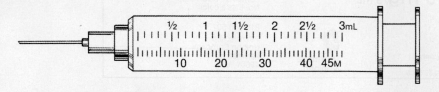

24. Order: cimetidine 1600 mg/day PO in two divided doses for gastroesophageal reflux disease

    ✳ **How many tablets per dose will you give?** _____

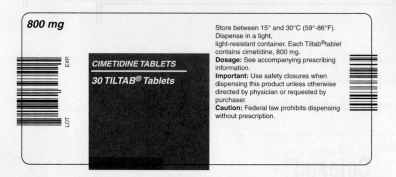

800 mg

EXP.

CIMETIDINE TABLETS

30 TILTAB® Tablets

LOT

Store between 15° and 30°C (59°-86°F).
Dispense in a tight,
light-resistant container. Each Tiltab® tablet
contains cimetidine, 800 mg.
Dosage: See accompanying prescribing
information.
Important: Use safety closures when
dispensing this product unless otherwise
directed by physician or requested by
purchaser.
Caution: Federal law prohibits dispensing
without prescription.

25. Order: chlorpromazine 1 g/day PO in three divided doses for psychoses

※ **How many milliliters per dose will you give?** _____

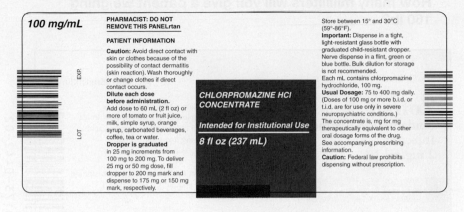

100 mg/mL

PHARMACIST: DO NOT
REMOVE THIS PANELrtan

PATIENT INFORMATION

Caution: Avoid direct contact with skin or clothes because of the possibility of contact dermatitis (skin reaction). Wash thoroughly or change clothes if direct contact occurs.
Dilute each dose before administration.
Add dose to 60 mL (2 fl oz) or more of tomato or fruit juice, milk, simple syrup, orange syrup, carbonated beverages, coffee, tea or water.
Dropper is graduated in 25 mg increments from 100 mg to 200 mg. To deliver 25 mg or 50 mg dose, fill dropper to 200 mg mark and dispense to 175 mg or 150 mg mark, respectively.

CHLORPROMAZINE HCl CONCENTRATE

Intended for Institutional Use

8 fl oz (237 mL)

Store between 15° and 30°C (59°-86°F).
Important: Dispense in a tight, light-resistant glass bottle with graduated child-resistant dropper. Nerve dispense in a flint, green or blue bottle. Bulk dilution for storage is not recommended.
Each mL contains chlorpromazine hydrochloride, 100 mg.
Usual Dosage: 75 to 400 mg daily. (Doses of 100 mg or more b.i.d. or t.i.d. are for use only in severe neuropsychiatric conditions.)
The concentrate is, mg for mg therapeutically equivalent to other oral dosage forms of the drug. See accompanying prescribing information.
Caution: Federal law prohibits dispensing without prescription.

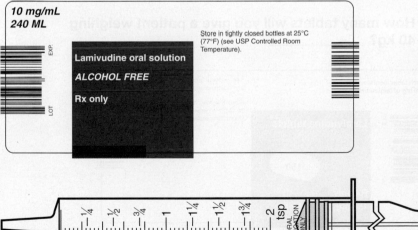

26. Order: lamivudine 4 mg/kg PO bid for treatment of HIV infection

※ **How many milliliters will you give a child weighing 20 kg?** _____

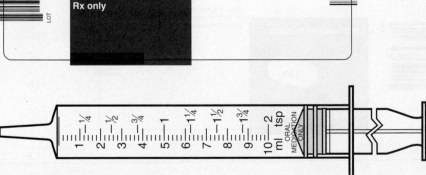

10 mg/mL
240 ML

Lamivudine oral solution

ALCOHOL FREE

Rx only

Store in tightly closed bottles at 25°C (77°F) (see USP Controlled Room Temperature).

(Practice Problems continue on page 196)

27. Order: Zofran 0.15 mg/kg IV 15 to 30 minutes before administration of chemotherapy for prevention of nausea and vomiting

   ✳ **How many milliliters will you give a patient weighing 160 lb?** _____

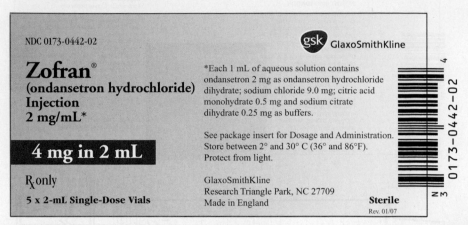

NDC 0173-0442-02

gsk GlaxoSmithKline

Zofran®
(ondansetron hydrochloride)
Injection
2 mg/mL*

4 mg in 2 mL

R only

5 x 2-mL Single-Dose Vials

*Each 1 mL of aqueous solution contains ondansetron 2 mg as ondansetron hydrochloride dihydrate; sodium chloride 9.0 mg; citric acid monohydrate 0.5 mg and sodium citrate dihydrate 0.25 mg as buffers.

See package insert for Dosage and Administration. Store between 2° and 30° C (36° and 86°F). Protect from light.

GlaxoSmithKline
Research Triangle Park, NC 27709
Made in England

Sterile
Rev. 01/07

Copyright GlaxoSmithKline. Used with permission.

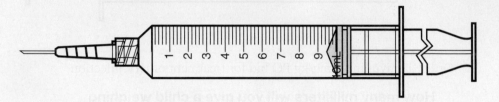

28. Order: lamivudine 2 mg/kg PO twice daily for treatment of HIV infection

   ✳ **How many tablets will you give a patient weighing 40 kg?** _____

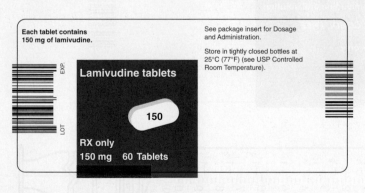

Each tablet contains 150 mg of lamivudine.

See package insert for Dosage and Administration.

Store in tightly closed bottles at 25°C (77°F) (see USP Controlled Room Temperature).

Lamivudine tablets

150

RX only
150 mg   60 Tablets

29. Order: Zovirax 20 mg/kg PO qid for 5 days for treatment of chicken pox

    ✳ **How many tablets will you give a child weighing 20 lb?** _____

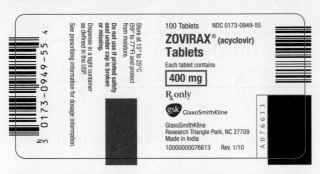

Copyright GlaxoSmithKline. Used with permission.

30. Order: Wellbutrin SR 450 mg/day PO in three divided doses for treatment of depression

    ✳ **How many tablets per dose will you give?** _____

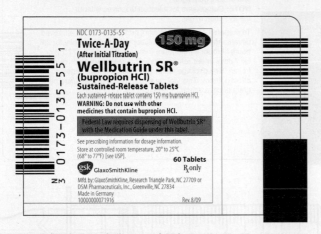

Copyright GlaxoSmithKline. Used with permission.

31. Order: Zantac 2.4 g/day PO in four divided doses for treatment of duodenal ulcer

    ✳ **How many tablets per dose will you give?** _____

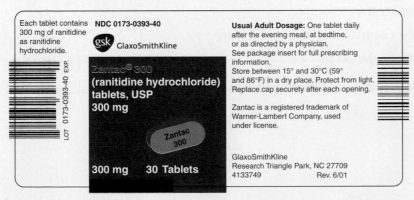

Copyright GlaxoSmithKline. Used with permission.

(Practice Problems continue on page 198)

32. Order: Zinacef 500 mg/day IV in two divided doses for urinary tract infection

    Supply: Zinacef 750 mg/8 mL

    ✳ **How many milliliters per dose will you give?** _____

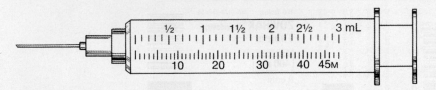

33. Order: ceftazidime 1000 mg/day IV in two divided doses for treatment of respiratory tract infection

    Nursing drug reference: Dilute each 1-g vial with 10 mL of normal saline.

    ✳ **How many milliliters per dose will you give?** _____

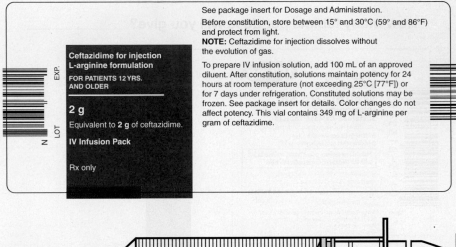

See package insert for Dosage and Administration.

Before constitution, store between 15° and 30°C (59° and 86°F) and protect from light.
NOTE: Ceftazidime for injection dissolves without the evolution of gas.

To prepare IV infusion solution, add 100 mL of an approved diluent. After constitution, solutions maintain potency for 24 hours at room temperature (not exceeding 25°C [77°F]) or for 7 days under refrigeration. Constituted solutions may be frozen. See package insert for details. Color changes do not affect potency. This vial contains 349 mg of L-arginine per gram of ceftazidime.

Ceftazidime for injection
L-arginine formulation

FOR PATIENTS 12 YRS.
AND OLDER

2 g

Equivalent to **2 g** of ceftazidime.

IV Infusion Pack

Rx only

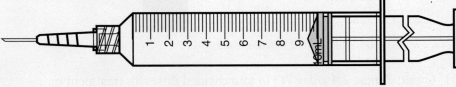

34. Order: gantrisin 150 mg/2.2 lb PO divided into five doses given over 24 hours for urinary tract infection

    Supply: Gantrisin 500 mg/5 mL (1 tsp)

    Child's weight: 30 kg

    ✳ **How many milliliters per dose will you give?** _____

35. Order: abacavir (Ziagen) 8 mg/kg PO bid for HIV-1 infection in combination with Zidovudine

    Supply: Ziagen 20 mg/mL oral solution

    Child's weight: 40 kg

    ✲ **How many milliliters will you give?** _____

Practice Problems	**Three-Factor Practice Problems**
	(See pages 214–217 for answers)

1. Order: cimetidine 40 mg/kg/day PO in four divided doses for treatment of active ulcer

   Child's weight: 60 kg

   ✲ **How many milliliters per day will you give?** _____

   ✲ **How many milliliters per dose will you give?** _____

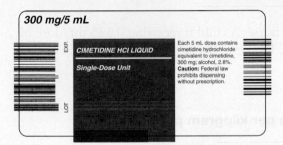

300 mg/5 mL

CIMETIDINE HCl LIQUID

Single-Dose Unit

Each 5 mL dose contains cimetidine hydrochloride equivalent to cimetidine, 300 mg; alcohol, 2.8%.
Caution: Federal law prohibits dispensing without prescription.

2. Order: furosemide 4 mg/kg/day IV for management of hypercalcemia of malignancy

   Child's weight: 60 lb

   ✲ **How many milliliters per day will you give?** _____

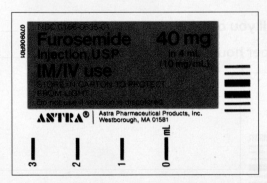

NDC 0186-0635-01

Furosemide   **40 mg**
Injection USP   in 4 mL
IM/IV use   (10 mg/mL)

STORE IN CARTON TO PROTECT FROM LIGHT

ASTRA® | Astra Pharmaceutical Products, Inc.
Westborough, MA 01581

3 2 1 0 mL

Courtesy of Astra Pharmaceutical Products.

(Practice Problems continue on page 200)

3. Order: Cleocin 30 mg/kg/day IV in divided doses every 8 hours for infection

   Child's weight: 50 kg

   ✳ **How many milliliters per day will you give?** _____

   ✳ **How many milliliters per dose will you give?** _____

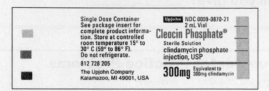

Single Dose Container	Upjohn NDC 0009-0870-21
See package insert for complete product informa-tion. Store at controlled room temperature 15° to 30° C (59° to 86° F). Do not refrigerate.	2 mL Vial
	Cleocin Phosphate®
	Sterile Solution
812 728 205	clindamycin phosphate injection, USP
The Upjohn Company Kalamazoo, MI 49001, USA	**300mg** Equivalent to 300mg clindamycin

Courtesy of the Upjohn Company.

4. Information obtained by the nurse: A child is receiving 0.575 mL/dose of gentamicin IV every 8 hours from a supply of gentamicin 40 mg/mL.

   Child's weight: 45 lb

   ✳ **How many milligrams per kilogram per day is the patient receiving?** _____

5. Information obtained by the nurse: A child is receiving 0.125 mL/dose of diphenhydramine (Benadryl) IV every 8 hours from a supply of Benadryl 50 mg/mL.

   Child's weight: 20 lb

   ✳ **How many milligrams per kilogram per day is the child receiving?** _____

6. Order: dopamine 5 mcg/kg/min IV for decreased cardiac output

   Supply: dopamine 400-mg vial

   Nursing drug reference: Dilute each 400-mg vial in 250 mL NS

   Patient's weight: 110 lb

   ✳ **How many milliliters will you draw from the vial?** _____

   ✳ **Calculate the milliliters per hour to set the IV pump.** _____

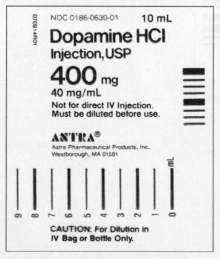

NDC 0186-0639-01   10 mL

Dopamine HCl
Injection, USP

400 mg
40 mg/mL

Not for direct IV Injection.
Must be diluted before use.

ASTRA®
Astra Pharmaceutical Products, Inc.
Westborough, MA 01581

CAUTION: For Dilution in
IV Bag or Bottle Only.

Courtesy of Astra Pharmaceutical Products.

7. Order: Nipride 0.8 mcg/kg/min IV for hypertensive crisis

   Supply: Nipride 50 mg/500 mL NS

   Patient's weight: 143 lb

   ✳ **Calculate the milliliters per hour to set the IV pump.** _____

8. Information obtained by the nurse: Nipride 50 mg in 250 mL NS is infusing at 68 mL/hr.

   Patient's weight: 250 lb

   ✳ **How many micrograms per kilogram per minute is the patient receiving?** _____

9. Order: Hydrea 30 mg/kg/day PO for ovarian carcinoma

   Patient's weight: 157 lb

   ✳ **How many grams per day is the patient receiving?** _____

10. Order: Venoglobulin-S 0.01 mL/kg/min for treatment of immunodeficiency syndrome

    Patient's weight: 180 lb

    ✳ **Calculate the milliliters per hour to set the IV pump.** _____

11. Information obtained by the nurse: dopamine 400 mg in 250 mL D5W is infusing at 28 mL/hr.

    Patient's weight: 15 kg

    ✳ **How many micrograms per kilogram per minute is the patient receiving?** _____

12. Order: Milrinone 50 mcg/kg over 10 minutes loading dose for congestive heart failure

    Supply: Milrinone 20 mg/100 mL of D5W

    Patient's weight: 160 lb

    ✳ **Calculate the milliliters per hour to set the IV pump.** _____

13. Order: Nipride 2 mcg/kg/min

    Supply: Nipride 50 mg/250 mL NS

    Patient's weight: 250 lb

    ✳ **Calculate the milliliters per hour to set the IV pump.** _____

(Practice Problems continue on page 202)

14. Order: Nipride 1 mcg/kg/min IV for hypertensive crisis

    Supply: Nipride 50 mg/250 mL NS

    Patient's weight: 160 lb

    ✳ **Calculate the milliliters per hour to set the IV pump.** _____

15. Order: dopamine 2.5 mcg/kg/min IV for hypotension

    Supply: dopamine 400 mg/500 mL D5W

    Patient's weight: 65 kg

    ✳ **Calculate the milliliters per hour to set the IV pump.** _____

16. Information obtained by the nurse: Isuprel 2 mg in 500 mL D5W is infusing at 15 mL/hr.

    Child's weight: 20 kg

    ✳ **How many micrograms per kilogram per minute is the child receiving?** _____

17. Order: Intropin 5 mcg/kg/min IV for treatment of oliguria after shock

    Supply: Intropin 400 mg/500 mL NS

    Patient's weight: 70 kg

    ✳ **Calculate the milliliters per minute.** _____

18. Order: vancomycin 40 mg/kg/day IV in three divided doses for infection

    Supply: vancomycin 500-mg vial

    Nursing drug reference: Reconstitute each 500-mg vial with 10 mL sterile water and further dilute in 100 mL of 0.9% NS to infuse over 60 minutes.

    Child's weight: 20 lb

    ✳ **How many milligrams per day is the child receiving?** _____

    ✳ **How many milligrams per dose is the child receiving?** _____

    ✳ **How many milliliters will you draw from the vial after reconstitution?** _____

    ✳ **Calculate the milliliters per hour to set the IV pump.** _____

19. Order: gentamicin 2 mg/kg/dose IV every 8 hours for infection

    Supply: gentamicin 40-mg/mL vial

    Nursing drug reference: Further dilute in 50 mL NS and infuse over 30 minutes.

    Child's weight: 40 kg

    ✳ **How many milligrams per dose is the child receiving?** _____

    ✳ **How many milliliters will you draw from the vial?** _____

    ✳ **Calculate the milliliters per hour to set the IV pump.** _____

20. Order: Cefazolin 25 mg/kg/day IV every 8 hours for infection

    Supply: Cefazolin 500-mg vial

    Nursing drug reference: Reconstitute each 500-mg vial with 10 mL of sterile water and further dilute in 50 mL NS to infuse over 30 minutes.

    Child's weight: 25 kg

    ✳ **How many milligrams per day is the child receiving?** _____

    ✳ **How many milligrams per dose is the child receiving?** _____

    ✳ **How many milliliters will you draw from the vial after reconstitution?** _____

    ✳ **Calculate the milliliters per hour to set the IV pump.** _____

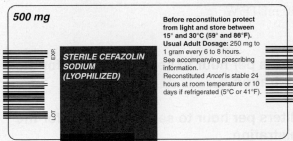

500 mg

EXP

STERILE CEFAZOLIN
SODIUM
(LYOPHILIZED)

LOT

Before reconstitution protect
from light and store between
15° and 30°C (59° and 86°F).
Usual Adult Dosage: 250 mg to
1 gram every 6 to 8 hours.
See accompanying prescribing
information.
Reconstituted *Ancef* is stable 24
hours at room temperature or 10
days if refrigerated (5°C or 41°F).

(Practice Problems continue on page 204)

21. Order: amikacin (Amikin) 12.5 mg/kg/day IV in two equally divided doses every 12 hours for 10 days for gram-negative bacterial infection

    Supply: Amikin 500 mg in 100 mL 0.9% Normal Saline to infuse over 60 minutes

    Patient's weight: 80 kg

    ✽ **How many milligrams per day is the patient receiving?** _____

    ✽ **How many milligrams per dose is the patient receiving?** _____

    ✽ **Calculate the milliliters per hour to set the IV pump.** _____

22. Order: dopamine (Intropin) 2 mcg/kg/minute IV for shock

    Supply: dopamine 200 mg/250 mL D5W

    Patient's weight: 175 lb

    ✽ **Calculate the milliliters per hour to set the IV pump.** _____

23. Order: epoetin (Procrit) 150 units/kg/day three times a week for chemotherapy-induced anemia

    Supply: Procrit 10,000 units/mL

    Patient's weight: 80 kg

    ✽ **How many milliliters per day will you give?** _____

24. Order: esmolol hydrochloride 500 mcg/kg/min for 1 minute then 50 mcg/kg/min for 4 minutes for supraventricular tachycardia in atrial fibrillation. Repeat after 5 minutes if SVT continues.

    Supply: esmolol 2.5 g/250 mL D5W

    Patient's weight: 90 kg

    ✽ **Calculate the milliliters per hour to set the IV pump for the one-minute administration.** _____

    ✽ **Calculate the milliliters per hour to set the IV pump for the four-minute administration.** _____

25. Order: prednisone 0.1 mg/kg/day for chronic obstructive pulmonary disease.

    Supply: prednisone 5 mg/5 mL oral solution

    Child's weight: 35 kg

    ✽ **How many milliliters per day will you give?** _____

Practice Problems **Comprehensive Practice Problems**

(See pages 217–218 for answers)

1. Order: digoxin 0.125 mg PO daily for congestive heart failure

   On hand: digoxin 0.25 mg/tablet

   ❋ **How many tablets will you give?** _____

2. Order: ascorbic acid 0.5 g PO daily for supplemental therapy

   On hand: ascorbic acid 500 mg/tablet

   ❋ **How many tablets will you give?** _____

3. Order: atropine gr 1/150 IM for on-call preanesthesia

   Supply: atropine 0.4 mg/mL

   ❋ **How many milliliters will you give?** _____

4. Order: Mycostatin oral suspension 500,000 units swish-and-swallow for oral thrush

   On hand: Mycostatin 100,000 units/mL

   ❋ **How many teaspoons will you give?** _____

5. Order: Demerol 50 mg IM every 4 hours for pain

   Supply: Demerol 100 mg/mL

   ❋ **How many milliliters will you give?** _____

6. Order: vancomycin 2 mg/kg IV every 12 hours for infection

   Supply: vancomycin 500 mg/10 mL

   Patient's weight: 75 kg

   ❋ **How many milliliters will you give?** _____

7. Order: ampicillin 2 mg/kg PO every 8 hours for infection

   Supply: ampicillin 500 mg/5 mL

   Patient's weight: 100 lb

   ❋ **How many milliliters will you give?** _____

8. Order: 1000 mL D5W to infuse in 12 hours

   Drop factor: 15 gtt/mL

   ❋ **Calculate the number of drops per minute.** _____

9. Order: 500 mL D5W

   Drop factor: 15 gtt/mL

   Infusion rate: 21 gtt/min

   ❋ **Calculate the hours to infuse.** _____

(Practice Problems continue on page 206)

10. Order: heparin 1500 units/hr

    Supply: 250-mL IV bag of D5W with 25,000 units of heparin

    ✳ **Calculate the milliliters per hour to set the IV pump. _____**

11. Order: 1000 mL NS IV

    Drop factor: 15 gtt/mL

    Infusion rate: 50 gtt/min

    ✳ **Calculate the hours to infuse. _____**

12. Order: regular insulin 8 units per hour IV for hyperglycemia

    Supply: 250 mL NS with 100 units of regular insulin

    ✳ **Calculate the milliliters per hour to set the IV pump. _____**

13. Order: 500 mL of 10% lipids to infuse in 8 hours

    Drop factor: 10 gtt/mL

    ✳ **Calculate the number of drops per minute. _____**

14. Order: KCl 2 mEq/100 mL of D5W for hypokalemia

    On hand: 20 mEq/10-mL vial

    Supply: 500 mL D5W

    ✳ **How many milliliters of KCl will you add to the IV bag? _____**

15. Order: aminophylline 44 mg/hr IV for bronchodilation

    Supply: 250 mL D5W with 1 g of aminophylline

    ✳ **Calculate the milliliters per hour to set the IV pump. _____**

16. Order: Dilaudid 140 mL/hr

    Supply: 1000 mL D5W/NS with 30 mg of Dilaudid

    ✳ **Calculate the milligrams per hour that the patient is receiving. _____**

17. Order: Staphcillin 750 mg IV every 4 hours for infection

    Supply: Staphcillin 6 g

    Nursing drug reference: Reconstitute with 8.6 mL of sterile water to yield 500 mg/mL and further dilute in 100 mL of NS to infuse over 30 minutes.

    ❋ **How many milliliters will you draw from the vial after reconstitution?** _____

    ❋ **Calculate the milliliters per hour to set the IV pump.** _____

    ❋ **Calculate the drops per minute with a drop factor of 10 gtt/mL.** _____

18. Order: Pipracil 1.5 g every 6 hours for uncomplicated urinary tract infection

    Supply: Pipracil 3-g vial

    Nursing drug reference: Reconstitute each 3-g vial with 5 mL of sterile water and further dilute in 50 mL of 0.9% NS to infuse over 20 minutes.

    ❋ **How many milliliters will you draw from the vial after reconstitution?** _____

    ❋ **Calculate the milliliters per hour to set the IV pump.** _____

    ❋ **Calculate the drops per minute with a drop factor of 20 gtt/mL.** _____

19. Order: dopamine 4 mcg/kg/min IV for decreased cardiac output

    Supply: 250 mL D5W with 400 mg of dopamine

    Patient's weight: 120 lb

    ❋ **Calculate the milliliters per hour to set the IV pump.** _____

20. Order: Nipride 0.8 mcg/kg/min IV for hypertension

    Supply: 500 mL D5W with 50 mg Nipride

    Patient's weight: 143 lb

    ❋ **Calculate the milliliters per hour to set the IV pump.** _____

21. Order: ampicillin (Principen) 500 mg PO every 6 hours for chronic infection

    Supply: 250 mg/5 mL

    ❋ **How many milliliters will you give?** _____

22. Order: atenolol (Tenormin) 50 mg PO per day for hypertension

    Supply: atenolol 100-mg tablets.

    ❋ **How many tablets will you give?** _____

(Practice Problems continue on page 208)

23. Order: amiodarone (Cordarone IV) 150 mg IV over 10 minutes

    Supply: amiodarone 150 mg in 100 mL D5W

    ❋ **Calculate the milliliters per hour to set the IV pump.** _____

24. Order: azithromycin (Zithromax) 30 mg/kg PO once a day for three days for otitis media

    Supply: azithromycin 100 mg/5 mL

    Child's weight: 15 kg

    ❋ **How many milliliters will you give?** _____

25. Order: amoxicillin 45 mg/kg/day in two divided doses for severe ear infection

    Supply: amoxicillin 400 mg/5 mL

    Child's weight: 35 kg

    ❋ **How many milligrams per day is the child receiving?** _____

    ❋ **How many milligrams per dose is the child receiving?** _____

    ❋ **How many milliliters per dose will you give?** _____

ANSWER KEY FOR SECTION 2: PRACTICE PROBLEMS

One-Factor Practice Problems

1

Sequential method:

$$\frac{200 \text{ mg}}{} \left| \frac{\text{mL}}{100 \text{ mg}} \right| \frac{2}{1} = 2 \text{ mL}$$

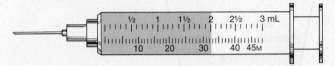

2

Sequential method:

$$\frac{30 \text{ mg}}{} \left| \frac{\text{tablet}}{30 \text{ mg}} \right| \frac{3}{3} = 1 \text{ tablet}$$

3

Sequential method:

$$\frac{7.5 \text{ mg}}{} \left| \frac{\text{tablet}}{2.5 \text{ mg}} \right| \frac{7.5}{2.5} = 3 \text{ tablets}$$

4

Sequential method:

$$\frac{160 \text{ mg}}{} \left| \frac{5 \text{ mL}}{160 \text{ mg}} \right| \frac{1 \text{ tsp}}{5 \text{ mL}} \left| 1 = 1 \text{ tsp} \right.$$

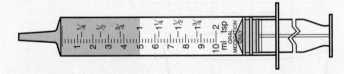

5

Sequential method:

$$\frac{0.5 \text{ mg}}{} \left| \frac{\text{tablet}}{1 \text{ mg}} \right| \frac{0.5}{1} = 0.5 \text{ tablet}$$

6

Sequential method:

$$\frac{60 \text{ mg}}{} \left| \frac{\text{tablet}}{60 \text{ mg}} \right| = 1 \text{ tablet}$$

7

Sequential method:

$$\frac{0.25 \text{ mg}}{} \left| \frac{\text{tablet}}{0.125 \text{ mg}} \right| \frac{0.25}{0.125} = 2 \text{ tablets}$$

8

Sequential method:

$$\frac{80 \text{ mg}}{} \left| \frac{\text{tablet}}{20 \text{ mg}} \right| \frac{8}{2} = 4 \text{ tablets}$$

9

Random method:

$$\frac{10 \text{ mg}}{\frac{1}{8} \text{ gr}} \left| \frac{\text{mL}}{60 \text{ mg}} \right| \frac{1 \text{ gr}}{\frac{1}{8} \times \frac{6}{1}} \left| \frac{1 \times 1}{\frac{6}{8}} \right| \frac{1}{0.75} = \frac{1.33 \text{ or}}{1.3 \text{ mL}}$$

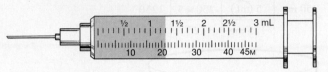

10

Random method:

$$\frac{100 \text{ mcg}}{0.4 \text{ mg}} \left| \frac{\text{mL}}{1000 \text{ mcg}} \right| \frac{1 \text{ mg}}{0.4 \times 10} \left| \frac{1 \times 1}{4} \right| = \frac{0.25 \text{ or}}{0.3 \text{ mL}}$$

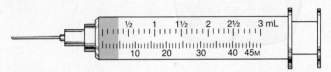

11

Sequential method:

$$\frac{80 \text{ mg}}{} \left| \frac{2 \text{ mL}}{125 \text{ mg}} \right| \frac{80 \times 2}{125} \left| \frac{160}{125} \right| = 1.28 \text{ or } 1.3 \text{ mL}$$

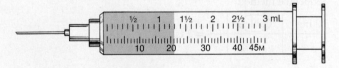

12

Sequential method:

$$\frac{20 \text{ g}}{} \left| \frac{15 \text{ mL}}{10 \text{ g}} \right| \frac{2 \times 15}{1} \left| \frac{30}{1} \right| = 30 \text{ mL}$$

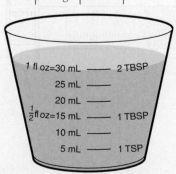

13

Sequential method:

$$\frac{5\ mg\ |\ \boxed{mL}}{|\ 5\ mg} = 1\ mL$$

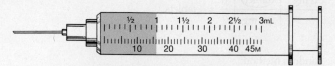

14

Sequential method:

$$\frac{250\ mg\ |\ 5\ \boxed{mL}\ |\ 250 \times 5\ |\ 1250}{|\ 125\ mg\ |\ 125\ |\ 125} = 10\ mL$$

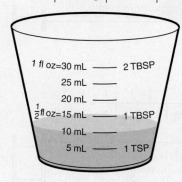

15

Sequential method:

$$\frac{200\ mg\ |\ \boxed{capsules}\ |\ 2}{|\ 100\ mg\ |\ 1} = 2\ capsules$$

16

Sequential method:

$$\frac{10\ mg\ |\ \boxed{tablet}\ |\ 10}{|\ 5\ mg\ |\ 5} = 2\ tablets$$

17

Sequential method:

$$\frac{3\ mg\ |\ \boxed{mL}\ |\ 3}{|\ 2\ mg\ |\ 2} = 1.5\ mL$$

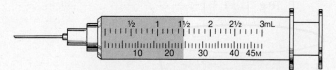

18

Sequential method:

$$\frac{400\ mg\ |\ 10.15\ \boxed{mL}\ |\ 400 \times 10.15\ |\ 4060}{|\ 325\ mg\ |\ 325\ |\ 325} = \begin{matrix} 12.49\ or \\ 12.5\ mL \end{matrix}$$

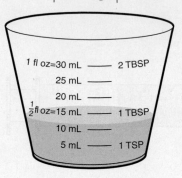

19

Random method:

$$\frac{1000\ mg\ |\ 2\ \boxed{mL}\ |\ 1\ g\ |\ 2 \times 1\ |\ 2}{|\ 1\ g\ |\ 1000\ mg\ |\ 1\ |\ 1} = 2\ mL$$

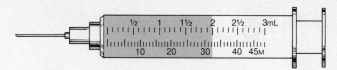

20

Sequential method:

$$\frac{10\ mg\ |\ 5\ mL\ |\ 1\ \boxed{tsp}\ |\ 10 \times 1\ |\ 10}{|\ 5\ mg\ |\ 5\ mL\ |\ 5\ |\ 5} = 2\ tsp$$

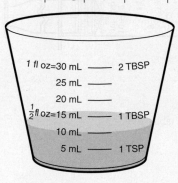

21

Random method:

$$\frac{0.25\ mg\ |\ \boxed{mL}\ |\ 1000\ mcg\ |\ 0.25 \times 100\ |\ 25}{|\ 250\ mcg\ |\ 1\ mg\ |\ 25 \times 1\ |\ 25} = 1\ mL$$

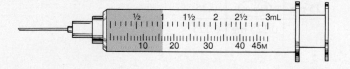

22

Sequential method:

$$\frac{500 \text{ mg}}{} \quad \frac{\text{mL}}{300 \text{ mg}} \quad \frac{5}{3} = 1.66 \text{ or } 1.7 \text{ mL}$$

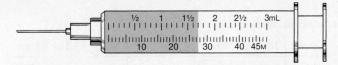

23

Sequential method:

$$\frac{2500 \text{ IU}}{} \quad \frac{0.2 \text{ mL}}{2500 \text{ IU}} \quad \frac{0.2}{} = 0.2 \text{ mL}$$

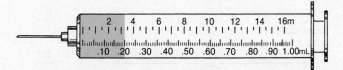

24

Sequential method:

$$\frac{200 \text{ mg}}{50 \text{ mg}} \quad \frac{5 \text{ mL}}{5} \quad \frac{20 \times 5}{5} \quad \frac{100}{5} = 20 \text{ mL}$$

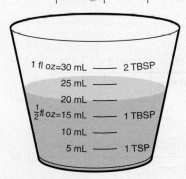

25

Sequential method:

$$\frac{300 \text{ mg}}{150 \text{ mg}} \quad \frac{\text{capsule}}{15} \quad \frac{30}{15} = 2 \text{ capsules}$$

26

Sequential method:

$$\frac{500 \text{ mg}}{500 \text{ mg}} \quad \frac{\text{tablets}}{500} \quad \frac{500}{500} = 1 \text{ tablet}$$

27

Sequential method:

$$\frac{0.25 \text{ mg}}{0.125 \text{ mg}} \quad \frac{\text{tablets}}{0.125} \quad \frac{0.25}{0.125} = 2 \text{ tablets}$$

28

Sequential method:

$$\frac{25 \text{ mg}}{50 \text{ mg}} \quad \frac{\text{tablets}}{50} \quad \frac{25}{50} = 0.5 \text{ tablet}$$

29

Sequential method:

$$\frac{5 \text{ mg}}{2.5 \text{ mg}} \quad \frac{\text{tablets}}{2.5} \quad \frac{5}{2.5} = 2 \text{ tablets}$$

30

Sequential method:

$$\frac{0.5 \text{ mg}}{0.25 \text{ mg}} \quad \frac{\text{tablets}}{0.25} \quad \frac{0.5}{0.25} = 2 \text{ tablets}$$

31

Sequential method:

$$\frac{150 \text{ mg}}{400 \text{ mg}} \quad \frac{\text{mL}}{40} \quad \frac{15}{40} = 0.375 \text{ or } 0.4 \text{ mL}$$

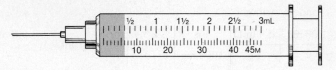

32

Sequential method:

$$\frac{600 \text{ mg}}{300 \text{ mg}} \quad \frac{\text{tablets}}{3} \quad \frac{6}{3} = 2 \text{ tablets}$$

33

Sequential method:

$$\frac{60 \text{ mg}}{20 \text{ mg}} \quad \frac{5 \text{ mL}}{2} \quad \frac{6 \times 5}{2} \quad \frac{30}{2} = 15 \text{ mL}$$

34

Sequential method:

$$\frac{600 \text{ mg}}{300 \text{ mg}} \quad \frac{\text{tablet}}{3} \quad \frac{6}{3} = 2 \text{ tablets}$$

35

Sequential method:

$$\frac{100 \text{ mg}}{10 \text{ mg}} \quad \frac{\text{mL}}{1} \quad \frac{10}{1} = 10 \text{ mL}$$

Two-Factor Practice Problems

1

Random method:

$$\frac{25 \text{ mcg}}{\text{kg}} \left| \frac{2.5 \text{ (mL)}}{0.125 \text{ mg}} \right| \frac{1 \text{ kg}}{2.2 \text{ lb}} \left| \frac{1 \text{ mg}}{1000 \text{ mcg}} \right| \frac{25 \text{ lb}}{} = \text{mL}$$

$$\frac{25 \times 2.5 \times 1 \times 1 \times 25}{0.125 \times 2.2 \times 1000} \left| \frac{1562.5}{275} \right. = 5.68 \text{ or } 5.7 \text{ mL}$$

2

Sequential method:

$$\frac{0.02 \text{ mg}}{\text{kg}} \left| \frac{\text{(mL)}}{0.1 \text{ mg}} \right| \frac{1 \text{ kg}}{2.2 \text{ lb}} \left| \frac{35 \text{ lb}}{} \right| \frac{0.02 \times 1 \times 35}{0.1 \times 2.2} \left| \frac{0.7}{0.22} \right. = \frac{3.18 \text{ or}}{3.2 \text{ mL}}$$

3

Random method:

$$\frac{2 \text{ mg}}{\text{min}} \left| \frac{500 \text{ (mL)}}{2 \text{ g}} \right| \frac{1 \text{ g}}{1000 \text{ mg}} \left| \frac{60 \text{ min}}{1 \text{ (hr)}} \right| \frac{5 \times 6}{1} \left| \frac{30}{1} \right. = \frac{30 \text{ mL}}{\text{hr}}$$

4

Random method:

$$\frac{500 \text{ mg}}{} \left| \frac{3.4 \text{ (mL)}}{1 \text{ g}} \right| \frac{1 \text{ g}}{1000 \text{ mg}} \left| \frac{5 \times 3.4}{10} \right| \frac{17}{10} = 1.7 \text{ mL}$$

Sequential method:

$$\frac{50 \text{ (mL)}}{30 \text{ min}} \left| \frac{60 \text{ min}}{1 \text{ (hr)}} \right| \frac{50 \times 6}{3 \times 1} \left| \frac{300}{3} \right. = 100 \frac{\text{mL}}{\text{hr}}$$

5

Sequential method:

$$\frac{1 \text{ mg}}{\text{kg}} \left| \frac{\text{(mL)}}{40 \text{ mg}} \right| \frac{1 \text{ kg}}{2.2 \text{ lb}} \left| \frac{94 \text{ lb}}{} \right| \frac{1 \times 1 \times 94}{40 \times 2.2} \left| \frac{94}{88} \right. = \frac{1.068 \text{ or}}{1.1 \text{ mL}}$$

6

Sequential method:

$$\frac{15 \text{ mg}}{\text{(hr)}} \left| \frac{500 \text{ (mL)}}{300 \text{ mg}} \right| \frac{15 \times 5}{3} \left| \frac{75}{3} \right. = 25 \frac{\text{mL}}{\text{hr}}$$

7

Sequential method:

$$\frac{25 \text{ mL}}{\text{(hr)}} \left| \frac{50 \text{ (mg)}}{250 \text{ mL}} \right| \frac{5}{} = 5 \frac{\text{mg}}{\text{hr}}$$

8

Sequential method:

$$\frac{10 \text{ mEq}}{} \left| \frac{20 \text{ (mL)}}{20 \text{ mEq}} \right| \frac{10}{} = 10 \text{ mL}$$

9

Sequential method:

$$\frac{3 \text{ mL}}{\text{hr}} \left| \frac{50 \text{ mg}}{500 \text{ mL}} \right| \frac{1000 \text{ (mcg)}}{1 \text{ mg}} \left| \frac{1 \text{ hr}}{60 \text{ (min)}} \right| \frac{3 \times 10}{6} \left| \frac{30}{6} \right. = 5 \frac{\text{mcg}}{\text{min}}$$

10

Sequential method:

$$\frac{100 \text{ mL}}{\text{(hr)}} \left| \frac{10 \text{ (mEq)}}{1000 \text{ mL}} \right| \frac{1}{} = 1 \frac{\text{mEq}}{\text{hr}}$$

11

Sequential method:

$$\frac{250 \text{ mL}}{\text{hr}} \left| \frac{20 \text{ (gtt)}}{\text{mL}} \right| \frac{1 \text{ hr}}{60 \text{ (min)}} \left| \frac{250 \times 2 \times 1}{6} \right| \frac{500}{6} = 83.3 \text{ or } 83 \frac{\text{gtt}}{\text{min}}$$

12

Sequential method:

$$\frac{750 \text{ mL}}{5 \text{ hr}} \left| \frac{10 \text{ (gtt)}}{\text{mL}} \right| \frac{1 \text{ hr}}{60 \text{ (min)}} \left| \frac{750 \times 1 \times 1}{5 \times 6} \right| \frac{750}{30} = 25 \frac{\text{gtt}}{\text{min}}$$

13

Sequential method:

$$\frac{500 \text{ mL}}{8 \text{ hr}} \left| \frac{60 \text{ (gtt)}}{\text{mL}} \right| \frac{1 \text{ hr}}{60 \text{ (min)}} \left| \frac{500 \times 1}{8} \right| \frac{500}{8} = 62.5 \text{ or } 63 \frac{\text{gtt}}{\text{min}}$$

14

Sequential method:

$$\frac{750 \text{ mL}}{} \left| \frac{15 \text{ gtt}}{\text{mL}} \right| \frac{\text{min}}{18 \text{ gtt}} \left| \frac{1 \text{ (hr)}}{60 \text{ min}} \right| \frac{750 \times 15 \times 1}{18 \times 60} \left| \frac{11250}{1080} \right. = \frac{10.41 \text{ or}}{10 \text{ hr}}$$

15

Sequential method:

$$\frac{250 \text{ mL}}{} \left| \frac{15 \text{ gtt}}{\text{mL}} \right| \frac{\text{min}}{50 \text{ gtt}} \left| \frac{1 \text{ (hr)}}{60 \text{ min}} \right| \frac{25 \times 15 \times 1}{50 \times 6} \left| \frac{375}{300} \right. = \frac{1.25 \text{ or}}{1 \text{ hr}}$$

16

Sequential method:

$$\frac{1000 \text{ mL}}{} \left| \frac{15 \text{ gtt}}{\text{mL}} \right| \frac{\text{min}}{25 \text{ gtt}} \left| \frac{1 \text{ (hr)}}{60 \text{ min}} \right| \frac{100 \times 15 \times 1}{25 \times 6} \left| \frac{1500}{150} \right. = 10 \text{ hr}$$

17

How many milliliters will you draw from the vial after reconstitution?

Sequential method:

$$\frac{1.25 \text{ g}}{} \left| \frac{10 \text{ (mL)}}{1 \text{ g}} \right| \frac{1.25 \times 10}{1} \left| \frac{12.5}{1} \right. = 12.5 \text{ mL}$$

Calculate the milliliters per hour to set the IV pump.

Sequential method:

$$\frac{112.5 \text{ (mL)}}{\text{(hr)}} = 112.5 \text{ or } 113 \frac{\text{mL}}{\text{hr}}$$

Calculate the drops per minute with a drop factor of 10 gtt/mL.

Sequential method:

$$\frac{112.5 \text{ mL}}{\text{hr}} \left| \frac{10 \text{ (gtt)}}{\text{mL}} \right| \frac{1 \text{ hr}}{60 \text{ (min)}} \left| \frac{112.5 \times 1 \times 1}{6} \right| \frac{112.5}{6} = 18.75 \text{ or } 19 \frac{\text{gtt}}{\text{min}}$$

18

How many milliliters will you draw from the vial after reconstitution?

Sequential method:

$$\frac{275 \text{ mg}}{} \left| \frac{10 \text{ (mL)}}{500 \text{ mg}} \right| \frac{275 \times 1}{50} \left| \frac{275}{50} = 5.5 \text{ mL} \right.$$

Calculate the milliliters per hour to set the IV pump.

Sequential method:

$$\frac{250 \text{ (mL)}}{\text{(hr)}} = \frac{250 \text{ mL}}{\text{hr}}$$

Calculate the drops per minute with a drop factor of 10 gtt/mL.

Sequential method:

$$\frac{250 \text{ mL}}{\text{hr}} \left| \frac{10 \text{ (gtt)}}{\text{mL}} \right| \frac{1 \text{ hr}}{60 \text{ (min)}} \left| \frac{250 \times 1 \times 1}{6} \right| \frac{250}{6} = 41.66 \text{ or } 42 \frac{\text{gtt}}{\text{min}}$$

19

Sequential method:

$$\frac{1 \text{ g}}{} \left| \frac{3.4 \text{ (mL)}}{1 \text{ g}} \right| \frac{3.4}{} = 3.4 \text{ mL}$$

Sequential method:

$$\frac{100 \text{ (mL)}}{60 \text{ min}} \left| \frac{60 \text{ min}}{1 \text{ (hr)}} \right| \frac{100}{1} = \frac{100 \text{ mL}}{\text{hr}}$$

Sequential method:

$$\frac{100 \text{ mL}}{\text{hr}} \left| \frac{20 \text{ (gtt)}}{\text{mL}} \right| \frac{1 \text{ hr}}{60 \text{ (min)}} \left| \frac{100 \times 2 \times 1}{6} \right| \frac{200}{6} = 33.3 \text{ or } 33 \frac{\text{gtt}}{\text{min}}$$

20

How many milliliters will you draw from the vial?

Sequential method:

$$\frac{23 \text{ mg}}{} \left| \frac{\text{(mL)}}{40 \text{ mg}} \right| \frac{23}{40} = 0.57 \text{ or } 0.6 \text{ mL}$$

Calculate the milliliters per hour to set the IV pump.

Sequential method:

$$\frac{100 \text{ (mL)}}{\text{(hr)}} = \frac{100 \text{ mL}}{\text{hr}}$$

Calculate the drops per minute with a drop factor of 15 gtt/mL.

$$\frac{100 \text{ mL}}{\text{hr}} \left| \frac{15 \text{ (gtt)}}{\text{mL}} \right| \frac{1 \text{ hr}}{60 \text{ (min)}} \left| \frac{100 \times 15 \times 1}{60} \right| \frac{1500}{60} = 25 \frac{\text{gtt}}{\text{min}}$$

21

Sequential method:

$$\frac{0.56 \text{ mg}}{\text{kg}} \left| \frac{18 \text{ kg}}{} \right| \frac{5 \text{ (mL)}}{10 \text{ mg}} \left| \frac{0.56 \times 18 \times 5}{10} \right| \frac{50.4}{10} = 5.04 \text{ or } 5 \text{ mL}$$

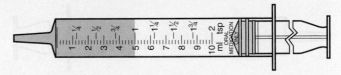

22

Random method:

$$\frac{30 \text{ g}}{\text{day}} \left| \frac{\text{day}}{4 \text{ (doses)}} \right| \frac{\text{(packet)}}{5 \text{ g}} \left| \frac{30}{4 \times 5} \right| \frac{30}{20} = 1.5 \frac{\text{packet}}{\text{dose}}$$

23

Random method:

$$\frac{10 \text{ mcg}}{\text{kg}} \left| \frac{2 \text{ (mL)}}{2 \text{ mg}} \right| \frac{50 \text{ kg}}{} \left| \frac{1 \text{ mg}}{1000 \text{ mcg}} \right| \frac{1 \times 2 \times 5 \times 1}{2 \times 10} \left| \frac{10}{20} = 0.5 \text{ mL} \right.$$

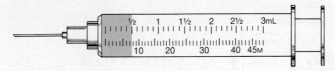

24

Sequential method:

$$\frac{1600 \text{ mg}}{\text{day}} \left| \frac{\text{(tablets)}}{800 \text{ mg}} \right| \frac{\text{day}}{2 \text{ (doses)}} \left| \frac{16}{8 \times 2} \right| \frac{16}{16} = 1 \frac{\text{tablet}}{\text{dose}}$$

25

Random method:

$$\frac{1 \text{ g}}{\text{day}} \left| \frac{\text{(mL)}}{100 \text{ mg}} \right| \frac{1000 \text{ mg}}{1 \text{ g}} \left| \frac{\text{day}}{3 \text{ (doses)}} \right| \frac{10}{1 \times 3} \left| \frac{10}{3} = 3.33 \text{ or } 3 \frac{\text{mL}}{\text{dose}} \right.$$

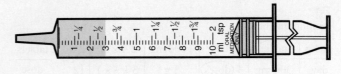

26

Sequential method:

$$\frac{4 \text{ mg}}{\text{kg}} \mid \frac{\text{mL}}{10 \text{ mg}} \mid \frac{20 \text{ kg}}{1} \mid \frac{4 \times 2}{1} \mid \frac{8}{1} = 8 \text{ mL}$$

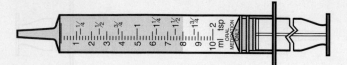

27

Sequential method:

$$\frac{0.15 \text{ mg}}{\text{kg}} \mid \frac{\text{mL}}{2 \text{ mg}} \mid \frac{1 \text{ kg}}{2.2 \text{ lb}} \mid \frac{160 \text{ lb}}{} \mid \frac{0.15 \times 1 \times 160}{2 \times 2.2} \mid \frac{24}{4.4} = \frac{5.45 \text{ or}}{5.5 \text{ mL}}$$

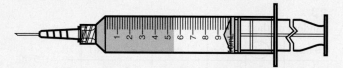

28

Sequential method:

$$\frac{2 \text{ mg}}{\text{kg}} \mid \frac{\text{tablet}}{150 \text{ mg}} \mid \frac{40 \text{ kg}}{} \mid \frac{2 \times 4}{15} \mid \frac{8}{15} = \frac{0.533 \text{ or}}{0.5 \text{ tablet}}$$

29

Sequential method:

$$\frac{20 \text{ mg}}{\text{kg}} \mid \frac{\text{tablet}}{400 \text{ mg}} \mid \frac{1 \text{ kg}}{2.2 \text{ lb}} \mid \frac{20 \text{ lb}}{} \mid \frac{2 \times 1 \times 2}{4 \times 2.2} \mid \frac{4}{8.8} = \frac{0.45 \text{ or}}{0.5 \text{ tablet}}$$

30

Sequential method:

$$\frac{450 \text{ mg}}{\text{day}} \mid \frac{\text{tablet}}{150 \text{ mg}} \mid \frac{\text{day}}{3 \text{ doses}} \mid \frac{45}{15 \times 3} \mid \frac{45}{45} = \frac{1 \text{ tablet}}{\text{dose}}$$

31

Random method:

$$\frac{2.4 \text{ g}}{\text{day}} \mid \frac{\text{tablet}}{300 \text{ mg}} \mid \frac{\text{day}}{4 \text{ doses}} \mid \frac{1000 \text{ mg}}{1 \text{ g}} \mid \frac{2.4 \times 10}{3 \times 4 \times 1} \mid \frac{24}{12} = \frac{2 \text{ tablets}}{\text{dose}}$$

32

Sequential method:

$$\frac{500 \text{ mg}}{\text{day}} \mid \frac{8 \text{ mL}}{750 \text{ mg}} \mid \frac{\text{day}}{2 \text{ doses}} \mid \frac{50 \times 8}{75 \times 2} \mid \frac{400}{150} = \frac{2.666 \text{ or } 2.7}{\text{dose}} \text{ mL}$$

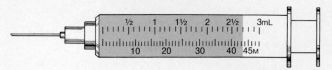

33

Random method:

$$\frac{1000 \text{ mg}}{\text{day}} \mid \frac{20 \text{ mL}}{2 \text{ g}} \mid \frac{1 \text{ g}}{1000 \text{ mg}} \mid \frac{\text{day}}{2 \text{ doses}} \mid \frac{20 \times 1}{2 \times 2} \mid \frac{20}{4} = \frac{5 \text{ mL}}{\text{dose}}$$

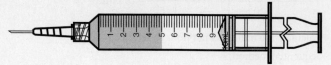

34

Sequential method:

$$\frac{150 \text{ mg}}{2.2 \text{ lb/5 doses}} \mid \frac{1 \text{ tsp}}{500 \text{ mg}} \mid \frac{2.2 \text{ lb}}{1 \text{ kg}} \mid \frac{30 \text{ kg}}{} \mid \frac{5 \text{ mL}}{1 \text{ tsp}} = \frac{\text{mL}}{\text{dose}}$$

$$\frac{15 \times 3}{5 \times 1} \mid \frac{45}{5} = \frac{9}{\text{dose}} \text{ mL}$$

35

Sequential method:

$$\frac{8 \text{ mg}}{\text{kg}} \mid \frac{\text{mL}}{20 \text{ mg}} \mid \frac{40 \text{ kg}}{} \mid \frac{8 \times 4}{2} \mid \frac{32}{2} = 16 \text{ mL}$$

Three-Factor Practice Problems

1

How many milliliters per day will you give?

Sequential method:

$$\frac{40 \text{ mg}}{\text{kg/day}} \mid \frac{5 \text{ mL}}{300 \text{ mg}} \mid \frac{60 \text{ kg}}{} \mid \frac{4 \times 5 \times 6}{3} \mid \frac{120}{3} = \frac{40 \text{ mL}}{\text{day}}$$

How many milliliters per dose will you give?

Sequential method:

$$\frac{40 \text{ mg}}{\text{kg/day}} \mid \frac{5 \text{ mL}}{300 \text{ mg}} \mid \frac{60 \text{ kg}}{} \mid \frac{\text{day}}{4 \text{ doses}} \mid \frac{4 \times 5 \times 6}{3 \times 4} \mid \frac{120}{12} = \frac{10 \text{ mL}}{\text{dose}}$$

2

Sequential method:

$$\frac{4 \text{ mg}}{\text{kg/day}} \mid \frac{\text{mL}}{10 \text{ mg}} \mid \frac{1 \text{ kg}}{2.2 \text{ lb}} \mid \frac{60 \text{ lb}}{} \mid \frac{4 \times 1 \times 6}{1 \times 2.2} \mid \frac{24}{2.2} = \frac{10.9 \text{ or } 11 \text{ mL}}{\text{day}}$$

3

How many milliliters per day will you give?

Sequential method:

$$\frac{30\ \text{mg}}{\text{kg/day}} \left| \frac{2\ \text{mL}}{300\ \text{mg}} \right| \frac{50\ \text{kg}}{} \left| \frac{2 \times 5}{} \right| \frac{10}{} = \frac{10}{} \frac{\text{mL}}{\text{day}}$$

How many milliliters per dose will you give?

Sequential method:

$$\frac{30\ \text{mg}}{\text{kg/day}} \left| \frac{2\ \text{mL}}{300\ \text{mg}} \right| \frac{50\ \text{kg}}{} \left| \frac{\text{day}}{3\ \text{doses}} \right| \frac{2 \times 5}{3} \left| \frac{10}{3} \right| = 3.33\ \text{or}\ 3.3\ \frac{\text{mL}}{\text{dose}}$$

4

Sequential method:

$$\frac{0.575\ \text{mL}}{\text{dose}} \left| \frac{40\ \text{mg}}{\text{mL}} \right| \frac{2.2\ \text{lb}}{1\ \text{kg}} \left| \frac{}{45\ \text{lb}} \right| \frac{3\ \text{doses}}{\text{day}} = \frac{\text{mg}}{\text{kg/day}}$$

$$\frac{0.575 \times 40 \times 2.2 \times 3}{1 \times 45} \left| \frac{151.8}{45} \right| = 3.37\ \text{or}\ 3.4\ \frac{\text{mg}}{\text{kg/day}}$$

5

Sequential method:

$$\frac{0.125\ \text{mL}}{\text{dose}} \left| \frac{50\ \text{mg}}{\text{mL}} \right| \frac{2.2\ \text{lb}}{1\ \text{kg}} \left| \frac{}{20\ \text{lb}} \right| \frac{3\ \text{doses}}{\text{day}} = \frac{\text{mg}}{\text{kg/day}}$$

$$\frac{0.125 \times 5 \times 2.2 \times 3}{1 \times 2} \left| \frac{4.125}{2} \right| = 2.06\ \text{or}\ 2.1\ \frac{\text{mg}}{\text{kg/day}}$$

6

How many milliliters will you draw from the vial?

Sequential method:

$$\frac{400\ \text{mg}}{} \left| \frac{10\ \text{mL}}{400\ \text{mg}} \right| \frac{10}{} = 10\ \text{mL}$$

Calculate the milliliters per hour to set the IV pump.

Random method:

$$\frac{5\ \text{mcg}}{\text{kg/min}} \left| \frac{260\ \text{mL}}{400\ \text{mg}} \right| \frac{1\ \text{mg}}{1000\ \text{mcg}} \left| \frac{1\ \text{kg}}{2.2\ \text{lb}} \right| \frac{110\ \text{lb}}{} \left| \frac{60\ \text{min}}{1\ \text{hr}} \right| = \frac{\text{mL}}{\text{hr}}$$

$$\frac{5 \times 26 \times 1 \times 11 \times 6}{4 \times 100 \times 2.2} \left| \frac{8580}{880} \right| = 9.75\ \text{or}\ 9.8\ \frac{\text{mL}}{\text{hr}}$$

7

Random method:

$$\frac{0.8\ \text{mcg}}{\text{kg/min}} \left| \frac{500\ \text{mL}}{50\ \text{mg}} \right| \frac{1\ \text{mg}}{1000\ \text{mcg}} \left| \frac{1\ \text{kg}}{2.2\ \text{lb}} \right| \frac{60\ \text{min}}{1\ \text{hr}} \left| \frac{143\ \text{lb}}{} \right| = \frac{\text{mL}}{\text{hr}}$$

$$\frac{0.8 \times 5 \times 1 \times 6 \times 143}{5 \times 10 \times 2.2} \left| \frac{3432}{110} \right| = 31.2\ \frac{\text{mL}}{\text{hr}}$$

8

Sequential method:

$$\frac{68\ \text{mL}}{\text{hr}} \left| \frac{50\ \text{mg}}{250\ \text{mL}} \right| \frac{1\ \text{hr}}{60\ \text{min}} \left| \frac{2.2\ \text{lb}}{1\ \text{kg}} \right| \frac{1000\ \text{mcg}}{1\ \text{mg}} \left| \frac{}{250\ \text{lb}} \right| = \frac{\text{mcg}}{\text{kg/min}}$$

$$\frac{68 \times 5 \times 1 \times 2.2 \times 10}{25 \times 6 \times 1 \times 1 \times 25} \left| \frac{7480}{3750} \right| = 1.99\ \text{or}\ 2\ \frac{\text{mcg}}{\text{kg/min}}$$

9

Random method:

$$\frac{30\ \text{mg}}{\text{kg/day}} \left| \frac{1\ \text{kg}}{2.2\ \text{lb}} \right| \frac{157\ \text{lb}}{} \left| \frac{1\ \text{g}}{1000\ \text{mg}} \right| \frac{3 \times 1 \times 157 \times 1}{2.2 \times 100} \left| \frac{471}{220} \right| = 2.14\ \text{or}\ 2.1\ \frac{\text{g}}{\text{day}}$$

10

Random method:

$$\frac{0.01\ \text{mL}}{\text{kg/min}} \left| \frac{1\ \text{kg}}{2.2\ \text{lb}} \right| \frac{180\ \text{lb}}{} \left| \frac{60\ \text{min}}{1\ \text{hr}} \right| \frac{0.01 \times 1 \times 180 \times 60}{2.2 \times 1} \left| \frac{108}{2.2} \right|$$

$$= 49.09\ \text{or}\ 49.1\ \frac{\text{mL}}{\text{hr}}$$

11

Random method:

$$\frac{28\ \text{mL}}{\text{hr}} \left| \frac{400\ \text{mg}}{250\ \text{mL}} \right| \frac{}{15\ \text{kg}} \left| \frac{1\ \text{hr}}{60\ \text{min}} \right| \frac{1000\ \text{mcg}}{1\ \text{mg}} = \frac{\text{mcg}}{\text{kg/min}}$$

$$\frac{28 \times 4 \times 1 \times 1000}{25 \times 15 \times 6 \times 1} \left| \frac{112,000}{2250} \right| = 49.77\ \text{or}\ 49.8\ \frac{\text{mcg}}{\text{kg/min}}$$

12

Sequential method:

$$\frac{50\ \text{mcg}}{\text{kg/10 min}} \left| \frac{60\ \text{min}}{1\ \text{hr}} \right| \frac{1\ \text{kg}}{2.2\ \text{lb}} \left| \frac{160\ \text{lb}}{} \right| \frac{1\ \text{mg}}{1000\ \text{mcg}} \left| \frac{100\ \text{mL}}{20\ \text{mg}} \right| \frac{50 \times 6 \times 16 \times 1}{10 \times 2.2 \times 2}$$

$$\frac{4800}{44} = 109\ \frac{\text{mL}}{\text{hr}}$$

13

Random method:

$$\frac{2\ \text{mcg}}{\text{kg/min}} \left| \frac{250\ \text{mL}}{50\ \text{mg}} \right| \frac{1\ \text{kg}}{2.2\ \text{lb}} \left| \frac{250\ \text{lb}}{} \right| \frac{1\ \text{mg}}{1000\ \text{mcg}} \left| \frac{60\ \text{min}}{1\ \text{hr}} \right| = \frac{\text{mL}}{\text{hr}}$$

$$\frac{2 \times 25 \times 1 \times 25 \times 6}{5 \times 2.2 \times 10} \left| \frac{7500}{110} \right| = 68.1\ \text{or}\ 68\ \frac{\text{mL}}{\text{hr}}$$

14

Random method:

$$\frac{1\ \text{mcg}}{\text{kg/min}} \left| \frac{250\ \text{mL}}{50\ \text{mg}} \right| \frac{1\ \text{kg}}{2.2\ \text{lb}} \left| \frac{60\ \text{min}}{1\ \text{hr}} \right| \frac{160\ \text{lb}}{} \left| \frac{1\ \text{mg}}{1000\ \text{mcg}} \right| = \frac{\text{mL}}{\text{hr}}$$

$$\frac{1 \times 25 \times 6 \times 16}{50 \times 2.2} \left| \frac{2400}{110} \right| = 21.81\ \text{or}\ 21.8\ \frac{\text{mL}}{\text{hr}}$$

15

Random method:

$$\frac{2.5 \text{ mcg}}{\text{kg/min}} \left| \frac{500 \text{ mL}}{400 \text{ mg}} \right| \frac{65 \text{ kg}}{} \left| \frac{60 \text{ min}}{1 \text{ hr}} \right| \frac{1 \text{ mg}}{1000 \text{ mcg}} = \frac{\text{mL}}{\text{hr}}$$

$$\frac{2.5 \times 5 \times 65 \times 6 \times 1}{4 \times 1 \times 100} \left| \frac{4875}{400} \right| = 12.18 \text{ or } 12.2 \frac{\text{mL}}{\text{hr}}$$

16

Random method:

$$\frac{15 \text{ mL}}{\text{hr}} \left| \frac{2 \text{ mg}}{500 \text{ mL}} \right| \frac{1 \text{ hr}}{60 \text{ min}} \left| \frac{}{20 \text{ kg}} \right| \frac{1000 \text{ mcg}}{1 \text{ mg}} = \frac{\text{mcg}}{\text{kg/min}}$$

$$\frac{15 \times 2 \times 1 \times 1}{5 \times 6 \times 20 \times 1} \left| \frac{30}{600} \right| = 0.05 \frac{\text{mcg}}{\text{kg/min}}$$

17

Random method:

$$\frac{5 \text{ mcg}}{\text{kg/min}} \left| \frac{500 \text{ mL}}{400 \text{ mg}} \right| \frac{70 \text{ kg}}{} \left| \frac{1 \text{ mg}}{1000 \text{ mcg}} \right| = \frac{\text{mL}}{\text{min}}$$

$$\frac{5 \times 5 \times 7 \times 1}{4 \times 100} \left| \frac{175}{400} \right| = 0.4375 \text{ or } 0.44 \frac{\text{mL}}{\text{min}}$$

18

How many milligrams per day is the child receiving?

Sequential method:

$$\frac{40 \text{ mg}}{\text{kg/day}} \left| \frac{1 \text{ kg}}{2.2 \text{ lb}} \right| \frac{20 \text{ lb}}{} \left| \frac{40 \times 1 \times 20}{2.2} \right| \frac{800}{2.2} = 363.63 \text{ or } 363.6 \frac{\text{mg}}{\text{day}}$$

How many milligrams per dose is the child receiving?

Sequential method:

$$\frac{363.6 \text{ mg}}{\text{day}} \left| \frac{\text{day}}{3 \text{ doses}} \right| \frac{363.6}{3} = 121.2 \frac{\text{mg}}{\text{dose}}$$

How many milliliters will you draw from the vial after reconstitution?

Sequential method:

$$\frac{121.2 \text{ mg}}{} \left| \frac{10 \text{ mL}}{500 \text{ mg}} \right| \frac{121.2 \times 10}{500} \left| \frac{1212}{500} \right| = 2.424 \text{ or } 2.4 \text{ mL}$$

Calculate the milliliters per hour to set the IV pump.

Sequential method:

$$\frac{100 \text{ mL}}{60 \text{ min}} \left| \frac{60 \text{ min}}{1 \text{ hr}} \right| \frac{100}{1} = 100 \frac{\text{mL}}{\text{hr}}$$

19

How many milligrams per dose is the child receiving?

Random method:

$$\frac{2 \text{ mg}}{\text{kg/dose}} \left| \frac{40 \text{ kg}}{} \right| \frac{2 \times 40}{} \left| \frac{80}{} \right| = 80 \frac{\text{mg}}{\text{dose}}$$

How many milliliters will you draw from the vial?

Sequential method:

$$\frac{80 \text{ mg}}{} \left| \frac{\text{mL}}{40 \text{ mg}} \right| \frac{8}{4} = 2 \text{ mL}$$

Calculate the milliliters per hour to set the IV pump.

Sequential method:

$$\frac{50 \text{ mL}}{30 \text{ min}} \left| \frac{60 \text{ min}}{1 \text{ hr}} \right| \frac{50 \times 6}{3 \times 1} \left| \frac{300}{3} \right| = 100 \frac{\text{mL}}{\text{hr}}$$

20

How many milligrams per day is the child receiving?

Sequential method:

$$\frac{25 \text{ mg}}{\text{kg/day}} \left| \frac{25 \text{ kg}}{} \right| \frac{25 \times 25}{} \left| \frac{625}{} \right| = 625 \frac{\text{mg}}{\text{day}}$$

How many milligrams per dose is the child receiving?

Sequential method:

$$\frac{625 \text{ mg}}{\text{day}} \left| \frac{\text{day}}{3 \text{ doses}} \right| \frac{625}{3} = 208.33 \text{ or } 208.3 \frac{\text{mg}}{\text{dose}}$$

How many milliliters will you draw from the vial after reconstitution?

Sequential method:

$$\frac{208.3 \text{ mg}}{} \left| \frac{10 \text{ mL}}{500 \text{ mg}} \right| \frac{208.3 \times 1}{50} \left| \frac{208.3}{50} \right| = 4.166 \text{ or } 4.2 \text{ mL}$$

Calculate the milliliters per hour to set the IV pump.

Sequential method:

$$\frac{50 \text{ mL}}{30 \text{ min}} \left| \frac{60 \text{ min}}{1 \text{ hr}} \right| \frac{50 \times 6}{3 \times 1} \left| \frac{300}{3} \right| = 100 \frac{\text{mL}}{\text{hr}}$$

21

Sequential method:

How many milligrams per day is the patient receiving?

$$\frac{12.5 \text{ mg}}{\text{kg/day}} \left| \frac{80 \text{ kg}}{} \right| \frac{12.5 \times 80}{} \left| \frac{1000}{} \right| = 1000 \frac{\text{mg}}{\text{day}}$$

How many milligrams per dose is the patient receiving?

$$\frac{1000 \text{ mg}}{\text{day}} \left| \frac{\text{day}}{2 \text{ doses}} \right| \frac{1000}{2} = 500 \frac{\text{mg}}{\text{dose}}$$

Calculate the milliliters per hour to set the IV pump.

$$\frac{500 \text{ mg}}{60 \text{ min}} \left| \frac{100 \text{ mL}}{500 \text{ mg}} \right| \frac{60 \text{ min}}{1 \text{ hr}} \left| \frac{100}{1} \right| = 100 \frac{\text{mL}}{\text{hr}}$$

22

Random method:

$$\frac{2\ \text{mcg}}{\text{kg/min}}\ \Big|\ \frac{250\ \text{mL}}{200\ \text{mg}}\ \Big|\ \frac{1\ \text{mg}}{1000\ \text{mcg}}\ \Big|\ \frac{1\ \text{kg}}{1\ \text{hr}}\ \Big|\ \frac{175\ \text{lb}}{2.2\ \text{lb}}\ =\ \frac{\text{mL}}{\text{hr}}$$

$$\frac{2 \times 25 \times 1 \times 6 \times 175}{20 \times 100 \times 2.2}\ \Big|\ \frac{52500}{4400}\ =\ 11.9\ \text{or}\ 12\ \frac{\text{mL}}{\text{hr}}$$

23

Sequential method:

$$\frac{150\ \text{units}}{\text{kg/day}}\ \Big|\ \text{mL}\ \Big|\ \frac{80\ \text{kg}}{10{,}000\ \text{units}}\ \Big|\ \frac{15 \times 8}{100}\ \Big|\ \frac{120}{100}\ =\ 1.2\ \frac{\text{mL}}{\text{day}}$$

24

Random method:

Calculate the milliliters per hour to set the IV pump for the one-minute administration.

$$\frac{500\ \text{mcg}}{\text{kg/min}}\ \Big|\ \frac{250\ \text{mL}}{2.5\ \text{g}}\ \Big|\ \frac{1\ \text{g}}{1000\ \text{mg}}\ \Big|\ \frac{1\ \text{mg}}{1000\ \text{mcg}}\ \Big|\ 90\ \text{kg}\ \Big|\ \frac{60\ \text{min}}{1\ \text{hr}}\ =\ \frac{\text{mL}}{\text{hr}}$$

$$\frac{5 \times 25 \times 1 \times 9 \times 6}{2.5 \times 10 \times 1}\ \Big|\ \frac{6750}{25}\ =\ 270\ \frac{\text{mL}}{\text{hr}}$$

Calculate the milliliters per hour to set the IV pump for the four-minute administration.

$$\frac{50\ \text{mcg}}{\text{kg/min}}\ \Big|\ \frac{250\ \text{mL}}{2.5\ \text{g}}\ \Big|\ \frac{1\ \text{g}}{1000\ \text{mg}}\ \Big|\ \frac{1\ \text{mg}}{1000\ \text{mcg}}\ \Big|\ 90\ \text{kg}\ \Big|\ \frac{60\ \text{min}}{1\ \text{hr}}\ =\ \frac{\text{mL}}{\text{hr}}$$

$$\frac{5 \times 25 \times 1 \times 9 \times 6}{2.5 \times 10 \times 10}\ \Big|\ \frac{6750}{250}\ =\ 27\ \frac{\text{mL}}{\text{hr}}$$

25

Sequential method:

$$\frac{0.1\ \text{mg}}{\text{kg/day}}\ \Big|\ \frac{5\ \text{mL}}{5\ \text{mg}}\ \Big|\ 35\ \text{kg}\ \Big|\ 0.1 \times 35\ =\ 3.5\ \frac{\text{mL}}{\text{day}}$$

Comprehensive Practice Problems

1

Sequential method:

$$\frac{0.125\ \text{mg}}{}\ \Big|\ \text{tablet}\ \Big|\ \frac{0.125}{0.25\ \text{mg}}\ \Big|\ \frac{0.125}{0.25}\ =\ 0.5\ \text{tablet}$$

2

Random method:

$$\frac{0.5\ \text{g}}{}\ \Big|\ \frac{\text{tablet}}{500\ \text{mg}}\ \Big|\ \frac{1000\ \text{mg}}{1\ \text{g}}\ \Big|\ \frac{0.5 \times 10}{5 \times 1}\ \Big|\ \frac{5}{5}\ =\ 1\ \text{tablet}$$

3

Random method:

$$\frac{\frac{1}{150}\ \text{gr}}{0.4\ \text{mg}}\ \Big|\ \frac{\text{mL}}{1\ \text{gr}}\ \Big|\ \frac{60\ \text{mg}}{0.4 \times 1}\ \Big|\ \frac{\frac{1}{150} \times \frac{60}{1}}{0.4}\ \Big|\ \frac{\frac{60}{150}}{0.4}\ \Big|\ \frac{0.4}{0.4}\ =\ 1\ \text{mL}$$

4

Sequential method:

$$\frac{500{,}000\ \text{units}}{}\ \Big|\ \frac{\text{mL}}{100{,}000\ \text{units}}\ \Big|\ \frac{1\ \text{tsp}}{5\ \text{mL}}\ \Big|\ \frac{5 \times 1}{1 \times 5}\ \Big|\ \frac{5}{5}\ =\ 1\ \text{tsp}$$

5

Sequential method:

$$\frac{50\ \text{mg}}{}\ \Big|\ \frac{\text{mL}}{100\ \text{mg}}\ \Big|\ \frac{5}{10}\ =\ 0.5\ \text{mL}$$

6

Sequential method:

$$\frac{2\ \text{mg}}{\text{kg}}\ \Big|\ \frac{10\ \text{mL}}{500\ \text{mg}}\ \Big|\ 75\ \text{kg}\ \Big|\ \frac{2 \times 1 \times 75}{50}\ \Big|\ \frac{150}{50}\ =\ 3\ \text{mL}$$

7

Sequential method:

$$\frac{2\ \text{mg}}{\text{kg}}\ \Big|\ \frac{5\ \text{mL}}{500\ \text{mg}}\ \Big|\ \frac{1\ \text{kg}}{2.2\ \text{lb}}\ \Big|\ 100\ \text{lb}\ \Big|\ \frac{2 \times 5 \times 1 \times 1}{5 \times 2.2}\ \Big|\ \frac{10}{11}\ =\ 0.9\ \text{mL}$$

8

Sequential method:

$$\frac{1000\ \text{mL}}{12\ \text{hr}}\ \Big|\ \frac{15\ \text{gtt}}{\text{mL}}\ \Big|\ \frac{1\ \text{hr}}{60\ \text{min}}\ \Big|\ \frac{100 \times 15 \times 1}{12 \times 6}\ \Big|\ \frac{1500}{72}\ =\ 20.8\ \text{or}\ 21\ \frac{\text{gtt}}{\text{min}}$$

9

Sequential method:

$$\frac{500\ \text{mL}}{}\ \Big|\ \frac{15\ \text{gtt}}{\text{mL}}\ \Big|\ \frac{\text{min}}{21\ \text{gtt}}\ \Big|\ \frac{1\ \text{hr}}{60\ \text{min}}\ \Big|\ \frac{50 \times 15 \times 1}{21 \times 6}\ \Big|\ \frac{750}{126}\ =\ 5.9\ \text{hr}$$

10

Sequential method:

$$\frac{1500\ \text{units}}{\text{hr}}\ \Big|\ \frac{250\ \text{mL}}{25{,}000\ \text{units}}\ \Big|\ \frac{15 \times 25}{25}\ \Big|\ \frac{375}{25}\ =\ 15\ \frac{\text{mL}}{\text{hr}}$$

11

Sequential method:

$$\frac{1000\ \text{mL}}{}\ \Big|\ \frac{15\ \text{gtt}}{\text{mL}}\ \Big|\ \frac{\text{min}}{50\ \text{gtt}}\ \Big|\ \frac{1\ \text{hr}}{60\ \text{min}}\ \Big|\ \frac{10 \times 15 \times 1}{5 \times 6}\ \Big|\ \frac{150}{30}\ =\ 5\ \text{hr}$$

12

Sequential method:

$$\frac{8\ \text{units}}{\text{hr}}\ \Big|\ \frac{250\ \text{mL}}{100\ \text{units}}\ \Big|\ \frac{8 \times 25}{10}\ \Big|\ \frac{200}{10}\ =\ 20\ \frac{\text{mL}}{\text{hr}}$$

13

Sequential method:

$$\frac{500\ \text{mL}}{8\ \text{hr}}\ \Big|\ \frac{10\ \text{gtt}}{\text{mL}}\ \Big|\ \frac{1\ \text{hr}}{60\ \text{min}}\ \Big|\ \frac{50 \times 10 \times 1}{8 \times 6}\ \Big|\ \frac{500}{48}\ =\ 10.4\ \text{or}\ 10\ \frac{\text{gtt}}{\text{min}}$$

14

Random method:

$$\frac{2 \text{ mEq}}{100 \text{ mL}} \left| \frac{10 \text{ mL}}{20 \text{ mEq}} \right| 500 \text{ mL} \left| \frac{2 \times 1 \times 5}{1 \times 2} \right| \frac{10}{2} = 5 \text{ mL}$$

15

Random method:

$$\frac{44 \text{ mg}}{\text{hr}} \left| \frac{250 \text{ mL}}{1 \text{ g}} \right| \frac{1 \text{ g}}{1000 \text{ mg}} \left| \frac{44 \times 25 \times 1}{1 \times 100} \right| \frac{1100}{100} = 11 \frac{\text{mL}}{\text{hr}}$$

16

Sequential method:

$$\frac{140 \text{ mL}}{\text{hr}} \left| \frac{30 \text{ mg}}{1000 \text{ mL}} \right| \frac{14 \times 3}{10} \left| \frac{42}{10} \right| = 4.2 \frac{\text{mg}}{\text{hr}}$$

17

How many milliliters will you draw from the vial after reconstitution?

Sequential method:

$$\frac{750 \text{ mg}}{} \left| \frac{\text{mL}}{500 \text{ mg}} \right| \frac{75}{50} = 1.5 \text{ mL}$$

Calculate the milliliters per hour to set the IV pump.

Sequential method:

$$\frac{100 \text{ mL}}{30 \text{ min}} \left| \frac{60 \text{ min}}{1 \text{ hr}} \right| \frac{100 \times 6}{3 \times 1} \left| \frac{600}{3} \right| = 200 \frac{\text{mL}}{\text{hr}}$$

Calculate the drops per minute with a drop factor of 10 gtt/mL.

Sequential method:

$$\frac{200 \text{ mL}}{\text{hr}} \left| \frac{10 \text{ gtt}}{\text{mL}} \right| \frac{1 \text{ hr}}{60 \text{ min}} \left| \frac{200 \times 1 \times 1}{6} \right| \frac{200}{6} = 33.33 \text{ or } 33 \frac{\text{gtt}}{\text{min}}$$

18

How many milliliters will you draw from the vial after reconstitution?

Sequential method:

$$\frac{1.5 \text{ g}}{} \left| \frac{5 \text{ mL}}{3 \text{ g}} \right| \frac{1.5 \times 5}{3} \left| \frac{7.5}{3} \right| = 2.5 \text{ mL}$$

Calculate the milliliters per hour to set the IV pump.

Sequential method:

$$\frac{50 \text{ mL}}{20 \text{ min}} \left| \frac{60 \text{ min}}{1 \text{ hr}} \right| \frac{50 \times 6}{2 \times 1} \left| \frac{300}{2} \right| = 150 \frac{\text{mL}}{\text{hr}}$$

Calculate the drops per minute with a drop factor of 20 gtt/mL.

Sequential method:

$$\frac{150 \text{ mL}}{\text{hr}} \left| \frac{20 \text{ gtt}}{\text{mL}} \right| \frac{1 \text{ hr}}{60 \text{ min}} \left| \frac{150 \times 2 \times 1}{6} \right| \frac{300}{6} = 50 \frac{\text{gtt}}{\text{min}}$$

19

Random method:

$$\frac{4 \text{ mcg}}{\text{kg/min}} \left| \frac{250 \text{ mL}}{400 \text{ mg}} \right| \frac{1 \text{ mg}}{1000 \text{ mcg}} \left| \frac{60 \text{ min}}{1 \text{ hr}} \right| \frac{1 \text{ kg}}{2.2 \text{ lb}} \left| 120 \text{ lb} \right| = \frac{\text{mL}}{\text{hr}}$$

$$\frac{4 \times 25 \times 1 \times 6 \times 1 \times 12}{40 \times 10 \times 1 \times 2.2} \left| \frac{7200}{880} \right| = 8.1 \text{ or } 8 \frac{\text{mL}}{\text{hr}}$$

20

Random method:

$$\frac{0.8 \text{ mcg}}{\text{kg/min}} \left| \frac{500 \text{ mL}}{50 \text{ mg}} \right| \frac{1 \text{ mg}}{1000 \text{ mcg}} \left| \frac{1 \text{ kg}}{2.2 \text{ lb}} \right| \frac{143 \text{ lb}}{} \left| \frac{60 \text{ min}}{1 \text{ hr}} \right| = \frac{\text{mL}}{\text{hr}}$$

$$\frac{0.8 \times 5 \times 1 \times 1 \times 143 \times 6}{5 \times 10 \times 2.2 \times 1} \left| \frac{3432}{110} \right| = 31.2 \text{ or } 31 \frac{\text{mL}}{\text{hr}}$$

21

Sequential method:

$$\frac{500 \text{ mg}}{} \left| \frac{5 \text{ mL}}{250 \text{ mg}} \right| \frac{50 \times 5}{25} \left| \frac{250}{25} \right| = 10 \text{ mL}$$

22

Sequential method:

$$\frac{50 \text{ mg}}{} \left| \frac{\text{tablets}}{100 \text{ mg}} \right| \frac{5}{10} = 0.5 \text{ tablet}$$

23

Sequential method:

$$\frac{150 \text{ mg}}{10 \text{ min}} \left| \frac{100 \text{ mL}}{150 \text{ mg}} \right| \frac{60 \text{ min}}{1 \text{ hr}} \left| \frac{100 \times 6}{1 \times 1} \right| \frac{600}{1} = 600 \frac{\text{mL}}{\text{hr}}$$

24

Sequential method:

$$\frac{30 \text{ mg}}{\text{kg}} \left| \frac{5 \text{ mL}}{100 \text{ mg}} \right| \frac{15 \text{ kg}}{} \left| \frac{3 \times 5 \times 15}{10} \right| \frac{225}{10} = 22.5 \text{ or } 23 \text{ mL}$$

25

Sequential method:

How many milligrams per day is the child receiving?

$$\frac{45 \text{ mg}}{\text{kg/day}} \left| \frac{35 \text{ kg}}{} \right| \frac{45 \times 35}{} \left| \frac{1575}{} \right| = 1575 \frac{\text{mg}}{\text{day}}$$

How many milligrams per dose is the child receiving?

$$\frac{1575 \text{ mg}}{\text{day}} \left| \frac{\text{day}}{2 \text{ doses}} \right| \frac{1575}{2} \left| \frac{787.5}{2} \right| = 787.5 \text{ or } 788 \frac{\text{mg}}{\text{dose}}$$

How many milliliters per dose will you give?

$$\frac{788 \text{ mg}}{\text{dose}} \left| \frac{5 \text{ mL}}{400 \text{ mg}} \right| \frac{788 \times 5}{400} \left| \frac{3940}{400} \right| = 9.85 \text{ or } 10 \frac{\text{mL}}{\text{dose}}$$

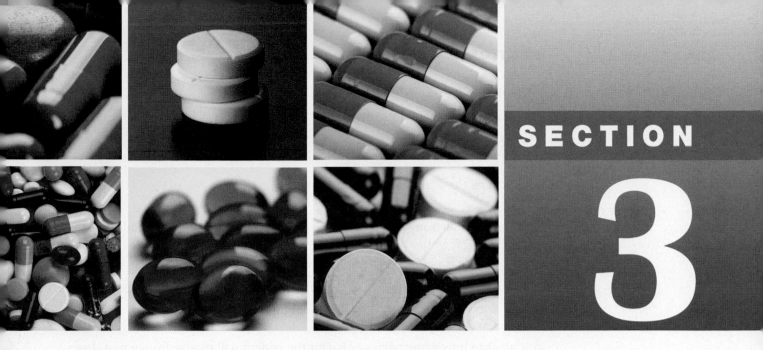

Case Studies

This section contains case studies simulating typical orders that might be written for patients with selected disorders. In each case, the orders include multiple situations that require the nurse to perform clinical calculations before being able to implement the order. After reading the short scenario, read through the list of orders.

Place a check mark in the box next to the physician's order that probably requires further calculations before implementing.

CASE STUDY 1 Congestive Heart Failure

A patient is admitted to the hospital with a diagnosis of dyspnea, peripheral edema with a 10-lb weight gain, and a history of congestive heart failure. The orders from the physician include:

- Bed rest in Fowler's position
- O_2 at 4 L/min per nasal cannula
- Chest x-ray, complete blood count, electrolyte panel, BUN, serum creatinine levels, and a digoxin level
- IV of D5W/$\frac{1}{2}$ NS at 50 mL/hr
- Daily AM weight
- Antiembolism stockings
- Furosemide 40 mg IV daily
- Digoxin 0.125 mg PO daily
- KCl 20 mEq PO tid
- Low-Na diet
- Restrict PO fluids to 1500 mL/day
- Vitals every 4h
- Accurate intake/output

Identify the orders that require calculations.

Set up and solve each problem using dimensional analysis.

1. Calculate gtt/min using microtubing (60 gtt/mL).

2. Calculate the weight gain in kilograms.

3. Calculate how many mL of Lasix the patient will receive IV from a multidose vial labeled 10 mg/mL.

4. Calculate how many tablets of digoxin the patient will receive from a unit dose of 0.25 mg/tablet.

5. Calculate how many tablets of K-Dur the patient will receive from a unit dose of 10 mEq/tablet.

CASE STUDY 2   COPD/Emphysema

A patient is admitted to the hospital with dyspnea and COPD exacerbation. The orders from the physician include:

- Stat ABGs, chest x-ray, complete blood count, and electrolytes
- IV D5W/½ NS 1000 mL/8 hr
- Aminophylline IV loading dose of 5.6 mg/kg over 30 minutes followed by 0.5 mg/kg/hr continuous IV
- O_2 at 2 L/min per nasal cannula
- Albuterol respiratory treatments every 4h
- Chest physiotherapy every 4h
- Erythromycin 800 mg IV every 6h
- Bed rest
- Accurate intake/output
- High-calorie, protein-rich diet in six small meals daily
- Encourage PO fluids to 3 L/day

Identify the orders that require calculations.

Set up and solve each problem using dimensional analysis.

1. Calculate mL/hr to set the IV pump.

2. Calculate mL/hr to set the IV pump for the loading dose of aminophylline for a patient weighing 140 lb. Aminophylline supply: 100 mg/100 mL D5W.

3. Calculate mL/hr to set the IV pump for the continuous dose of aminophylline for a patient weighing 140 lb. Aminophylline supply: 1 g/250 mL D5W.

4. Calculate mL/hr to set the IV pump to infuse erythromycin 800 mg. Erythromycin supply: 1-g vial to be reconstituted with 20 mL sterile water and further diluted in 250 mL NS to infuse over 1 hr.

5. Calculate the PO fluids in mL/shift for an 8-hour shift.

CASE STUDY 3   Small-Cell Lung Cancer

A patient with small-cell lung cancer is admitted to the hospital with fever and dehydration. The orders from the physician include:

- O$_2$ at 2 L/min per nasal cannula
- Chest x-ray; complete blood count; electrolytes; blood, urine, and sputum cultures; BUN and serum creatinine levels; type and cross for 2 units of PRBCs
- IV D5W/$\frac{1}{2}$ NS 1000 mL with 10 mEq KCl at 125 mL/hr
- 2 units of PRBCs if Hg is below 8
- 6 packs of platelets if under 20,000
- Neupogen 5 mcg/kg SQ daily
- Gentamicin 80 mg IV every 8h
- Decadron 8 mg IV daily
- Fortaz 1 g IV every 8h
- Accurate intake/output
- Encourage PO fluids
- Vitals every 4h (call for temperature above 102°F)

Identify the orders that require calculations.

Set up and solve each problem using dimensional analysis.

1. Calculate gtt/min using macrotubing (20 gtt/mL).

2. Calculate how many mcg of Neupogen will be given SQ to a patient weighing 160 lb.

3. Calculate mL/hr to set the IV pump to infuse gentamicin. The vial is labeled 40 mg/mL and is to be further diluted in 100 mL D5W to infuse over 1 hr.

4. Calculate how many mL of Decadron the patient will receive from a vial labeled dexamethasone 4 mg/mL.

5. Calculate mL/hr to set the IV pump to infuse Fortaz 1 g over 30 minutes. Supply: Fortaz 1 g/50 mL.

CASE STUDY 4   **Acquired Immunodeficiency Syndrome (AIDS)**

A patient who is HIV+ and a Jehovah's Witness is admitted to the hospital with anemia, fever of unknown origin, and wasting syndrome with dehydration. The orders from the physician include:

- O_2 at 4 L/min per nasal cannula
- IV D5W/$\frac{1}{2}$NS at 150 mL/hr
- CD4 and CD8 T-cell subset counts; erythrocyte sedimentation rate; complete blood count; urine, sputum, and stool cultures; chest x-ray
- Acyclovir 350 mg IV every 8h
- Neupogen 300 mcg SQ daily
- Epogen 100 units/kg SQ three times a week
- Megace 40 mg PO tid
- Zidovudine 100 mg PO every 4h
- Vancomycin 800 mg IV every 6h
- Respiratory treatments with pentamidine
- High-calorie, protein-rich diet in six small meals daily
- Encourage PO fluids to 3 L/day
- Accurate intake/output
- Daily AM weight

Identify the orders that require calculations.

Set up and solve each problem using dimensional analysis.

1. Calculate gtt/min using macrotubing (20 gtt/mL).

2. Calculate mL/hr to set the IV pump to infuse acyclovir 350 mg. Supply: 500-mg vial to be reconstituted with 10 mL sterile water and further diluted in 100 mL D5W to infuse over 1 hr.

3. Calculate how many mL of Neupogen will be given SQ. The vial is labeled 300 mcg/mL.

4. Calculate how many mL of Epogen will be given SQ to the patient weighing 100 lb. The vial is labeled 4000 units/mL.

5. Calculate how many mL/hr to set the IV pump to infuse vancomycin 800 mg. Supply: 1-g vials to be reconstituted with 10 mL NS and further diluted in 100 mL D5W to infuse over 60 min.

CASE STUDY 5   Sickle Cell Anemia

A patient is admitted to the hospital in sickle cell crisis. The orders from the physician include:

- Bed rest with joint support
- O_2 at 2 L/min per nasal cannula

- Complete blood count, erythrocyte sedimentation rate, serum iron levels, and chest x-ray
- IV D5W/½ NS at 150 mL/hr
- Zofran 8 mg IV every 8h
- Morphine sulfate 5 mg IV prn
- Hydrea 10 mg/kg/day PO
- Folic acid 0.5 mg daily PO
- Encourage 3000 mL/daily PO

Identify the orders that require calculations.

Set up and solve each problem using dimensional analysis.

1. Calculate gtt/min using macrotubing (10 gtt/mL).

2. Calculate mL/hr to set the IV pump to infuse Zofran 8 mg. Supply: Zofran 8 mg in 50 mL D5W to infuse over 15 min.

3. Calculate how many mL of morphine sulfate will be given IV. The syringe is labeled 10 mg/mL.

4. Calculate how many mg/day of Hydrea will be given PO to the patient weighing 125 lb.

5. Calculate how many tablets of folic acid will be given PO. Supply: 1 mg/tablet.

CASE STUDY 6   Deep Vein Thrombosis

A patient is admitted to the hospital with right leg erythema and edema to R/O DVT. The orders from the physician include:

- Bed rest with right leg elevated
- Warm, moist heat to right leg with Aqua-K pad
- Doppler ultrasonography
- Partial thromboplastin time (PTT) and prothrombin time (PT)
- IV D5W/½ NS with 20 mEq KCl at 50 mL/hr
- Heparin 5000 units IV push followed by continuous IV infusion of 1000 units/hr
- Lasix 20 mg IV bid
- Morphine 5 mg IV every 4h

Identify the orders that require calculations.

Set up and solve each problem using dimensional analysis.

1. Calculate gtt/min using microtubing (60 gtt/mL).

2. Calculate how many mL of heparin the patient will receive IV from a multidose vial labeled 10,000 units/mL.

3. Calculate mL/hr to set the IV pump for the continuous dose of heparin. Heparin supply: 25,000 units/250 mL D5W.

4. Calculate how many mL of Lasix the patient will receive IV from a multidose vial labeled 10 mg/mL.

5. Calculate how many mL of morphine the patient will receive from a syringe labeled 10 mg/mL.

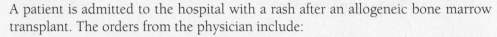

CASE STUDY 7 | **Bone Marrow Transplant**

A patient is admitted to the hospital with a rash after an allogeneic bone marrow transplant. The orders from the physician include:

- IV 1000 mL D5W/½ NS with 20 mEq KCL per liter at 80 mL/hr
- Complete blood count; electrolytes; sputum, urine, and stool cultures; blood cultures ×3; liver panel; BUN; and creatinine
- Vitals every 4h
- Strict intake/output
- Fortaz 2 g IV every 8h
- Vancomycin 1 g IV every 6h
- Claforan 1 g IV every 12h
- Erythromycin 800 mg IV every 6h

Identify the orders that require calculations.

Set up and solve each problem using dimensional analysis.

1. Calculate how many mEq/hr of KCl the patient will receive IV.

2. Calculate mL/hr to set the IV pump to infuse Fortaz 2 g. Supply: Fortaz 2-g vial to be reconstituted with 10 mL of sterile water and further diluted in 50 mL D5W to infuse over 30 min.

3. Calculate mL/hr to set the IV pump to infuse vancomycin 1 g. Supply: vancomycin 500-mg vial to be reconstituted with 10 mL of sterile water and further diluted in 100 mL of D5W to infuse over 60 min.

4. Calculate mL/hr to set the IV pump to infuse Claforan 1 g. Supply: Claforan 600 mg/4 mL to be further diluted with 100 mL D5W to infuse over 1 hr.

5. Calculate mL/hr to set the IV pump to infuse erythromycin 800 mg. Supply: erythromycin 1-g vial to be diluted with 20 mL sterile water and further diluted in 250 mL of NS to infuse over 60 min.

CASE STUDY 8   Pneumonia

A patient is admitted to the hospital with fever, cough, chills, and dyspnea to rule out pneumonia. The orders from the physician include:

- IV 600 mL D5W every 8h
- Intake/output
- Vitals every 4h
- Complete blood count, electrolytes, chest x-ray, ABGs, sputum specimen, blood cultures, and bronchoscopy
- Bed rest
- Humidified O_2 at 4 L/min per nasal cannula
- High-calorie diet
- Encourage oral fluids of 2000 to 3000 mL/day
- Pulse oximetry every AM
- Clindamycin 400 mg IV every 6h
- Albuterol respiratory treatments
- Guaifenesin 200 mg PO every 4h
- Terbutaline 2.5 mg PO tid
- MS Contrin 30 mg PO every 4h prn

Identify the orders that require calculations.

Set up and solve each problem using dimensional analysis.

1. Calculate mL/hr to set the IV pump to infuse clindamycin 400 mg. Supply: clindamycin 600 mg/4 mL to be further diluted with 50 mL D5W to infuse over 1 hr.

2. Calculate gtt/min to infuse the clindamycin using macrotubing (20 gtt/mL).

3. Calculate how many mL of guaifenesin the patient will receive from a stock bottle labeled 30 mg/tsp.

4. Calculate how many tablets of terbutaline the patient will receive from a unit dose of 5 mg/tablet.

5. Calculate how many tablets of MS Contrin the patient will receive from a unit dose of 30 mg/tablet.

CASE STUDY 9   Pain

A patient is admitted to the hospital with intractable bone pain secondary to prostate cancer. The orders from the physician include:

- IV 1000 mL D5W/$\frac{1}{2}$ NS with 20 mEq KCL per liter at 60 mL/hr
- IV 500 mL NS with 25 mg Dilaudid and 50 mg Thorazine at 21 mL/hr
- Heparin 25,000 units/250 mL D5W at 11 mL/hr

- Bed rest
- Do not resuscitate
- O$_2$ at 2 L/min per nasal cannula
- Bumex 2 mg IV every AM after albumin infusion
- Albumin 12.5 g IV every AM

Identify the orders that require calculations.

Set up and solve each problem using dimensional analysis.

1. Calculate how many mEq/hr of KCl the patient is receiving.

2. Calculate how many mg/hr of Dilaudid the patient is receiving.

3. Calculate how many mg/hr of Thorazine the patient is receiving.

4. Calculate how many units/hr of heparin the patient is receiving.

5. Calculate how many mL of Bumex the patient will receive from a stock dose of 0.25 mg/mL.

CASE STUDY 10   Cirrhosis

A patient is admitted to the hospital with ascites, stomach pain, dyspnea, and a history of cirrhosis of the liver. The orders from the physician include:

- IV D5W/$\frac{1}{2}$ NS with 20 mEq KCl at 125 mL/hr
- IV Zantac 150 mg/250 mL NS at 11 mL/hr
- O$_2$ at 2 L/min per nasal cannula
- Type and crossmatch for 2 units of packed red blood cells, complete blood count, liver panel, PT/PTT, SMA-12
- Carafate 1 g every 4h PO
- Vitamin K 10 mg SQ every AM
- Spironolactone 50 mg PO bid
- Lasix 80 mg IV every AM
- Measure abdominal girth every AM
- Sodium restriction to 500 mg/day
- Fluid restriction to 1500 mL/day

Identify the orders that require calculations.

Set up and solve each problem using dimensional analysis.

1. Calculate the gtt/min using macrotubing (20 gtt/mL).

2. Calculate the mg/hr of Zantac the patient is receiving.

3. Calculate how many mL of vitamin K the patient will receive SQ from a unit dose labeled 10 mg/mL.

4. Calculate how many tablets of spironolactone the patient will receive from a unit dose labeled 25 mg/tablet.

5. Calculate how many mL of Lasix the patient will receive from a unit dose labeled 10 mg/mL.

CASE STUDY 11 | **Hyperemesis Gravidarum**

A 14-year-old patient is admitted to the hospital with weight loss and dehydration secondary to hyperemesis gravidarum. The orders from the physician include:

- Bed rest with bathroom privileges
- Obtain weight daily
- Vital every 4h
- Test urine for ketones
- Urinalysis, complete blood count, electrolytes, liver enzymes, and bilirubin
- NPO for 48 hr, then advance diet to clear liquid, full liquid, and as tolerated
- IV D5$\frac{1}{2}$NS at 150 mL/hr for 8 hr, then decrease to 100 mL/hr
- Observe for signs of metabolic acidosis, jaundice, or hemorrhage
- Monitor intake and output
- Droperidol (Inapsine) 1 mg IV every 4h prn for nausea
- Metoclopramide (Reglan) 20 mg IV in 50 mL of D5W to infuse over 15 min
- Diphenhydramine (Benadryl) 25 mg IV every 3h prn for nausea
- Dexamethasone (Decadron) 4 mg IV every 6h

Identify the orders that require calculations.

Set up and solve each problem using dimensional analysis.

1. Calculate gtt/min using macrotubing (20 gtt/mL) to infuse 150 mL/hr, then 100 mL/hr.

2. Calculate how many mL of droperidol the patient will receive IV. Supply: 2.5 mg/mL

3. Calculate mL/hr to set the IV pump to infuse metoclopramide (Reglan) 20 mg in 50 mL of D5W to infuse over 15 min.

4. Calculate how many mL of diphenhydramine (Benadryl) the patient will receive IV. Supply: 10 mg/mL.

5. Calculate how many mL of dexamethasone (Decadron) the patient will receive IV. Supply: 4 mg/mL.

CASE STUDY 12 | Preeclampsia

A nulliparous female is admitted to the hospital with pregnancy-induced hypertension. The orders from the physician include:

- Complete bed rest in left lateral position
- Insert Foley catheter and check hourly for protein and specific gravity
- Daily weight
- Methyldopa (Aldomet) 250 mg PO tid
- Hydralazine (Apresoline) 5 mg IV every 20 min for blood pressure over 160/100
- Complete blood count, liver enzymes, chemistry panel, clotting studies, type and crossmatch, and urinalysis
- Magnesium sulfate 4 g in 250 mL D5LR loading dose to infuse over 30 min
- Magnesium sulfate 40 g in 1000 mL LR to infuse at 1 g/hr
- Keep calcium gluconate and intubation equipment at the bedside
- Nifedipine (Procardia) 10 mg sublingual for blood pressure over 160/100 and repeat in 15 min if needed.
- Keep lights dimmed and maintain a quiet environment
- Monitor blood pressure, pulse, and respiratory rate, fetal heart rate (FHR) contractions every 15 to 30 min, and deep tendon reflexes (DTR) hourly
- Monitor intake and output, proteinuria, presence of headache, visual disturbances, and epigastric pain hourly
- Restrict hourly fluid intake to 100 to 125 mL/hr

Identify the orders that require calculations.

Set up and solve each problem using dimensional analysis.

1. Calculate how many tablets of methyldopa (Aldomet) will be given PO. Supply: 500 mg/tablet.

2. Calculate how many mL of hydralazine (Apresoline) will be given IV. Supply: 20 mg/mL.

3. Calculate mL/hr to set the IV pump to infuse magnesium sulfate 4 g in 250 mL D5W loading dose to infuse over 30 min.

4. Calculate mL/hr to set the IV pump to infuse magnesium sulfate 40 g in 1000 mL LR to infuse at 1 g/hr.

5. Calculate how many capsules of nifedipine (Procardia) will be needed to give the sublingual dose. Supply: 10 mg/capsule.

CASE STUDY 13   Premature Labor

A 35-year-old female in the 30th week of gestation is admitted to the hospital in premature labor. The orders from the physician include:

- Bed rest in left lateral position
- Monitor intake and output
- Daily weights
- Continuous fetal monitoring
- Monitor blood pressure, pulse rate, respirations, fetal heart rate, uterine contraction pattern, and neurologic reflexes
- Keep calcium gluconate at the bedside
- Initiate magnesium sulfate 4 g in 250 mL LR loading dose over 20 min, then 2 g in 250 mL LR at 2 g/hr until contractions stop
- Continue tocolytic therapy with terbutaline (Brethine) 0.25 mg SQ every 30 min for 2 hr after contractions stop
- Give nifedipine (Procardia) 10 mg sublingual now, then 20 mg PO every 6h after infusion of magnesium sulfate and contractions have stopped
- Betamethasone 12 mg IM × 2 doses 12 hr apart
- IV LR 1000 mL over 8 hr

Identify the orders that require calculations.

Set up and solve each problem using dimensional analysis.

1. Calculate mL/hr to set the IV pump to infuse the loading dose magnesium sulfate 4 g in 250 mL LR over 20 min and the 2 g/hr maintenance dose.

2. Calculate how many mL of terbutaline (Brethine) will be given SQ. Supply: 1 mg/mL.

3. Calculate how many capsules of nifedipine (Procardia) will be given PO every 6h. Supply: 10 mg/capsule.

4. Betamethasone 12 mg IM × 2 doses 12 hr apart. Supply: 6 mg/mL.

5. Calculate mL/hr to set the IV pump to infuse LR 1000 mL over 8 hr.

CASE STUDY 14   Cystic Fibrosis

A 10-year-old child weighing 65 lb is admitted to the hospital with pulmonary exacerbation. The orders from the physician include:

- Complete blood count with differential, ABGs, chest x-ray, urinalysis, chemistry panel, and sputum culture
- IV 0.9% normal saline at 75 mL/hr
- Daily weights
- Monitor vitals every 4h

- Oxygen at 2 L/min with pulse oximetry checks to maintain oxygen saturation above 92%
- Pancrease 2 capsules PO with meals and snacks
- High-calorie, high-protein diet
- Multivitamin 1 tablet PO daily
- Tagamet 30 mg/kg/day PO in four divided doses with meals and HS with a snack
- Clindamycin 10 mg/kg IV every 6h
- Postural drainage and percussion after aerosolized treatments
- Albuterol treatments with 2 inhalations every 4h to 6h
- Terbutaline PO 2.5 mg every 6h
- Tobramycin 1.5 mg/kg every 6h
- Tobramycin peak and trough levels after fourth dose

Identify the orders that require calculations.

Set up and solve each problem using dimensional analysis.

1. Calculate gtt/min using macrotubing (15 gtt/mL).

2. Calculate how many tablets of Tagamet will be given PO with meals and HS snack. Supply: 200 mg/tablet.

3. Calculate how many mg of clindamycin the patient will receive, how many mL to draw from the vial, and mL/hr to set the IV pump. Supply: 150 mg/mL vial to be further diluted in 50 mL of NS and infused over 20 min.

4. Calculate how many tablets of terbutaline will be given PO. Supply: 2.5 mg/tablet.

5. Calculate how many mg of tobramycin the patient will receive, how many mL to draw from the vial, and mL/hr to set the IV pump. Supply: 40 mg/mL vial to be further diluted in 50 mL of NS and infused over 30 min.

CASE STUDY 15   Respiratory Syncytial Virus (RSV)

A 2-year-old child weighing 30 lb is admitted to the hospital for severe respiratory distress. The orders from the physician include:

- Complete blood count with differential, electrolytes, blood culture, chest x-ray, and nasal washing
- Humidified oxygen therapy to keep oxygen saturation >92%
- Continuous pulse oximetry
- IV D5W$\frac{1}{2}$NS at 50 mL/hr
- Elevate HOB
- Vitals every 2h
- Contact isolation
- Cardiorespiratory monitor
- Strict intake and output with urine specific gravities

- Acetaminophen elixir 120 mg every 4h prn for temperature above 101°F
- Aminophylline loading dose of 5 mg/kg to infuse over 30 min and maintenance dose of 0.8 mg/kg/hr
- Ribavirin (Virazole) inhalation therapy × 12 hr/day
- NPO with respiratory rate above 60
- RespiGam 750 mg/kg IV monthly
- Pediapred 1.5 mg/kg/day in three divided doses
- Ampicillin 100 mg/kg/day in divided doses every 6h

Identify the orders that require calculations.

Set up and solve each problem using dimensional analysis.

1. Calculate how many mL of acetaminophen elixir the patient will receive. Supply: 120 mg/5 mL.

2. Calculate how many mg of aminophylline the patient will receive and the mL/hr to set the IV pump for the loading dose, then calculate the mL/hr to set the IV pump for the maintenance dose. Supply: 250 mg/100 mL.

3. Calculate how many mg of RespiGam the patient will receive IV on a monthly infusion.

4. Calculate how many mL/dose of Pediapred the patient will receive. Supply: 15 mg/5 mL.

5. Calculate how many mg/dose of ampicillin the patient will receive IV, how many mL to draw from the vial, and mL/hr to set the IV pump. Supply: 1-g vials to be diluted with 10 mL of NS and further diluted in 50 mL NS to infuse over 30 min.

CASE STUDY 16   Leukemia

A 14-year-old child is admitted to the hospital with fever of unknown origin (FUO) after chemotherapy administration. The orders from the physician include:

- Complete blood count with differential, bone marrow aspiration, chemistry panel, PT/PTT, blood cultures, urinalysis, and type and crossmatch
- Regular diet as tolerated
- Vitals every 4h
- Daily weights
- Monitor intake and output
- Type and cross for 2 units PRBCs
- Irradiate all blood products
- Infuse 6 pack of platelets for counts under 20,000
- IV D5W/NS with 20 mEq KCl 1000 mL/8 hr
- Allopurinol 200 mg PO tid
- Fortaz 1 g IV every 6h
- Aztreonam (Azactam) 2 g IV every 12h

- Flagyl 500 mg IV every 8h
- Acetaminophen two tablets every 4h prn

Identify the orders that require calculations.

Set up and solve each problem using dimensional analysis.

1. Calculate mL/hr to set the IV pump.

2. Calculate how many tablets of allopurinol will be given PO. Supply: 100 mg/tablet.

3. Calculate how many mL/hr to set the IV pump to infuse Fortaz. Supply: 1-g vial to be diluted with 10 mL of sterile water and further diluted in 50 mL NS to infuse over 30 min.

4. Calculate how many mL of aztreonam to draw from the vial. Supply: 2-g vial to be diluted with 10 mL of sterile water and further diluted in 100 mL NS to infuse over 60 min.

5. Calculate how many mL/hr to set the IV pump to infuse Flagyl. Supply: 500 mg/100 mL to infuse over 1 hr.

CASE STUDY 17   Sepsis

A neonate born at 32 weeks' gestation (weight 2005 g) is admitted to the Neonatal Intensive Care Unit (NICU) with a diagnosis of sepsis. The orders from the physician include:

- Admit to NICU with continuous cardiorespiratory monitoring
- Complete blood counts, blood and urine cultures, chest x-ray, bilirubin, ABGs, theophylline levels, and lumbar puncture
- Strict intake and output
- Daily weight
- Vitals every 3h
- NG breast milk diluted with sterile water 120 mL/day with feedings every 3h
- IV D10 and 20% lipids 120 mL/kg/day
- Aminophylline 5 mg/kg IV every 6h
- Cefotaxime (Claforan) 50 mg/kg every 12h
- Vancomycin 10 mg/kg/dose every 12h

Identify the orders that require calculations.

Set up and solve each problem using dimensional analysis.

1. Calculate how many mL the child will receive with every feeding.

2. Calculate how many mL/hr the child will receive IV.

3. Calculate how many mg of aminophylline the child will receive every 6h. Calculate how many mL/hr you will set the IV pump. Supply: 50 mg/10 mL to infuse over 5 min.

4. Calculate how many mg of cefotaxime the child will receive every 12 hr. Calculate how many mL/hr you will set the IV pump. Supply: 40 mg/mL to infuse over 30 min.

5. Calculate how many mg of vancomycin the child will receive every 12 hr. Calculate how many mL/hr you will set the IV pump. Supply: 5 mg/mL to infuse over 1 hr.

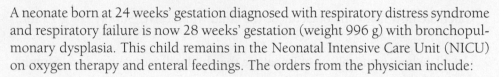

CASE STUDY 18   Bronchopulmonary Dysplasia

A neonate born at 24 weeks' gestation diagnosed with respiratory distress syndrome and respiratory failure is now 28 weeks' gestation (weight 996 g) with bronchopulmonary dysplasia. This child remains in the Neonatal Intensive Care Unit (NICU) on oxygen therapy and enteral feedings. The orders from the physician include:

- Complete blood count, chemistry panel, ABGs, chest x-ray, CPPD with nebulizations, glucose monitoring, caffeine citrate levels, and newborn screen
- NG feedings with Special Care with Iron 120 kcal/kg/day
- Chlorothiazide (Diuril) 10 mg/kg/day PO
- Fer-In-Sol 2 mg/kg/day
- Vitamin E 25 units/kg/day in divided doses every 12h
- Caffeine citrate 5 mg/kg/dose daily

Identify the orders that require calculations.

Set up and solve each problem using dimensional analysis.

1. Calculate how many total calories the child will receive daily. Calculate how many mL/day the child will receive. Supply: 24 kcal/oz.

2. Calculate how many mg of chlorothiazide the child will receive daily. Calculate how many mL/day the child will receive. Supply: 250 mg/5 mL.

3. Calculate how many mg of Fer-In-Sol the child will receive daily. Calculate how many mL/day the child will receive. Supply: 15 mg/0.6 mL.

4. Calculate how many units/dose of vitamin E the child will receive every 12 hr. Calculate how many mL/dose the child will receive. Supply: 67 units/mL.

5. Calculate how many mg of caffeine citrate the child will receive daily. Supply: 10 mg/mL.

CASE STUDY 19   Cerebral Palsy

A 13-year-old child (weight 38 kg) with cerebral palsy being cared for in a children's facility is admitted to the hospital for seizure evaluation. The orders from the physician include:

- Complete blood count, chemistry panel, urinalysis, dilantin levels, EEG, and CT scan
- Vitals every 4h
- Seizure precautions
- Lactulose 3 g PO tid
- Valproic acid (Depakote) 30 mg/kg/day PO in three divided doses
- Diazepam (Valium) 2.5 mg PO daily
- Chlorothiazide (Thiazide) 250 mg PO daily
- Phenytoin (Dilantin) 5 mg/kg/day PO in three divided doses

Identify the orders that require calculations.

Set up and solve each problem using dimensional analysis.

1. Calculate how many mL of lactulose the child will receive. Supply: 10 g/15 mL.

2. Calculate how many tablets of Depakote the child will receive per dose. Supply: 125 mg/tablet.

3. Calculate how many tablets of diazepam the child will receive per dose. Supply: 5 mg/tablet.

4. Calculate how many tablets of chlorothiazide the child will receive per dose. Supply: 250 mg/tablet.

5. Calculate how many mL of Dilantin the child will receive per dose. Supply: 125 mg/5 mL.

CASE STUDY 20   Hyperbilirubinemia

A 4-day-old neonate born at 35 weeks' gestation (weight 2210 g) is readmitted to the hospital for treatment of dehydration and jaundice with a bilirubin level of 21 mg/dL. The orders from the physician include:

- Phototherapy and exchange transfusion through an umbilical venous catheter
- Total and indirect bilirubin levels, electrolytes, complete blood count, and type and crossmatch
- Continuous cardiorespiratory monitoring
- Vitals every 2h
- Monitor intake and output
- Albumin 5% infusion 1 g/kg 1 hr before exchange

- Ampicillin 100 mg/kg/dose IV every 12h
- Gentamicin 4 mg/kg/dose IV every 12h
- NPO before exchange, then 120 mL/kg/day formula
- IV D10W 120 mL/kg/day

Identify the orders that require calculations.

Set up and solve each problem using dimensional analysis.

1. Calculate how many g of albumin the infant will receive before exchange therapy.

2. Calculate how many mg/dose of ampicillin the infant will receive every 12 hr. Calculate how many mL the infant will receive. Supply: 250 mg/5 mL IV push over 5 min.

3. Calculate how many mg/dose of gentamicin the infant will receive every 12 hr. Calculate how many mL the infant will receive. Supply: 2 mg/mL.

4. Calculate how many mL/day of formula the infant will receive.

5. Calculate how many mL/hr to set the IV pump.

CASE STUDY 21   Spontaneous Abortion

A 31-year-old female is admitted to the hospital to control severe hemorrhage after a spontaneous abortion. The orders from the physician include:

- CBC to determine blood loss
- WBC with differential to rule out infection
- Type and crossmatch for 2 units of blood
- Obtain Coombs' test to determine Rh status
- Administer Rhogam 300 mcg IM if patient is Rh-negative with a negative indirect Coombs' test
- IV D5/0.9% NS at 100 mL/hr
- IV oxytocin (Pitocin) 10 units infused at 20 mU/min
- Prepare for a dilatation and curettage (D&C)
- Complete bed rest. Monitor bedpan for contents for intrauterine material
- Administer meperidine (Demerol) 50 mg IM every 4h for severe discomfort
- Administer ibuprofen 400 mg PO every 6h for mild discomfort
- Monitor vital signs every 4h for 24 hr
- Monitor urine output
- Note the amount, color, and odor of vaginal bleeding

Identify the orders that require calculations.

Set up and solve each problem using dimensional analysis.

1. Calculate how many mL of Rhogam the patient will receive. Supply: Rhogam 300 mcg/mL vial. Administer into the deltoid muscle within 72 hr of abortion.

2. Calculate gtt/min using macrotubing (15 gtt/mL).

3. Calculate how many mL/hr to set the IV pump to infuse oxytocin 10 units. Supply: oxytocin 10 units in 500 mL D5/NS.

4. Calculate how many mL of meperidine (Demerol) will be given IM. The pre-filled syringe is labeled 100 mg/mL.

5. Calculate how many tablets of ibuprofen will be given PO. Supply: 200 mg/tablet.

CASE STUDY 22   Bipolar Disorder

A 25-year-old female is brought to the hospital by her friends after she fainted at the PowerShop. Her friends reported that she has been very sad, withdrawn, and not involved in any of her usual activities for some time but had suddenly become "full of energy" at the PowerShop. The orders from the physician include:

- CBC and electrolytes
- WBC with differential
- BUN and creatinine
- Liver panel
- Lithium levels
- IV 0.9% NS at 75 mL/hr
- Lithium 300 mg PO tid
- Clonazepam 0.5 mg PO bid; increase to 1 mg PO bid after 3 days
- Doxepin 50 mg PO tid
- Intake and output

Identify the orders that require calculations.

Set up and solve each problem using dimensional analysis.

1. Calculate the gtt/min using macrotubing (20 gtt/mL).

2. Calculate how many capsules of lithium will be given PO. Supply: 150 mg/capsule.

3. Calculate how many tablets of clonazepam will be given PO. Supply: 0.5-mg tablets.

4. Calculate how many tablets of clonazepam will be given PO after 3 days. Supply: 0.5-mg tablets.

5. Calculate how many tablets of doxepin will be given PO. Supply: 25-mg tablets.

CASE STUDY 23   Anorexia Nervosa

A 17-year-old female high school student is admitted by her parents for self-induced starvation, vomiting, and laxative abuse. The 12-week hospital stay is for management of diet with a 1- to 2-lb/week weight gain goal. The orders from the physician include:

- DSM-IV evaluation
- Nutritional consult for 1500-calorie diet advance to 3500 calories over 12 weeks
- CBC, platelet count, and sedimentation rate
- WBC with differential
- Electrolytes, BUN, and creatinine
- Liver enzymes
- Urinalysis
- ECG
- Daily weight
- Intake and output
- 1000 mL IV D5/LR with 20 mEq K+ to infuse over 8 hr
- Olanzapine (Zyprexa) 10 mg PO HS
- Fluoxetine (Prozac) 60 mg/day PO every AM
- Amitriptyline 25 mg PO qid
- Cyproheptadine 32 mg/day PO in four divided doses

Identify the orders that require calculations.

Set up and solve each problem using dimensional analysis.

1. Calculate how many mL/hr to set the IV pump.

2. Calculate how many tablets of olanzapine (Zyprexa) will be given at HS. Supply: 5-mg tablets.

3. Calculate how many mL of fluoxetine (Prozac) will be given PO. Supply: 20 mg/5 mL.

4. Calculate how many tablets of amitriptyline will be given PO. Supply: 10 mg/5 mL.

5. Calculate how many mL of cyproheptadine will be given PO. Supply: 2 mg/5 mL.

CASE STUDY 24   Clinical Depression

A 44-year-old successful businessman with a wife and two children, and diagnosed with clinical depression, has received several months of treatment with antidepressants and psychotherapy. The depression has not responded to therapy. He has become suicidal, and he has agreed to try electroconvulsive therapy (also called ECT). The orders from the physician include:

- Admit for ECT
- CBC and urinalysis
- ECG
- NPO after midnight
- Obtain AM weight
- Obtain baseline vitals 60 min before procedure
- Start IV D5/0.45% at 100 mL/hr
- Administer glycopyrrolate (Robinul) 4.4 mcg/kg IM 30 min preoperatively
- Zoloft 50 mg PO every AM
- Sinequan 25 mg PO tid
- Parnate 30 mg/day PO in two divided doses

Identify the orders that require calculations.

Set up and solve each problem using dimensional analysis.

1. Calculate the gtt/min using macrotubing (10 gtt/mL).

2. Calculate how many mL of glycopyrrolate (Robinul) will be given IM. Supply: 200 mcg/mL. Patient weight: 175 lb.

3. Calculate how many tablets of sertraline (Zoloft) will be given PO. Supply: 50-mg tablets.

4. Calculate how many capsules of doxepin (Sinequan) will be given PO. Supply: 25-mg capsules.

5. Calculate how many tablets of tranylcypromine (Parnate) will be given PO. Supply: 10-mg tablets.

CASE STUDY 25   Alzheimer's Disease

A 62-year-old executive is experiencing difficulty remembering and performing familiar tasks, problems with abstract thinking, and changes in mood and behavior. He is hospitalized for evaluation. The orders from the physician include:

- CT of the brain
- EEG and cerebral blood flow studies
- CBC and electrolytes
- Cerebrospinal fluid analysis
- Urinalysis

- 1000 mL IV D5/0.45% NS to infuse over 8 hr
- Donepezil (Aricept) 5 mg PO HS
- Thioridazine (Mellaril) 25 mg PO tid
- Imipramine (Tofranil) 50 mg PO qid
- Temazepam (Restoril) 7.5 mg PO HS

Identify the orders that require calculations.

Set up and solve each problem using dimensional analysis.

1. Calculate gtt/min using macrotubing (10 gtt/mL).

2. Calculate how many tablets of donepezil (Aricept) will be given PO. Supply: 5-mg tablets.

3. Calculate how many tablets of thioridazine (Mellaril) will be given PO. Supply: 25-mg tablets.

4. Calculate how many tablets of imipramine (Tofranil) will be given PO. Supply: 25-mg tablets.

5. Calculate how many tablets of temazepam (Restoril) will be given PO. Supply: 15-mg tablets.

CASE STUDY 26   Otitis Media

An 18-month-old child is seen in the nurse practitioner's office for reoccurring otitis media and fever. The child's weight is 23 lb. The orders from the nurse practitioner include:

- Amoxicillin 45 mg/kg/day PO in divided doses every 12h
- Acetaminophen (Tylenol) 120 mg PO every 4h alternating with ibuprofen 5 mg/kg PO every 6h if temperature is 102.5°F or below and 10 mg/kg if temperature is greater than 102.5°F
- Cetirizine (Zyrtec) 2.5 mg PO every 12h
- Pedialyte 75 mL per kg PO not to exceed more than 100 mL in any 20-minute period during the first 8 hr

Identify the orders that require calculations.

Set up and solve each problem using dimensional analysis.

1. Calculate how many mL/dose of amoxicillin will be given PO. Supply: amoxicillin 125 mg/5 mL solution.

2. Calculate how many mL of acetaminophen (Tylenol) will be given PO for a temperature of 102°. Supply: acetaminophen 100 mg/mL solution.

3. Calculate how many mL of ibuprofen will be given PO for a temperature of 102°. Supply: ibuprofen 100 mg/5 mL solution.

4. Calculate how many mL of Zyrtec will be given PO. Supply: Zyrtec 1 mg/mL.

5. Calculate how many mL/hr/8 hr of Pedialyte the patient will receive PO during the first 8 hr.

CASE STUDY 27   Seizures

An 8-year-old child is admitted to the pediatric hospital with seizures secondary to a head injury following a fall on the playground. The child's weight is 60 lb. The orders from the physician include:

- Admit to pediatric intensive care
- Bed rest in quiet, darken environment
- Complete blood count, chemistry panel, urinalysis, EEG, skull and neck x-ray and CT scan
- Vitals every 2h
- Monitor intake and output
- Seizure precautions
- IV D5W/0.45% NS at 500 mL/8 hr
- Phenytoin (Dilantin) 2 mg/kg/min IV
- Diazapam (Valium) 0.3 mg/kg IV push given over 3 minutes every 15–30 min to a total dose of 10 mg, repeat every 2–4 hr for seizure activity following Dilantin administration
- Acetaminophen (Tylenol) 320 mg PO every 4 hours alternating with ibuprofen 7.5 mg/kg PO every 6 hours

Identify the orders that require calculations.

Set up and solve each problem using dimensional analysis.

1. Calculate how many mL/hr to set the IV pump. Supply: D5W/0.45% NS 500 mL.

2. Calculate how many mL/hr to set the IV pump to administer Dilantin. Supply: Dilantin 100 mg/50 mL to be administered over 15 minutes.

3. Calculate how many mL of diazepam will be given IV push over 3 minutes. Supply: diazepam 5 mg/mL.

4. Calculate how many mL of acetaminophen will be given every 4 hours PO. Supply: acetaminophen 100 mg/mL.

5. Calculate how many mL of ibuprofen will be given PO every 6 hours. Supply: ibuprofen 100 mg/5 mL.

CASE STUDY 28   Fever of Unknown Origin

A 10-year-old child is admitted to the pediatric hospital with fever of unknown origin. The child's weight is 80 lb. The orders from the physician include:

- Admit to the Pediatric Unit
- Complete blood count with differential, chest x-ray, urinalysis, chemistry panel, and sputum culture
- Vitals every 4 hours
- Monitor intake and output
- Acetaminophen (Tylenol) 400 mg PO every 4h alternating with ibuprofen 7.5 mg/kg PO every 6h
- IV D5W/0.45% NS at 500 mL/4 hr
- Unasyn 1500 mg IV every 6h

Identify the orders that require calculations.

Set up and solve each problem using dimensional analysis.

1. Calculate how many mL of acetaminophen will be given every 4 hours PO. Supply: acetaminophen 500 mg/15 mL.

2. Calculate how many mL of ibuprofen will be given every 6h PO. Supply: ibuprofen 100 mg/5 mL.

3. Calculate how many mL/hr to set the IV pump. Supply: D5W/0.45% NS 500 mL.

4. Calculate the gtt/min using a microtubing (60 gtt/mL).

5. Calculate how many mL/hr to set the IV pump to administer Unasyn. Supply: Unasyn 1.5 g/50 mL over 30 minutes.

CASE STUDY 29   TURP with CBI

A 58-year-old male is admitted to the medical/surgical unit following surgery for transurethral resection of prostate. The physician's postoperative orders include:

- Admit to the medical/surgical unit
- Monitor intake and output
- Monitor urinary output hourly
- Vitals every 2 hr
- Monitor for symptoms of TURP syndrome
- Adjust rate of continuous bladder irrigation, 3-liter bags of sterile normal saline to maintain a patent catheter, adjust rate to maintain pink to clear urine, and maintain urinary catheter traction
- IV D5W/0.45% normal saline 1000 mL/8 hr
- Ciprofloxacin (Cipro) 400 mg IV every 12 hr

- Docusate sodium (Colace) 100 mg PO bid
- Dimenhydrinate 25 mg IV every 4 hr prn
- Acetaminophen (Tylenol) 300 mg with 30 mg of codeine PO 1 to 2 tablets every 4 to 6 hr prn
- Discontinue IV when drinking well
- Complete blood count, electrolytes, creatinine in AM

Identify the orders that require calculations.

Set up and solve each problem using dimensional analysis.

1. Calculate how many mL/hr to set the IV pump. Supply: D5W/0.45% NS 1000 mL bag.

2. Calculate how many gtt/min using 20 gtt/mL IV tubing.

3. Calculate how many mL/hr to set the IV pump to deliver the Cipro. Supply: ciprofloxacin 400 mg/200 mL D5W to infuse over 60 min.

4. Calculate how many capsules to give of Colace. Supply: docusate sodium 100 mg/capsule.

5. Calculate how many mL will be given of dimenhydrinate. Supply: dimenhydrinate 50 mg/mL.

CASE STUDY 30   Hypercholesterolemia

A 40-year-old male returns to his nurse practitioner's office after 3 months for a cholesterol level of 240 mg/dL. The nurse practitioner's orders include:

- Continue low-fat, high-fiber diet
- Continue to briskly walk 3 to 4 times weekly for 30 minutes
- Stop smoking and begin Chantix 0.5 mg PO once daily for days 1–3 then 0.5 mg PO bid for days 4–7, then 1 mg PO for day 8
- Atorvastatin (Lipitor) 20 mg PO daily
- Cholestyramine resin 4 g/dose PO bid to be taken 1 hr before Lipitor
- Niacin 1.5 g/day PO
- Return appointment in 4 weeks for lipid levels.

Identify the orders that require calculations.

Set up and solve each problem using dimensional analysis.

1. Calculate how many tablets of Chantix the patient will be taking on days 1–3. Supply: Chantix 0.5-mg tablets.

2. Calculate how many tablets of Chantix the patient will be taking on day 8. Supply: Chantix 0.5-mg tablets.

3. Calculate how many tablets of Lipitor the patient will be taking. Supply: Lipitor 10-mg tablets.

4. Calculate how many g/day of cholestyramine resin the patient will be taking. Supply: cholestyramine resin 4 g/dose powder to be mixed with 4 to 6 oz of fluid.

5. Calculate how many tablets/day of niacin the patient is taking. Supply: niacin 500-mg tablets.

CASE STUDY 31   Hypertension

A 60-year-old male returns to his nurse practitioner's office after 3 months for elevated blood pressure. Patient's weight: 90 kg. The nurse practitioner's orders include:

- Continue on low-sodium diet
- Continue to briskly walk 3 to 4 times weekly for 30 minutes
- Maintain a fluid intake of 2 L/day
- Nifedipine (Procardia XL) 60 mg PO once daily for 14 days then return to the office for reevaluation
- Docusate sodium (Colace) 100 mg PO bid
- Hydrochlorothiazide (HydroDIURIL) 25 mg daily PO in AM with a glass of orange juice
- Report any weight gain of greater than 2 lb/day
- Return appointment in 14 days for reevaluation of blood pressure

Identify the orders that require calculations.

Set up and solve each problem using dimensional analysis.

1. Calculate how many mL/meal the patient will need to consume.

2. Calculate how many tablets of nifedipine the patient is taking. Supply: Procardia XL 30 mg/tablets.

3. Calculate how many capsules of docusate sodium the patient is taking. Supply: Colace 100 mg/capsule.

4. Calculate how many tablets of hydrochlorothiazide the patient is taking. Supply: HydroDIURIL 50 mg/tablets.

5. Calculate the weight gain from 90 kg to 95 kg that will be reported to the nurse practitioner in lb.

CASE STUDY 32   Diabetic Ketoacidosis

A 16-year-old is admitted to the medical intensive care unit with diabetic ketoacidosis secondary to fever. The patient weighs 125 lbs. The orders from the physician include:

- Admit to the medical intensive care unit
- Complete blood count, electrolytes, blood sugar, ABGs, and ECG
- Blood, urine, and sputum cultures
- Electrolytes and blood sugars hourly until stable
- Strict intake and output
- Daily weight
- Vitals hourly × 4, then every 2 hours × 4, then every 4 hr
- IV 0.9% NS 1000 mL/8 hr
- Regular insulin 0.15 unit/kg IV bolus followed by the continuous intravenous infusion of regular insulin 0.1 unit/kg/hr in 0.9% NS
- Change IV fluids to D5W/0.45% NS when plasma glucose falls to under 250 mg/dL at 10 mL/kg/hr
- Ampicillin sodium 500 mg every 6 hr IVPB for 3 days

Identify the orders that require calculations.

Set up and solve each problem using dimensional analysis.

1. Calculate the mL/hr to set the IV pump to 1000 mL/8 hr. Supply: 0.9% NS 1000 mL.

2. Calculate the mL for the IV bolus to infuse regular insulin at 0.15 unit/kg. Supply: 250 mL 0.9% NS with 250 units regular insulin.

3. Calculate the mL/hr to set the IV pump for the continuous infusion of regular insulin at 0.1 unit/kg/hr in 0.9% NS. Supply: 250 mL 0.9% NS with 250 units regular insulin.

4. Calculate the mL/hr to set the IV pump after the plasma glucose falls to under 250 mg/dL. Supply: D5W/0.45% NS 1000 mL.

5. Calculate the mL/hr to set the IV pump to infuse ampicillin sodium. Supply: ampicillin sodium 1 g/100 mL over 30 min.

CASE STUDY 33   End-Stage Renal Failure

A 60-year-old patient is seen at the dialysis center for weekly dialysis treatment. The patient weighs 140 lbs after dialysis. The orders from the physician include:

- Obtain weight three times weekly prior to and after dialysis treatment
- Furosemide 120 mg PO bid
- Metolazone (Zaroxolyn) 10 mg PO daily
- Enalapril maleate (Vasotec) 2.5 mg PO bid

- Epogen 100 units/kg IV three times weekly in venous line following dialysis
- Calcium carbonate 10 g/day in divided doses with meals

Identify the orders that require calculations.

Set up and solve each problem using dimensional analysis.

1. Calculate how many tablets of furosemide the patient is taking. Supply: furosemide 80 mg/tablets.

2. Calculate how many tablets of Zaroxolyn the patient is taking. Supply: metolazone 5 mg/tablet.

3. Calculate how many tablets of Vasotec the patient is taking. Supply: enalapril maleate 2.5 mg/tablets.

4. Calculate how many mL of Epogen the patient should receive three times weekly. Supply: Epogen 4000 units/mL.

5. Calculate how many tablets/meal of calcium carbonate the patient will receive. Supply: calcium carbonate 1500 mg/tablets.

CASE STUDY 34   Fluid Volume Deficit

A 5-year old child is admitted to the pediatric unit for fluid volume deficit secondary to gastroenteritis. The child's weight is 35 lb. The orders from the physician include:

- Admit to pediatric unit for 24-hour observation
- Monitor intake and output
- IV 50 mL/kg 0.9% NS/2.5% dextrose over 4 hr
- Discontinue IV when taking PO fluids without emesis
- Acetaminophen (Tylenol) 400 mg/dose PO every 4 hours alternating with ibuprofen 7.5 mg/kg PO every 6 hours
- Encourage sips of fluids every 10 minutes if not vomiting, repeated every 15 minutes until able to consume 30 mL then fluids as tolerated at 1.5 oz/lb/24 hr
- Pedialyte 53 oz/24 hr when tolerating fluids

Identify the orders that require calculations.

Set up and solve each problem using dimensional analysis.

1. Calculate the mL/hr to set the IV pump to infuse 50 mL/kg/4 hr. Supply: 1000 mL 0.9% NS/2.5% dextrose.

2. Calculate how many mL of acetaminophen will be given PO. Supply: acetaminophen 100 mg/mL solution.

3. Calculate how many mL of ibuprofen per dose will be given PO. Supply: ibuprofen 100 mg/5 mL solution.

4. Calculate how many mL/hr of fluids the child will receive.

5. Calculate how many mL/hr of Pedialyte the child will receive.

CASE STUDY 35   Increased Intracranial Pressure

A 35-year-old male is admitted to the hospital with signs and symptoms of increased intracranial pressure secondary to brain metastasis. The patient weighs 75 kg. The orders from the physician include:

- Admit to oncology unit
- IV 0.9% NS 1000 mL/10 hr
- Loading dose of phenytoin (Dilantin) 10 mg/kg IV push (50 mg/min) then Dilantin 100 mg IV every 8 hr
- Mannitol 0.5 g/kg/10 min IV initial dose followed by mannitol 0.25 g/kg IV every 4 hr
- Dexamethasone 10 mg IV
- Furosemide 0.5 mg/kg IV push
- Elevate HOB 25–30 degrees to promote intracranial drainage
- Bed rest in a quiet, darkened environment

Identify the orders that require calculations.

Set up and solve each problem using dimensional analysis.

1. Calculate the mL/hr to set the IV pump to infuse 0.9% NS. Supply: 1000 mL 0.9% NS.

2. Calculate how many mL of Dilantin the patient will receive as a loading dose. Supply: Dilantin 1000 mg/20 mL 0.9% NS.

3. Calculate the mL/hr to set the IV pump to infuse the mannitol ordered every 4 h. Supply: mannitol 100 g/500 mL D5W.

4. Calculate how many mL of dexamethasone will be given IV push. Supply: Decadron 120 mg/5 mL.

5. Calculate how many mL of furosemide will be given IV push. Supply: furosemide 10 mg/mL.

CASE STUDY 36   Breast Cancer

A patient is admitted to the hospital with nausea, shortness of breath, and fatigue 10 days after receiving chemotherapy for breast cancer. The orders from the physician include:

- Admit to Oncology Unit
- O_2 at 2 L/min per nasal cannula
- Complete blood cell count (CBC) with differential, chest x-ray, urinalysis, chemistry panel, and sputum culture
- Vitals every 4 hours (call if temperature above 102°F)
- Bed rest with BRP
- Monitor intake/output
- Type and crossmatch for 1 unit of PRBC for Hg 8 g/dL or below
- Filgrastim (Neupogen) 5 mcg/kg/day IV until the ANC reaches 10,000/mm^3
- 6 pack of platelets if count under 20,000
- Premedicate prior to blood transfusion with acetaminophen (Tylenol) 650 mg PO and diphenhydramine (Benadryl) 25 mg IV
- Metoclopramide (Reglan) 2 mg/kg IV every 2 hours for two doses
- IV D5W at 100 mL/hr

Identify the orders that require calculations.

Set up and solve each problem using dimensional analysis.

1. Calculate gtt/min using macrotubing (15 gtt/mL).

2. Calculate how many mL per day of filgrastim (Neupogen) will be given for a patient weighing 150 lb. Supply: Neupogen 300 mcg/mL.

3. Calculate how many mg of metoclopramide (Reglan) the patient will receive IV. Patient weighs 150 lb. Supply: metoclopramide 5 mg/mL.

4. Calculate mL/hr to set the IV pump to infuse 1 unit of PRBC over 3 hours. Supply: PRBC 1 unit = 450 mL.

   *Preventing Medication Errors: Before administration of the PRBC, the nurse must change the IV to 0.9% NS and strictly follow the protocol for administration of blood or blood components. Use of other IV solutions will damage the blood components: D5W solutions will cause red blood cells to aggregate and lyse and Lactated Ringers will cause blood to clot.

5. Calculate how many mL of diphenhydramine (Benadryl) the patient will receive from a vial labeled diphenhydramine 50 mg/mL to be administrated over 1 minute IV push.

CASE STUDY 37   Severe Abdominal Pain

A 12-year-old patient is admitted to the hospital with severe abdominal pain in the right lower quadrant. The orders from the physician include:

- Admit to Pediatric Unit
- Weight 88 lb
- Vitals every 2 hours until stable, then every 4 hours
- Ultrasound for possible ruptured appendix
- CBC with differential
- IV D5W/0.45% NS @ 1000 mL/8 hr
- Clindamycin (Cleocin) 300 mg IV every 6 hours
- Cefotaxime (Claforan) 50 mg/kg IV every 12 hours
- Morphine sulfate 3 mg IV push every 3 to 4 hours prn for severe pain

Identify the orders that require calculations.

Set up and solve each problem using dimensional analysis.

1. Calculate the weight of the patient in kilograms.

2. Calculate mL/hr to set the IV pump.

3. Calculate mL/hr to set the IV pump to infuse clindamycin 300 mg. Supply: Cleocin 300 mg/50 mL NS to infuse over 20 minutes.

4. Supply: Claforan 2-g vial to be reconstituted with 10 mL sterile water and further diluted in 50 mL NS to infuse over 30 minutes. Calculate mL to draw from the vial to mix with 50 mL NS and calculate mL/hr to set the IV pump to infuse cefotaxime.

5. Calculate the mL of morphine sulfate to be given IV push. Supply: morphine sulfate 4 mg/mL to be further diluted in 5 mL sterile water or NS and administered over 4 to 5 minutes.

CASE STUDY 38   Acute Asthma Attack

A patient is admitted to the hospital during an acute asthma attack. The orders from the physician include:

- Admit to the Pulmonary Unit
- O$_2$ at 2 L/min per nasal cannula
- Vitals every 2 hours until stable, then every 4 hours
- CBC with differential, chemistry panel, and blood gases
- Bed rest in high Fowler's position
- IV D5W/1/2 NS at 1000 mL/10 hr
- Levalbuterol (Xopenex) 1.25 mg administered every 4 hours via nebulizer for wheezing (1.25 vials)

- Fluticasone and salmeterol (Advair) 250/50 inhaler every 12 hours
- Weight 176 lb
- Methylprednisolone (Solu-Medrol) 80 mg infused IV push over 3 minutes every 6 hours
- Azithromycin (Zithromax) 500 mg PO on day, 1 followed by 250 mg PO daily on days 2 to 5 for a total dose of 1.5 g
- Cimetidine (Tagamet) 300 mg IV every 6 hours

Identify the orders that require calculations.

Set up and solve each problem using dimensional analysis.

1. Calculate mL/hr to set the IV pump.

2. Calculate the weight of the patient in kilograms.

3. Calculate how many mL of Solu-Medrol the patient will receive IV push from an Act-O-Vial System labeled 125 mg/2 mL.

4. Calculate how many tablets of azithromycin the patient will receive from a unit dose of 250 mg/capsular for the initial dose of 500 mg.

5. Calculate mL/hr to set the IV pump to infuse cimetidine 300 mg IV. Supply: Tagamet 300 mg/50 mL of D5W and infused over 20 minutes.

CASE STUDY 39   Right Total Hip Replacement

A patient is admitted to the hospital for a right total hip replacement. The orders from the physician include:

- Admit to Orthopedic Unit
- IV D5W/NS at 100 mL/hr
- CBC with differential, chemistry panel, BUN, creatinine, and urinalysis
- Monitor intake/output
- Atenolol 50 mg PO daily
- Lisinopril 5 mg PO daily
- Enoxaparin (Lovenox) 40 mg SQ every 12 hours
- Dimenhydrinate 50 mg IV every 4 hours for nausea and vomiting
- Morphine 10 mg IV every 4 hours prn for pain

Identify the orders that require calculations.

Set up and solve each problem using dimensional analysis.

1. Calculate how many tablets of atenolol the patient will receive from a unit dose of 25 mg/tablet.

2. Calculate how many tablets of lisinopril the patient will receive from a unit dose of 2.5 mg/tablet.

3. Calculate how many mL of Lovenox the patient will receive SQ from a vial labeled enoxaparin 80 mg/0.8 mL.

4. Calculate the mL of dimenhydrinate to be given IV. Supply: dimenhydrinate 50 mg/mL to be further diluted in 10 mL NS and administered slowly over 2 minutes.

5. Calculate the mL of morphine sulfate to be given IV. Supply: morphine sulfate 8 mg/mL to be further diluted in 5 mL sterile water or NS and administered over 4 to 5 minutes.

CASE STUDY 40   Colon Resection

A patient is admitted to the hospital for a colon resection. The orders from the physician include:

- Admit to Medical/Surgical Unit
- IV NS with KCl 20 mEq/L 1000 mL/12 hr
- CBC, electrolytes, urea, glucose, creatinine
- Enoxaparin (Lovenox) 40 mg SQ daily
- Cefoxitin 1 g IV every 8 hours
- Ranitidine 50 mg IV every 8 hours
- Tamsulosin (Flomax) 0.8 mg PO daily PC
- Calcium carbonate (Os-Cal) 1.25 g PO daily (1250 mg/tablet)

Identify the orders that require calculations.

Set up and solve each problem using dimensional analysis.

1. Calculate mL/hr to set the IV pump.

2. Calculate mL/hr to set the IV pump to infuse cefoxitin (Mefoxin) 1 g IV. Supply: cefoxitin 1 g in 50 mL 0.9% NS to infuse over 30 minutes.

3. Calculate mL/hr to set the IV pump to infuse ranitidine 50 mg IV. Supply: ranitidine (Zantac) 50 mg/100 mL D5W to be administered over 20 minutes.

4. Calculate how many capsules of Flomax the patient will receive from a unit dose of 0.4 mg/capsule.

5. Calculate how many tablets of Os-Cal the patient will receive from a unit dose of 1250 mg/tablet.

CASE STUDY 41   Left Total Knee Replacement

A patient is admitted to the hospital for a left total knee replacement. The orders from the physician include:

- Admit to Orthopedic Unit
- IV D5/LR with 20 mEq KCl 1000 mL every 8 hours
- CBC with differential, chemistry panel, and blood gases
- Cefazolin 1 g IV 1 hour prior to surgery and 500 mg every 8 hours post-operation
- Enoxaparin (Lovenox) 30 mg SQ daily
- Ferrous sulfate 0.3 g PO daily
- Docusate sodium 100 mg PO bid

Identify the orders that require calculations.

Set up and solve each problem using dimensional analysis.

1. Calculate mL/hr to set the IV pump.

2. Calculate mL/hr to set the IV pump to infuse cefazolin 1 g IV. Supply: cefazolin (Ancef) 1 g/100 mL D5W to be administered over 30 minutes.

3. Calculate mL/hr to set the IV pump to infuse cefazolin 500 mg IV. Supply: cefazolin (Ancef) 500 mg/50 mL D5W to be administered over 30 minutes.

4. Calculate how many mL of Lovenox the patient will receive SQ from a vial labeled enoxaparin 40 mg/0.4 mL.

5. Calculate how many tablets of ferrous sulfate the patient will receive from a unit dose of 300 mg/tablet.

CASE STUDY 42   Chest Pain

A patient is admitted to the hospital for chest pain. The orders from the physician include:

- Admit to intensive care unit (ICU)
- IV nitroglycerin 10 mcg/min and increase infusion rate by 10 mcg/min every 10 minutes until relief of pain (NTG 50 mg/250 mL D5W)
- CK/CKMB and Troponin I at 6 and 10 hours
- CBC, electrolytes, urea, creatinine, and ABGs
- O_2 per nasal cannula
- Accurate intake/output
- Chest x-ray
- ECG at 6 and 10 hours
- Vitals every 2 hours until stable and then every 4 hours
- ASA 160 mg PO × 1 (80-mg tablet)

- Morphine 2.5 mg IV administered every 5 minutes until pain subsides (up to a maximum of 20 mg can be given)

Identify the orders that require calculations.

Set up and solve each problem using dimensional analysis.

1. Calculate mL/hr to set the IV pump to infuse nitroglycerin 10 mcg/min. Supply: nitroglycerin 50 mg/250 mL D5W.

2. The patient is now receiving 15 mL/hr of nitroglycerin. How many mcg/min is the patient receiving?

3. Calculate how many tablets of ASA the patient will receive from a unit dose of 80 mg/tablet.

4. Calculate how many mL of morphine the patient will receive IV from a vial labeled morphine 5 mg/mL. Mix with 5 mL sterile water for injection and administer over 5 minutes.

5. The patient is still reporting pain at 8 on a scale of 1 to 10 and a third dose of morphine is to be given. Calculate how many mL of morphine the patient has now received with three doses.

CASE STUDY 43 Pneumococcal Meningitis

A child with pneumococcal meningitis is admitted to the hospital. The orders from the physician include:

- Admit to the Pediatric ICU
- CBC, electrolytes, urea, creatinine, liver enzymes, bilirubin, and urinalysis
- Vital signs every 2 hours until stable, then every 4 hours
- Daily weight (44 lb when admitted)
- Accurate intake/output
- IV 0.9% normal saline bolus 10 mL/kg followed by D5W/0.45% NS at 50 mL/hr
- Acetaminophen 15 mg/kg/dose PO every 4 hours prn for fever or mild pain
- Ceftriaxone (Rocephin) 50 mg/kg/dose IV every 12 hours three times, then every 24 hours
- Vancomycin 60 mg/kg/day IV divided in four equal doses every 6 hours

Identify the orders that require calculations.

Set up and solve each problem using dimensional analysis.

1. Calculate the weight of the child in kilograms.

2. Calculate how many mL the child will receive IV bolus.

3. Calculate how many mL/dose of acetaminophen the child will receive from a stock bottle of elixir labeled acetaminophen 80 mg/2.5 mL.

4. Calculate how many mg/dose of ceftriaxone the child will receive and then calculate mL/hr to set the IV pump to infuse ceftriaxone. Supply: Premixed IV Rocephin 1 g/50 mL to be administered over 30 minutes.

5. Calculate how many mg/dose of vancomycin the child will receive and then calculate mL/hr to set the IV pump to infuse vancomycin. Supply: Premixed IV vancomycin 500 mg/100 mL to be administered over 30 minutes.

CASE STUDY 44   Diabetic Ketoacidosis

A child is admitted to the hospital in diabetic ketoacidosis with dehydration and vomiting. The orders from the physician include:

- Admit to Pediatric ICU
- Blood sugar, electrolytes, urea, creatinine, CBC, HgA$_{1C}$, and urinalysis
- Vitals every 1 hour
- NPO
- Accurate intake/output
- Hourly blood glucose
- Weigh daily (54 lb when admitted)
- NS IV bolus 10 mL/kg
- NS IV 3.5 mL/kg/hr with KCl 20 mEq/L
- 25 units regular insulin/250 mL NS at 0.1 unit/kg/hr
- Ondansetron (Zofran) IV push 0.1 mg/kg over 2 minutes

Identify the orders that require calculations.

Set up and solve each problem using dimensional analysis.

1. Calculate the weight of the child in kilograms.

2. Calculate how many mL the child will receive IV bolus.

3. Calculate mL/hr to set the IV pump to infuse the IV NS with KCl 20 mEq/L.

4. Calculate mL/hr to set the IV pump to infuse regular insulin 0.1 unit/kg/hr. Supply: regular insulin 25 units/250 mL NS.

5. Calculate how many mL of ondansetron 0.1 mg/kg will be given IV push over 2 minutes. Supply: Zofran 2 mg/mL.

CASE STUDY 45   C-Section Delivery

An HIV+ patient is admitted to the hospital for C-section delivery. The orders from the physician include:

- Admit to OB in private room
- NPO
- Up ad lib
- CBC and electrolytes
- Type and crossmatch for 2 units of blood
- Admission weight 164 lb
- Lactated Ringers IV at 100 mL/hr
- Zidovudine 2 mg/kg IV over 1 hour on admission to labor and delivery then zidovudine 1 mg/kg/hr continuous IV infusion beginning 3 hours prior to C-section
- Cefazolin 1 g IVPB × 1 dose 1 hour prior to C-section
- Metoclopramide (Reglan) 10 mg IV push every 6 hours prn for nausea and vomiting
- Hydrocodone 5 mg and acetaminophen 325 mg PO two tablets every 4 hours prn for moderate to severe pain
- Docusate sodium 100 mg PO two capsules bid

Identify the orders that require calculations.

Set up and solve each problem using dimensional analysis.

1. Calculate the weight of the patient in kilograms.

2. Calculate how many mL/hr to set the IV pump to infuse zidovudine 2 mg/kg over 1 hour. Supply: Zidovudine 200 mg/50 mL D5W.

3. Calculate mL/hr to set the IV pump to infuse zidovudine 1 mg/kg/hr. Supply: zidovudine 400 mg/100 mL D5W.

4. Calculate mL/hr to set the IV pump to infuse cefazolin 1 g IV. Supply: cefazolin (Ancef) 1000 mg/100 mL D5W to be administered over 30 minutes.

5. Calculate how many mL of metoclopramide 10 mg will be given IV push over 2 minutes. Supply: Reglan 5 mg/mL.

CASE STUDY 46   Iron Deficiency Anemia

A pregnant teenager with iron deficiency anemia and hyperemesis gravidarum is seen in the nurse practitioner's office for her 2-month follow-up. The nurse practitioner's orders include:

- Hematocrit and hemoglobin
- RBC indices
- Serum electrolytes

- Serum iron and ferritin levels
- UA for ketones and specific gravity
- Ferrous sulfate 325 mg daily PO with food
- Ascorbic acid 1500 mg PO per day in three divided doses
- Folic acid (Folate) 400 mcg PO once daily
- Vitamin B6 25 mg PO three times daily
- Doxylamine 12.5 mg PO three times daily

Identify the orders that require calculations.

Set up and solve each problem using dimensional analysis.

1. Calculate how many tablets of ferrous sulfate the patient will be taking PO per dose. Supply: ferrous sulfate 325 mg coated tablets.

2. Calculate how many tablets of ascorbic acid the patient will be taking PO per dose. Supply: ascorbic acid 500 mg/tablet.

3. Calculate how many tablets of folic acid (Folate) the patient will be taking PO per dose. Supply: folic acid 0.4 mg/tablet.

4. Calculate how many tablets of vitamin B6 the patient will take PO per dose. Supply: vitamin B6 50 mg/scored tablet.

5. Calculate how many tablets of doxylamine the patient will be taking PO per dose. Supply: doxylamine 25 mg/scored tablet.

CASE STUDY 47   Lyme Disease

A 12-year-old boy returning from Boy Scouts Camp is admitted to the hospital with fever, rash, and headache. The hospitalist's orders include:

- ELISA
- Western blot testing if ELISA is positive
- ECG to rule out Lyme carditis
- CBS and sed rate
- UA
- Weight 40 kg
- IV 0.9% NS infusing at 100 mL/hr
- Ceftriaxone (Rocephin) 50 mg/kg/day (up to 2 g) in two divided doses every 12 hours IV
- Amoxicillin 25 mg/kg/day in two divided doses every 12 hours PO
- Accurate intake/output
- Encourage PO fluids
- Bed rest

Identify the orders that require calculations.

Set up and solve each problem using dimensional analysis.

1. Calculate the gtt/min using macrotubing (20 gtt/mL).

2. Calculate how many mg of ceftriaxone the child will receive per dose. Supply from pharmacy: ceftriaxone (Rocephin) 1 g in 100 mL.

3. Calculate the mL/hr to set the IV pump to infuse ceftriaxone. Supply from pharmacy: Ceftriaxone (Rocephin) 1 g in 100 mL to infuse over 30 minutes.

4. Calculate how many mg of amoxicillin the child will receive per day. Supply: amoxicillin 250 mg/5 mL suspension.

5. Calculate how many mL of amoxicillin the child will receive per dose. Supply: amoxicillin 250 mg/5 mL.

CASE STUDY 48   Infectious Mononucleosis

A female college student is seen by the nurse practitioner complaining of sore throat, fatigue, and low-grade fever. The nurse practitioner's orders include:

- Heterophile antibody test
- EBV serologic testing
- CBC
- Supportive care including rest during the acute phase
- Avoid heavy lifting or contact sports for 1 month to prevent splenic rupture
- Acyclovir (Zovirax) 400 mg PO tid for 10 days
- Prednisone 40 mg PO every 12 hours for a short-course 5-day burst
- Ibuprofen >102.5°F 400 mg PO every 6 hours prn not to exceed 3.2 g/day to alternate with acetaminophen 1000 mg PO every 8 hours prn not to exceed 4 g/day
- Encourage fluid intake to 2400 mL/day

Identify the orders that require calculations.

Set up and solve each problem using dimensional analysis.

1. Calculate how many capsules of Zovirax the patient will be taking daily PO per dose. Supply: acyclovir (Zovirax) 200 mg/capsule.

2. Calculate how many tablets of prednisone the patient will be taking PO per day. Supply: prednisone 20 mg/tablet.

3. Calculate how many tablets of ibuprofen you will give the patient PO per day. Supply: ibuprofen 200 mg/tablets.

4. Calculate how many tablets of acetaminophen the patient will be taking daily. Supply: Acetaminophen Extra Strength 500 mg/tablets.

5. Calculate how many mg of ibuprofen per day and how many mg of acetaminophen per day the patient is taking. Does this dosage fall within the
safe dosage range?
Supply: Ibuprofen 200 mg/tablets.
Supply: Acetaminophen Extra Strength 500 mg/tablets.

CASE STUDY 49   H1N1 Influenza (Swine Flu)

A 40-year-old man is admitted to the hospital 24 hours after onset of fever, cough,
sore throat, chills, fatigue, body aches, and headache. He reports that he did not
have time to get a flu shot this year. The hospitalist's orders include:

- Human Influenza Virus Real-Time RT-PCR Detection and Characterization
  Panel (rRT-PCR Flu Panel)
- CBC
- Serum electrolytes
- Chest x-ray to rule out pneumonia
- IV D5W/0.9 NS 1000 mL/8 hr
- O_2 at 2 L/min per nasal cannula
- Bed rest
- Accurate intake/output
- Encourage PO fluids to 2 L/day
- Oseltamivir (Tamiflu) 75 mg PO every 12 hours × 5 days (75-mg capsules)
- Acetaminophen 650 mg PO every 8 hours prn not to exceed 4 g/day
- Ibuprofen 400 mg PO for fever >102.5°F 400 mg PO every 6 hours prn not
  to exceed 3.2 g/day
- Promethazine with codeine 10 mg PO every 4 hours prn not to exceed
  30 mL/24 hr

Identify the orders that require calculations.

Set up and solve each problem using dimensional analysis.

1. Calculate the milliliters per hour to set the IV pump.

2. Calculate the total micrograms of oseltamivir the patient will be receiving over
   5 days.

3. Calculate how many tablets of acetaminophen the patient will be taking PO per
   dose. Supply: acetaminophen 325-mg tablets.

4. Calculate how many tablets of ibuprofen the patient will be taking PO per dose.
   Supply: ibuprofen 200-mg tablets.

5. Calculate how many milliliters of promethazine with codeine the patient will
   be taking PO per dose. Supply: promethazine with codeine 10 mg/5 mL.

CASE STUDY 50   Bronchiolitis

A 12-month-old boy is admitted to the hospital with a low-grade fever, congestion, profuse coryza, wheezing, and feeding difficulties. The hospitalist suspects respiratory syncytial virus (RSV). The hospitalist's orders include:

- WBC count and differential
- Serum electrolytes
- C-reactive protein
- Viral antigen testing of nasopharyngeal secretions
- Chest x-ray
- Monitor intake/output and specific gravity
- O_2 therapy nasal cannula if pulse oximetry is below 90%
- Albuterol nebulizer treatments every 4 hours
- Weight 20 kg
- IV therapy 500 mL 0.9% NS over 8 hours
- Unasyn 300 mg per kg of body weight per day administered via intravenous infusion in equally divided doses every 6 hours
- Acetaminophen 80 mg per dose PO every 6 hours (160 mg/5 mL infants suspension drops)

Identify the orders that require calculations.

Set up and solve each problem using dimensional analysis.

1. Calculate the milliliters per hour to set the IV pump.

2. Calculate how many milligrams of Unasyn the child will receive per dose every 6 hours.

3. How many milliliters per dose of Unasyn will the child receive every 6 hours? Supply: Unasyn 1.5 g/50 mL.

4. Calculate the milliliters per hour to set the IV pump to infuse the Unasyn. Supply: Unasyn 1.5 g/50 mL to infuse over 30 minutes.

5. Calculate how many milliliters of acetaminophen the child will receive per dose.

References

Davis Drug Guide for Nurses (14th ed.). F. A. Davis Company (2015).
GlobalRPh.com http://www.globalrph.com/
Medscape.com http://www.medscape.com/
Merck Manual online http://www.merck.com/mmpe/index.html
WebMD.com http://www.webmd.com/

ANSWER KEY FOR SECTION 3: CASE STUDIES

Case Study 1 — Congestive Heart Failure

Orders requiring calculations: IV of D5W/½ NS at 50 mL/hr; weight gain; furosemide 40 mg IV every day digoxin 0.125 mg PO qd; KCl 20 mEq PO tid

1

$$\frac{50 \text{ mL}}{\text{hr}} \left| \frac{60 \text{ gtt}}{\text{mL}} \right| \frac{1 \text{ hr}}{60 \text{ min}} \left| \frac{50 \times 1}{60} \right. = \frac{50}{\ } \frac{\text{gtt}}{\text{min}}$$

2

$$\frac{10 \text{ lb}}{\ } \left| \frac{1 \text{ kg}}{2.2 \text{ lb}} \right| \frac{10 \times 1}{2.2} \left| \frac{10}{2.2} \right. = 4.5 \text{ kg}$$

3

$$\frac{40 \text{ mg}}{\ } \left| \frac{\text{mL}}{10 \text{ mg}} \right| \frac{4}{1} = 4 \text{ mL}$$

4

$$\frac{0.125 \text{ mg}}{\ } \left| \frac{\text{tablet}}{0.25 \text{ mg}} \right| \frac{0.125}{0.25} = 0.5 \text{ tablet}$$

5

$$\frac{20 \text{ mEq}}{\ } \left| \frac{\text{tablet}}{10 \text{ mEq}} \right| \frac{2}{1} = 2 \text{ tablets}$$

Case Study 2 — COPD/Emphysema

Orders requiring calculations: IV of D5W/½ NS 1000 mL/8 hr; aminophylline IV loading dose of 5.6 mg/kg over 30 min followed by 0.5 mg/kg/hr continuous IV; erythromycin 800 mg IV every 6h; accurate intake/output.

1

$$\frac{1000 \text{ mL}}{8 \text{ hr}} \left| \frac{1000}{8} \right. = 125 \frac{\text{mL}}{\text{hr}}$$

2

$$\frac{5.6 \text{ mg}}{\text{kg/30 min}} \left| \frac{100 \text{ mL}}{100 \text{ mg}} \right| \frac{1 \text{ kg}}{2.2 \text{ lb}} \left| \frac{140 \text{ lb}}{\ } \right| \frac{60 \text{ min}}{1 \text{ hr}} \left| \frac{5.6 \times 140 \times 6}{3 \times 2.2} \right.$$

$$\frac{4704}{6.6} = 712.2 \frac{\text{mL}}{\text{hr}} \text{ or } 713 \frac{\text{mL}}{\text{hr}}$$

3

$$\frac{0.5 \text{ mg}}{\text{kg/hr}} \left| \frac{250 \text{ mL}}{\frac{1}{2} \text{ g}} \right| \frac{\frac{1}{2} \text{ g}}{1000 \text{ mg}} \left| \frac{1 \text{ kg}}{2.2 \text{ lb}} \right| \frac{140 \text{ lb}}{\ } \left| \frac{0.5 \times 25 \times 1 \times 14}{10 \times 2.2} \right.$$

$$\frac{175}{22} = 7.9 \frac{\text{mL}}{\text{hr}} \text{ or } 8 \frac{\text{mL}}{\text{hr}}$$

4

$$\frac{800 \text{ mg}}{\ } \left| \frac{20 \text{ mL}}{\frac{1}{2} \text{ g}} \right| \frac{\frac{1}{2} \text{ g}}{1000 \text{ mg}} \left| \frac{8 \times 2}{1} \right. = 16 \text{ mL}$$

$$\frac{266 \text{ mL}}{1 \text{ hr}} = \frac{266 \text{ mL}}{\text{hr}}$$

5

$$\frac{3 \text{ L}}{\text{day}} \left| \frac{\text{day}}{3 \text{ shifts}} \right| \frac{1000 \text{ mL}}{1 \text{ L}} \left| \frac{1000}{1} \right. = \frac{1000 \text{ mL}}{\text{shift}}$$

Case Study 3 — Small-Cell Lung Cancer

Orders requiring calculations: IV D5W/½ NS 1000 mL with 10 mEq KCl at 125 mL/hr; Neupogen 5 mcg/kg SQ daily; gentamicin 80 mg IV every 8h; Decadron 8 mg IV daily; Fortaz 1 g IV every 8h

1

$$\frac{125 \text{ mL}}{\text{hr}} \left| \frac{20 \text{ gtt}}{\text{mL}} \right| \frac{1 \text{ hr}}{60 \text{ min}} \left| \frac{125 \times 2 \times 1}{6} \right| \frac{250}{6} = 41.6 \text{ or } 42 \frac{\text{gtt}}{\text{min}}$$

2

$$\frac{5 \text{ mcg}}{\text{kg}} \left| \frac{1 \text{ kg}}{2.2 \text{ lb}} \right| \frac{160 \text{ lb}}{\ } \left| \frac{5 \times 1 \times 160}{2.2} \right| \frac{800}{2.2} = 363.6 \text{ mcg or } 364 \text{ mcg}$$

3

$$\frac{80 \text{ mg}}{\ } \left| \frac{\text{mL}}{40 \text{ mg}} \right| \frac{8}{4} = 2 \text{ mL}$$

$$\frac{100 \text{ mL}}{1 \text{ hr}} = \frac{100 \text{ mL}}{\text{hr}}$$

4

$$\frac{8 \text{ mg}}{\ } \left| \frac{\text{mL}}{4 \text{ mg}} \right| \frac{8}{4} = 2 \text{ mL}$$

5

$$\frac{50 \text{ mL}}{30 \text{ min}} \left| \frac{60 \text{ min}}{1 \text{ hr}} \right| \frac{50 \times 6}{3 \times 1} \left| \frac{300}{3} \right. = 100 \frac{\text{mL}}{\text{hr}}$$

Case Study 4 — Acquired Immunodeficiency Syndrome (AIDS)

Orders requiring calculations: IV D5W/$\frac{1}{2}$ NS at 150 mL/hr; acyclovir 350 mg IV every 8h; Neupogen 300 mcg SQ daily; Epogen 100 units/kg SQ three times a week; vancomycin 800 mg IV every 6h

1

$$\frac{150\ \text{mL}}{\text{hr}}\ \Big|\ \frac{20\ \text{gtt}}{\text{mL}}\ \Big|\ \frac{1\ \text{hr}}{60\ \text{min}}\ \Big|\ \frac{150\times2\times1}{6}=\frac{300}{6}=\frac{50}{}\ \frac{\text{gtt}}{\text{min}}$$

2

$$\frac{350\ \text{mg}}{}\ \Big|\ \frac{10\ \text{mL}}{500\ \text{mg}}\ \Big|\ \frac{35\times1}{5}=\frac{35}{5}=7\ \text{mL}$$

$$\frac{100\ \text{mL}}{1\ \text{hr}}\ \Big|\ \frac{100}{1}=\frac{100}{}\ \frac{\text{mL}}{\text{hr}}$$

3

$$\frac{300\ \text{mcg}}{}\ \Big|\ \frac{1\ \text{mL}}{300\ \text{mcg}}=1\ \text{mL}$$

4

$$\frac{100\ \text{units}}{\text{kg}}\ \Big|\ \frac{\text{mL}}{4000\ \text{units}}\ \Big|\ \frac{1\ \text{kg}}{2.2\ \text{lb}}\ \Big|\ \frac{100\ \text{lb}}{}\ \Big|\ \frac{10\times1\times1}{4\times2.2}=\frac{10}{8.8}=1.1\ \text{mL or 1 mL}$$

5

$$\frac{800\ \text{mg}}{}\ \Big|\ \frac{10\ \text{mL}}{1\ \text{g}}\ \Big|\ \frac{1\ \text{g}}{1000\ \text{mg}}\ \Big|\ \frac{8\times1}{10}=\frac{80}{10}=8\ \text{mL}$$

$$\frac{100\ \text{mL}}{60\ \text{min}}\ \Big|\ \frac{60\ \text{min}}{1\ \text{hr}}\ \Big|\ \frac{100}{1}=\frac{100}{}\ \frac{\text{mL}}{\text{hr}}$$

Case Study 5 — Sickle Cell Anemia

Orders requiring calculations: IV D5W/$\frac{1}{2}$ NS at 150 mL/hr; Zofran 8 mg IV every 8h; morphine sulfate 5 mg IV prn; Hydrea 10 mg/kg/day PO; folic acid 0.5 mg daily PO

1

$$\frac{150\ \text{mL}}{\text{hr}}\ \Big|\ \frac{10\ \text{gtt}}{\text{mL}}\ \Big|\ \frac{1\ \text{hr}}{60\ \text{min}}\ \Big|\ \frac{150\times1\times1}{6}=\frac{150}{6}=25\ \frac{\text{gtt}}{\text{min}}$$

2

$$\frac{50\ \text{mL}}{15\ \text{min}}\ \Big|\ \frac{60\ \text{min}}{1\ \text{hr}}\ \Big|\ \frac{50\times60}{15\times1}=\frac{3000}{15}=200\ \frac{\text{mL}}{\text{hr}}$$

3

$$\frac{5\ \text{mg}}{}\ \Big|\ \frac{\text{mL}}{10\ \text{mg}}\ \Big|\ \frac{5}{10}=0.5\ \text{mL}$$

Case Study 6 — Deep Vein Thrombosis

4

$$\frac{10\ \text{mg}}{\text{kg/day}}\ \Big|\ \frac{1\ \text{kg}}{2.2\ \text{lb}}\ \Big|\ \frac{125\ \text{lb}}{}\ \Big|\ \frac{10\times1\times125}{2.2}=\frac{1250}{2.2}=568\ \frac{\text{mg}}{\text{day}}$$

5

$$\frac{0.5\ \text{mg}}{}\ \Big|\ \frac{\text{tablet}}{1\ \text{mg}}\ \Big|\ \frac{0.5}{1}=0.5\ \text{tablet}$$

Orders requiring calculations: IV D5W/$\frac{1}{2}$ NS with 20 mEq KCl at 50 mL/hr; heparin 5000 units IV push followed by continuous IV infusion of 1000 units/hr; Lasix 20 mg IV bid; morphine 5 mg IV every 4h

1

$$\frac{50\ \text{mL}}{\text{hr}}\ \Big|\ \frac{60\ \text{gtt}}{\text{mL}}\ \Big|\ \frac{1\ \text{hr}}{60\ \text{min}}\ \Big|\ \frac{50\times1}{60}=\frac{50}{}=50\ \frac{\text{gtt}}{\text{min}}$$

2

$$\frac{5000\ \text{units}}{}\ \Big|\ \frac{\text{mL}}{10{,}000\ \text{units}}\ \Big|\ \frac{5}{10}=0.5\ \text{mL}$$

3

$$\frac{1000\ \text{units}}{\text{hr}}\ \Big|\ \frac{250\ \text{mL}}{25{,}000\ \text{units}}\ \Big|\ \frac{10}{}=\frac{10}{}\ \frac{\text{mL}}{\text{hr}}$$

4

$$\frac{20\ \text{mg}}{}\ \Big|\ \frac{\text{mL}}{10\ \text{mg}}\ \Big|\ \frac{2}{1}=2\ \text{mL}$$

5

$$\frac{5\ \text{mg}}{}\ \Big|\ \frac{\text{mL}}{10\ \text{mg}}\ \Big|\ \frac{5}{10}=0.5\ \text{mL}$$

Case Study 7 — Bone Marrow Transplant

Orders requiring calculations: IV D5W/$\frac{1}{2}$ NS with 20 mEq KCl/L at 80 mL/hr; Fortaz 2 g IV every 8h; vancomycin 1 g IV every 6h; Claforan 1 g IV every 12h; erythromycin 800 mg IV every 6h

1

$$\frac{80\ \text{mL}}{\text{hr}}\ \Big|\ \frac{20\ \text{mEq}}{1\ \text{L}}\ \Big|\ \frac{1\ \text{L}}{1000\ \text{mL}}\ \Big|\ \frac{8\times2}{10}=\frac{16}{10}=1.6\ \frac{\text{mEq}}{\text{hr}}$$

2

$$\frac{2\ \text{g}}{}\ \Big|\ \frac{10\ \text{mL}}{2\ \text{g}}\ \Big|\ \frac{10}{}=10\ \text{mL}$$

$$\frac{60\ \text{mL}}{30\ \text{min}}\ \Big|\ \frac{60\ \text{min}}{1\ \text{hr}}\ \Big|\ \frac{60\times6}{3\times1}=\frac{360}{3}=120\ \frac{\text{mL}}{\text{hr}}$$

3

$$\frac{\frac{1}{2}\,g}{} \left| \frac{10\,(mL)}{500\,mg} \right| \frac{1000\,mg}{\frac{1}{2}\,g} \left| \frac{10\times10}{5} \right| \frac{100}{5} = 20\,mL$$

$$\frac{120\,(mL)}{60\,min} \left| \frac{60\,min}{1\,(hr)} \right| \frac{120}{1} = 120\,\frac{mL}{hr}$$

4

$$\frac{\frac{1}{2}\,g}{} \left| \frac{4\,(mL)}{600\,mg} \right| \frac{1000\,mg}{\frac{1}{2}\,g} \left| \frac{4\times10}{6} \right| \frac{40}{6} = 6.7\,mL\ or\ 7\,mL$$

$$\frac{100\,(mL)}{1\,(hr)} \left| \frac{100}{1} \right. = 100\,\frac{mL}{hr}$$

5

$$\frac{800\,mg}{} \left| \frac{20\,(mL)}{\frac{1}{2}\,g} \right| \frac{\frac{1}{2}\,g}{1000\,mg} \left| \frac{8\times2}{1} \right| \frac{16}{1} = 16\,mL$$

$$\frac{266\,(mL)}{60\,min} \left| \frac{60\,min}{1\,(hr)} \right| \frac{266}{1} = 266\,\frac{mL}{hr}$$

Case Study 8   Pneumonia

Orders requiring calculations: clindamycin 400 mg IV every 6h; guaifenesin 200 mg PO every 4h; terbutaline 2.5 mg PO tid; MS Contin 30 mg PO every 4h prn

1

$$\frac{400\,mg}{} \left| \frac{4\,(mL)}{600\,mg} \right| \frac{4\times4}{6} \left| \frac{16}{6} \right. = 2.7\,mL\ or\ 3\,mL$$

$$\frac{53\,(mL)}{(hr)} \left| \frac{53}{} \right. = 53\,\frac{mL}{hr}$$

2

$$\frac{53\,mL}{hr} \left| \frac{20\,(gtt)}{mL} \right| \frac{1\,hr}{60\,(min)} \left| \frac{53\times2\times1}{6} \right| \frac{106}{6} = 18\,\frac{gtt}{min}$$

3

$$\frac{200\,mg}{30\,mg} \left| \frac{tsp}{1\,tsp} \right| \frac{5\,(mL)}{3\times1} \left| \frac{20\times5}{3} \right| \frac{100}{3} = 33\,mL$$

4

$$\frac{2.5\,mg}{5\,mg} \left| \frac{(tablet)}{5} \right| \frac{2.5}{5} = 0.5\,tablet$$

5

$$\frac{30\,mg}{30\,mg} \left| \frac{(tablet)}{30} \right| \frac{30}{30} = 1\,tablet$$

Case Study 9   Pain

Orders requiring calculations: IV D5W/$\frac{1}{2}$ NS with 20 mEq KCl/L at 60 mL/hr; IV 500 mL NS with 25 mg Dilaudid and 50 mg Thorazine at 21 mL/hr; Bumex 2 mg IV every AM after albumin infusion

1

$$\frac{60\,mL}{(hr)} \left| \frac{20\,(mEq)}{1\,L} \right| \frac{1\,L}{1000\,mL} \left| \frac{6\times2}{10} \right| \frac{12}{10} = 1.2\,\frac{mEq}{hr}$$

2

$$\frac{21\,mL}{(hr)} \left| \frac{25\,(mg)}{500\,mL} \right| \frac{21\times25}{500} \left| \frac{525}{500} \right. = 1.05\,\frac{mg}{hr}$$

3

$$\frac{21\,mL}{(hr)} \left| \frac{50\,(mg)}{500\,mL} \right| \frac{21\times5}{50} \left| \frac{105}{50} \right. = 2.1\,\frac{mg}{hr}$$

4

$$\frac{11\,mL}{(hr)} \left| \frac{25,000\,(units)}{250\,mL} \right| \frac{11\times2500}{25} \left| \frac{27,500}{25} \right. = 1100\,\frac{units}{hr}$$

5

$$\frac{2\,mg}{} \left| \frac{(mL)}{0.25\,mg} \right| \frac{2}{0.25} = 8\,mL$$

Case Study 10   Cirrhosis

Orders requiring calculations: IV D5W/$\frac{1}{2}$ NS with 20 mEq KCl at 125 mL/hr; IV Zantac 150 mg/250 mL NS at 11 mL/hr; vitamin K 10 mg SQ every AM; Spironolactone 50 mg PO bid; Lasix 80 mg IV every AM

1

$$\frac{125\,mL}{hr} \left| \frac{20\,(gtt)}{mL} \right| \frac{1\,hr}{60\,(min)} \left| \frac{125\times2\times1}{6} \right| \frac{250}{6} = 41.66\ or\ 42\,\frac{gtt}{min}$$

2

$$\frac{11\,mL}{(hr)} \left| \frac{150\,(mg)}{250\,mL} \right| \frac{11\times15}{25} \left| \frac{165}{25} \right. = 6.6\,\frac{mg}{hr}$$

3

$$\frac{10\,mg}{10\,mg} \left| \frac{(mL)}{10} \right| \frac{10}{10} = 1\,mL$$

4

$$\frac{50\,mg}{25\,mg} \left| \frac{(tablet)}{25} \right| \frac{50}{25} = 2\,tablets$$

5

$$\frac{80\,mg}{10\,mg} \left| \frac{(mL)}{1} \right| \frac{8}{1} = 8\,mL$$

Case Study 11 Hyperemesis Gravidarum

Orders requiring calculations: IV D5½ NS at 150 mL/hr and 100 mL/hr; droperidol (Inapsine) 1 mg IV; metoclopramide (Reglan) 20 mg IV in 50 mL of D5W to infuse over 15 min; diphenhydramine (Benadryl) 25 mg; dexamethasone (Decadron) 4 mg IV

1

$$\frac{150 \text{ mL}}{\text{hr}} \left| \frac{20 \text{ gtt}}{\text{mL}} \right| \frac{1 \text{ hr}}{60 \text{ min}} \left| \frac{150 \times 2 \times 1}{6} \right| \frac{300}{6} = \frac{50}{\text{min}} \frac{\text{gtt}}{\text{min}}$$

$$\frac{100 \text{ mL}}{\text{hr}} \left| \frac{20 \text{ gtt}}{\text{mL}} \right| \frac{1 \text{ hr}}{60 \text{ min}} \left| \frac{100 \times 2 \times 1}{6} \right| \frac{200}{6} = 33.3 \text{ or } 33 \frac{\text{gtt}}{\text{min}}$$

2

$$\frac{1 \text{ mg}}{} \left| \frac{\text{mL}}{2.5 \text{ mg}} \right| \frac{1}{2.5} = 0.4 \text{ mL}$$

3

$$\frac{50 \text{ mL}}{15 \text{ min}} \left| \frac{60 \text{ min}}{1 \text{ hr}} \right| \frac{50 \times 60}{15 \times 1} \left| \frac{3000}{15} \right| = 200 \frac{\text{mL}}{\text{hr}}$$

4

$$\frac{25 \text{ mg}}{} \left| \frac{\text{mL}}{10 \text{ mg}} \right| \frac{25}{10} = 2.5 \text{ mL}$$

5

$$\frac{4 \text{ mg}}{} \left| \frac{\text{mL}}{4 \text{ mg}} \right| \frac{4}{4} = 1 \text{ mL}$$

Case Study 12 Preeclampsia

Orders requiring calculations: methyldopa (Aldomet) 250 mg; hydralazine (Apresoline) 5 mg IV; magnesium sulfate 4 g in 250 mL D5W loading dose to infuse over 30 min; magnesium sulfate 40 g in 1000 mL LR to infuse at 1 g/hr; nifedipine (Procardia) 10 mg sublingual

1

$$\frac{250 \text{ mg}}{} \left| \frac{\text{tablet}}{500 \text{ mg}} \right| \frac{25}{50} = 0.5 \text{ tablet}$$

2

$$\frac{5 \text{ mg}}{} \left| \frac{\text{mL}}{20 \text{ mg}} \right| \frac{5}{20} = 0.25 \text{ mL}$$

3

$$\frac{250 \text{ mL}}{30 \text{ min}} \left| \frac{60 \text{ min}}{1 \text{ hr}} \right| \frac{250 \times 6}{3 \times 1} \left| \frac{1500}{3} \right| = 500 \frac{\text{mL}}{\text{hr}}$$

4

$$\frac{1 \text{ g}}{\text{hr}} \left| \frac{1000 \text{ mL}}{40 \text{ g}} \right| \frac{1 \times 100}{4} \left| \frac{100}{4} \right| = 25 \frac{\text{mL}}{\text{hr}}$$

5

$$\frac{10 \text{ mg}}{} \left| \frac{\text{capsule}}{10 \text{ mg}} \right| \frac{10}{10} = 1 \text{ capsule}$$

Case Study 13 Premature Labor

Orders requiring calculations: magnesium sulfate at 2 g/hr; terbutaline (Brethine) 0.25 mg SQ; nifedipine (Procardia) 20 mg; betamethasone 12 mg IM; LR 1000 mL over 8 hr

1

$$\frac{250 \text{ mL}}{20 \text{ min}} \left| \frac{60 \text{ min}}{1 \text{ hr}} \right| \frac{250 \times 6}{2 \times 1} \left| \frac{1500}{2} \right| = 750 \frac{\text{mL}}{\text{hr}}$$

$$\frac{2 \text{ g}}{\text{hr}} \left| \frac{250 \text{ mL}}{4 \text{ g}} \right| \frac{2 \times 250}{4} \left| \frac{500}{4} \right| = 125 \frac{\text{mL}}{\text{hr}}$$

2

$$\frac{0.25 \text{ mg}}{} \left| \frac{\text{mL}}{1 \text{ mg}} \right| \frac{0.25}{1} = 0.25 \text{ mL}$$

3

$$\frac{20 \text{ mg}}{} \left| \frac{\text{capsule}}{10 \text{ mg}} \right| \frac{2}{1} = 2 \text{ capsules}$$

4

$$\frac{12 \text{ mg}}{} \left| \frac{\text{mL}}{6 \text{ mg}} \right| \frac{12}{6} = 2 \text{ mL}$$

5

$$\frac{1000 \text{ mL}}{8 \text{ hr}} \left| \frac{1000}{8} \right| = 125 \frac{\text{mL}}{\text{hr}}$$

Case Study 14 Cystic Fibrosis

Orders requiring calculations: IV 0.9% normal saline at 75 mL/hr; Tagamet 30 mg PO; clindamycin 10 mg/kg IV; terbutaline 2.5 mg PO; tobramycin 1.5 mg/kg IV

1

$$\frac{75 \text{ mL}}{\text{hr}} \left| \frac{15 \text{ gtt}}{\text{mL}} \right| \frac{1 \text{ hr}}{60 \text{ min}} \left| \frac{75 \times 15 \times 1}{60} \right| \frac{1125}{60} = 18.75 \text{ or } 19 \frac{\text{gtt}}{\text{min}}$$

2

$$\frac{30 \text{ mg}}{\text{kg/day}} \left| \frac{\text{tablet}}{200 \text{ mg}} \right| \frac{1 \text{ kg}}{2.2 \text{ lb}} \left| \frac{65 \text{ lb}}{} \right| \frac{\text{day}}{4 \text{ doses}} \left| \frac{3 \times 1 \times 65}{20 \times 2.2 \times 4} \right| \frac{195}{176} = 1.1 \text{ or } 1 \frac{\text{tablet}}{\text{dose}}$$

3

$$\frac{10 \ \boxed{mg}}{kg} \left| \frac{1 \ kg}{2.2 \ lb} \right| \frac{65 \ lb}{} \left| \frac{10 \times 1 \times 65}{2.2} \right| \frac{650}{2.2} = 295.45 \text{ or } 295 \text{ mg}$$

$$\frac{295 \ mg}{} \left| \frac{\boxed{mL}}{150 \ mg} \right| \frac{295}{150} = 1.96 \text{ or } 2 \text{ mL}$$

$$\frac{50 \ \boxed{mL}}{20 \ min} \left| \frac{60 \ min}{1 \ \boxed{hr}} \right| \frac{50 \times 6}{2 \times 1} \left| \frac{300}{2} \right| = \frac{150}{hr} \text{ mL}$$

4

$$\frac{2.5 \ mg}{} \left| \frac{\boxed{tablet}}{2.5 \ mg} \right| \frac{2.5}{2.5} = 1 \text{ tablet}$$

5

$$\frac{1.5 \ \boxed{mg}}{kg} \left| \frac{1 \ kg}{2.2 \ lb} \right| \frac{65 \ lb}{} \left| \frac{1.5 \times 1 \times 65}{2.2} \right| \frac{97.5}{2.2} = 44.31 \text{ or } 44 \text{ mg}$$

$$\frac{44 \ mg}{} \left| \frac{\boxed{mL}}{40 \ mg} \right| \frac{44}{40} = 1.1 \text{ or } 1 \text{ mL}$$

$$\frac{50 \ \boxed{mL}}{30 \ min} \left| \frac{60 \ min}{1 \ \boxed{hr}} \right| \frac{50 \times 6}{3 \times 1} \left| \frac{300}{3} \right| = \frac{100}{hr} \text{ mL}$$

Case Study 15 — Respiratory Syncytial Virus (RSV)

Orders requiring calculations: acetaminophen elixir 120 mg PO; aminophylline 5 mg/kg to infuse over 30 min and 0.8 mg/kg/hr IV; RespiGam 750 mg/kg IV; Pediapred 1.5 mg/kg/day in three divided doses PO; ampicillin 100 mg/kg/day in divided doses every 6h IV

1

$$\frac{120 \ mg}{} \left| \frac{5 \ \boxed{mL}}{120 \ mg} \right| \frac{5}{} = 5 \text{ mL}$$

2

$$\frac{5 \ \boxed{mg}}{kg} \left| \frac{1 \ kg}{2.2 \ lb} \right| \frac{30 \ lb}{} \left| \frac{5 \times 1 \times 30}{2.2} \right| \frac{150}{2.2} = 68.18 \text{ or } 68.2 \text{ mg}$$

$$\frac{68.2 \ mg}{30 \ min} \left| \frac{100 \ \boxed{mL}}{250 \ mg} \right| \frac{60 \ min}{1 \ \boxed{hr}} \left| \frac{68.2 \times 10 \times 6}{3 \times 25 \times 1} \right| \frac{4092}{75} = \frac{54.56 \text{ or } 54.6}{hr} \text{ mL}$$

$$\frac{0.8 \ mg}{kg \ \boxed{hr}} \left| \frac{100 \ \boxed{mL}}{250 \ mg} \right| \frac{1 \ kg}{2.2 \ lb} \left| \frac{30 \ lb}{} \right| \frac{0.8 \times 100 \times 1 \times 3}{25 \times 2.2} \left| \frac{240}{55} \right| = \frac{4.36 \text{ or } 4.4}{hr} \text{ mL}$$

3

$$\frac{750 \ \boxed{mg}}{kg} \left| \frac{1 \ kg}{2.2 \ lb} \right| \frac{30 \ lb}{} \left| \frac{750 \times 1 \times 30}{2.2} \right| \frac{22,500}{2.2} = \frac{10,227.27}{\text{or } 10,227.3 \text{ mg}}$$

4

$$\frac{1.5 \ mg}{kg/day} \left| \frac{5 \ \boxed{mL}}{15 \ mg} \right| \frac{1 \ kg}{2.2 \ lb} \left| \frac{30 \ lb}{} \right| \frac{day}{3 \ \boxed{doses}} \left| \frac{1.5 \times 5 \times 1 \times 30}{15 \times 2.2 \times 3} \right| \frac{225}{99} = \frac{2.27 \text{ or } 2.3 \text{ mL}}{hr}$$

5

$$\frac{100 \ \boxed{mg}}{kg/day} \left| \frac{1 \ kg}{2.2 \ lb} \right| \frac{30 \ lb}{} \left| \frac{day}{4 \ \boxed{doses}} \right| \frac{100 \times 1 \times 30}{2.2 \times 4} \left| \frac{3000}{8.8} \right| = \frac{340.9 \text{ or } 341 \text{ mg}}{dose}$$

$$\frac{341 \ mg}{} \left| \frac{10 \ \boxed{mL}}{1 \ g} \right| \frac{1 \ g}{1000 \ mg} \left| \frac{341 \times 1 \times 1}{1 \times 100} \right| \frac{341}{100} = 3.41 \text{ or } 3.4 \text{ mL}$$

$$\frac{50 \ \boxed{mL}}{30 \ min} \left| \frac{60 \ min}{1 \ \boxed{hr}} \right| \frac{50 \times 6}{3 \times 1} \left| \frac{300}{3} \right| = \frac{100}{hr} \text{ mL}$$

Case Study 16 — Leukemia

Orders requiring calculations: IV D5W/NS with 20 mEq KCl 1000 mL over 8 h; allopurinol 200 mg PO; Fortaz 1 g IV; aztreonam 2 g IV; Flagyl 500 mg IV

1

$$\frac{1000 \ \boxed{mL}}{8 \ \boxed{hr}} \left| \frac{1000}{8} \right| = \frac{125}{hr} \text{ mL}$$

2

$$\frac{200 \ mg}{} \left| \frac{\boxed{tablet}}{100 \ mg} \right| \frac{2}{1} = 2 \text{ tablets}$$

3

$$\frac{1 \ g}{} \left| \frac{10 \ \boxed{mL}}{1 \ g} \right| = 10 \text{ mL}$$

$$\frac{60 \ \boxed{mL}}{30 \ min} \left| \frac{60 \ min}{1 \ \boxed{hr}} \right| \frac{60 \times 6}{3 \times 1} \left| \frac{360}{3} \right| = \frac{120}{hr} \text{ mL}$$

4

$$\frac{2 \ g}{} \left| \frac{10 \ \boxed{mL}}{2 \ g} \right| = 10 \text{ mL}$$

$$\frac{110 \ \boxed{mL}}{60 \ min} \left| \frac{60 \ min}{1 \ \boxed{hr}} \right| \frac{110}{1} = \frac{110}{hr} \text{ mL}$$

5

$$\frac{500 \ mg}{1 \ \boxed{hr}} \left| \frac{100 \ \boxed{mL}}{500 \ mg} \right| \frac{100}{1} = \frac{100}{hr} \text{ mL}$$

Case Study 17   Sepsis

Orders requiring calculations: NG breast milk with sterile water 120 mL per feeding; IV D10 and 20% lipids 120 mL/kg/day; aminophylline 5 mg/kg IV every 6h; cefotaxime 50 mg/kg every 12h; vancomycin 10 mg/kg/dose every 12h

1

$$\frac{120 \text{ mL}}{\text{day}} \cdot \frac{\text{day}}{24 \text{ hr}} \cdot \frac{3 \text{ hr}}{\text{feeding}} = \frac{120 \times 3}{24} = \frac{360}{24} = 15 \frac{\text{mL}}{\text{feeding}}$$

2

$$\frac{120 \text{ mL}}{\text{kg/day}} \cdot \frac{\text{day}}{24 \text{ hr}} \cdot \frac{1 \text{ kg}}{1000 \text{ g}} \cdot \frac{2005 \text{ g}}{} = \frac{12 \times 1 \times 2005}{24 \times 100} = \frac{24{,}060}{2400} = 10.025 \text{ or } 10 \frac{\text{mL}}{\text{hr}}$$

3

$$\frac{5 \text{ mg}}{\text{kg}} \cdot \frac{1 \text{ kg}}{1000 \text{ g}} \cdot \frac{2005 \text{ g}}{} = \frac{5 \times 1 \times 2005}{1000} = \frac{10025}{1000} = 10.025 \text{ or } 10 \text{ mg}$$

$$\frac{10 \text{ mg}}{5 \text{ min}} \cdot \frac{10 \text{ mL}}{50 \text{ mg}} \cdot \frac{60 \text{ min}}{1 \text{ hr}} = \frac{10 \times 10 \times 6}{5 \times 5 \times 1} = \frac{600}{25} = 24 \frac{\text{mL}}{\text{hr}}$$

4

$$\frac{50 \text{ mg}}{\text{kg}} \cdot \frac{1 \text{ kg}}{1000 \text{ g}} \cdot \frac{2005 \text{ g}}{} = \frac{5 \times 1 \times 2005}{100} = \frac{10025}{100} = 100.25 \text{ or } 100 \text{ mg}$$

$$\frac{100 \text{ mg}}{30 \text{ min}} \cdot \frac{\text{mL}}{40 \text{ mg}} \cdot \frac{60 \text{ min}}{1 \text{ hr}} = \frac{10 \times 6}{3 \times 4 \times 1} = \frac{60}{12} = 5 \frac{\text{mL}}{\text{hr}}$$

5

$$\frac{10 \text{ mg}}{\text{kg/dose}} \cdot \frac{1 \text{ kg}}{1000 \text{ g}} \cdot \frac{2005 \text{ g}}{} = \frac{1 \times 1 \times 2005}{100} = \frac{2005}{100} = 20.05 \text{ or } 20 \frac{\text{mg}}{\text{dose}}$$

$$\frac{20 \text{ mg}}{1 \text{ hr}} \cdot \frac{1 \text{ mL}}{5 \text{ mg}} = \frac{20 \times 1}{1 \times 5} = \frac{20}{5} = 4 \frac{\text{mL}}{\text{hr}}$$

Case Study 18   Bronchopulmonary Dysplasia

Orders requiring calculations: NG feedings with Special Care with Iron 120 KCal/kg/day; chlorothiazide 10 mg/kg/day; Fer-In-Sol 2 mg/kg/day; vitamin E 25 units/kg/day in divided doses every 12h; caffeine citrate 5 mg/kg/dose daily

1

$$\frac{120 \text{ kcal}}{\text{kg/day}} \cdot \frac{1 \text{ kg}}{1000 \text{ g}} \cdot \frac{996 \text{ g}}{} = \frac{12 \times 1 \times 996}{100} = \frac{11{,}952}{100} = 119.52 \text{ or } 120 \frac{\text{kcal}}{\text{day}}$$

$$\frac{120 \text{ kcal}}{\text{day}} \cdot \frac{\text{oz}}{24 \text{ kcal}} \cdot \frac{30 \text{ mL}}{1 \text{ oz}} = \frac{120 \times 30}{24 \times 1} = \frac{3600}{24} = 150 \frac{\text{mL}}{\text{day}}$$

2

$$\frac{10 \text{ mg}}{\text{kg/day}} \cdot \frac{1 \text{ kg}}{1000 \text{ g}} \cdot \frac{996 \text{ g}}{} = \frac{1 \times 1 \times 996}{100} = \frac{996}{100} = 9.96 \text{ or } 10 \frac{\text{mg}}{\text{day}}$$

$$\frac{10 \text{ mg}}{\text{day}} \cdot \frac{5 \text{ mL}}{250 \text{ mg}} = \frac{1 \times 5}{25} = \frac{5}{25} = 0.2 \frac{\text{mL}}{\text{day}}$$

3

$$\frac{2 \text{ mg}}{\text{kg/day}} \cdot \frac{1 \text{ kg}}{1000 \text{ g}} \cdot \frac{996 \text{ g}}{} = \frac{2 \times 1 \times 996}{1000} = \frac{1992}{1000} = 1.99 \text{ or } 2 \frac{\text{mg}}{\text{day}}$$

$$\frac{2 \text{ mg}}{\text{day}} \cdot \frac{0.6 \text{ mL}}{15 \text{ mg}} = \frac{2 \times 0.6}{15} = \frac{1.2}{15} = 0.08 \frac{\text{mL}}{\text{day}}$$

4

$$\frac{25 \text{ units}}{\text{kg/day}} \cdot \frac{1 \text{ kg}}{1000 \text{ g}} \cdot \frac{996 \text{ g}}{} \cdot \frac{\text{day}}{2 \text{ doses}} = \frac{25 \times 1 \times 996}{1000 \times 2} = \frac{24{,}900}{2000} = 12.45 \text{ or } 12.5 \frac{\text{units}}{\text{dose}}$$

$$\frac{12.5 \text{ units}}{\text{dose}} \cdot \frac{\text{mL}}{67 \text{ units}} = \frac{12.5}{67} = 0.18 \text{ or } 0.2 \frac{\text{mL}}{\text{dose}}$$

5

$$\frac{5 \text{ mg}}{\text{kg/day}} \cdot \frac{1 \text{ kg}}{1000 \text{ g}} \cdot \frac{996 \text{ g}}{} = \frac{5 \times 1 \times 996}{1000} = \frac{4980}{1000} = 4.98 \text{ or } 5 \frac{\text{mg}}{\text{day}}$$

$$\frac{1.2 \text{ mg}}{\text{dose}} \cdot \frac{\text{mL}}{10 \text{ mg}} = \frac{1.2}{10} = 0.12 \text{ or } 0.1 \frac{\text{mL}}{\text{dose}}$$

Case Study 19   Cerebral Palsy

Orders requiring calculations: Lactulose 3 g PO tid; Depakote 30 mg/kg/day PO in three divided doses; diazapam 2.5 mg PO daily; chlorothiazide 250 mg PO daily; Dilantin 5 mg/kg/day PO in three divided doses

1

$$\frac{3 \text{ g}}{} \cdot \frac{15 \text{ mL}}{10 \text{ g}} = \frac{3 \times 15}{10} = \frac{45}{10} = 4.5 \text{ or } 5 \text{ mL}$$

2

$$\frac{30 \text{ mg}}{\text{kg/day}} \cdot \frac{38 \text{ kg}}{} \cdot \frac{\text{day}}{3 \text{ doses}} = \frac{30 \times 38}{3} = \frac{1140}{3} = 380 \frac{\text{mg}}{\text{dose}}$$

$$\frac{380 \text{ mg}}{} \cdot \frac{\text{tablet}}{125 \text{ mg}} = \frac{380}{125} = 3.04 \text{ or } 3 \text{ tablets}$$

3

$$\frac{2.5 \text{ mg}}{} \cdot \frac{\text{tablet}}{5 \text{ mg}} = \frac{2.5}{5} = 0.5 \text{ tablet}$$

4

$$\frac{250 \text{ mg}}{} \left| \frac{\text{tablet}}{250 \text{ mg}} \right| \frac{250}{250} = 1 \text{ tablet}$$

5

$$\frac{5 \text{ mg}}{\text{kg/day}} \left| \frac{38 \text{ kg}}{} \right| \frac{\text{day}}{3 \text{ dose}} \left| \frac{5 \text{ mL}}{125 \text{ mg}} \right| \frac{5 \times 38 \times 5}{3 \times 125} \left| \frac{950}{375} = 2.53 \text{ or } 2.5 \frac{\text{mL}}{\text{dose}} \right.$$

Case Study 20   Hyperbilirubinemia

Orders requiring calculations: albumin 5% infusion 1 g/kg 1 hr before exchange; ampicillin 100 mg/kg/dose IV every 12h; gentamicin 2.5 mg/kg/dose IV every 12h; 120 mL/kg/day formula; IV D10W 120 mL/kg/day

1

$$\frac{1 \text{ g}}{\text{kg}} \left| \frac{1 \text{ kg}}{1000 \text{ g}} \right| \frac{2210 \text{ g}}{} \left| \frac{1 \times 1 \times 221}{100} \right| \frac{221}{100} = 2.21 \text{ or } 2.2 \text{ g}$$

2

$$\frac{100 \text{ mg}}{\text{kg/dose}} \left| \frac{1 \text{ kg}}{1000 \text{ g}} \right| \frac{2210 \text{ g}}{} \left| \frac{1 \times 221}{1} \right| \frac{221}{1} = 221 \frac{\text{mg}}{\text{dose}}$$

$$\frac{221 \text{ mg}}{} \left| \frac{5 \text{ mL}}{250 \text{ mg}} \right| \frac{221 \times 5}{250} \left| \frac{1105}{250} = 4.42 \text{ or } 4.4 \text{ mL} \right.$$

3

$$\frac{4 \text{ mg}}{\text{kg/dose}} \left| \frac{1 \text{ kg}}{1000 \text{ g}} \right| \frac{2210 \text{ g}}{} \left| \frac{4 \times 1 \times 221}{100} \right| \frac{884}{100} = 8.84 \text{ or } 8.8 \frac{\text{mg}}{\text{dose}}$$

$$\frac{8.8 \text{ mg}}{} \left| \frac{\text{mL}}{2 \text{ mg}} \right| \frac{8.8}{2} = 4.4 \text{ mL}$$

4

$$\frac{120 \text{ mL}}{\text{kg/day}} \left| \frac{1 \text{ kg}}{1000 \text{ g}} \right| \frac{2210 \text{ g}}{} \left| \frac{12 \times 1 \times 221}{10} \right| \frac{2652}{10} = 265.2 \text{ or } 265 \frac{\text{mL}}{\text{day}}$$

5

$$\frac{120 \text{ mL}}{\text{kg/day}} \left| \frac{1 \text{ kg}}{1000 \text{ g}} \right| \frac{2210 \text{ g}}{} \left| \frac{\text{day}}{24 \text{ hr}} \right| \frac{12 \times 1 \times 221}{10 \times 24} \left| \frac{2652}{240} = 11.05 \text{ or } 11 \frac{\text{mL}}{\text{hr}} \right.$$

Case Study 21   Spontaneous Abortion

Orders requiring calculations: Rhogam 300 mcg IM; IV D5/0.9% NS at 100 mL/hr; oxytocin (Pitocin) 10 units infused at 20 mL/min; meperidine 50 mg IM every 4h; ibuprofen 400 mg PO

1

$$\frac{300 \text{ mcg}}{} \left| \frac{1 \text{ mL}}{300 \text{ mcg}} \right| \frac{1}{} = 1 \text{ mL}$$

2

$$\frac{100 \text{ mL}}{\text{hr}} \left| \frac{15 \text{ gtt}}{\text{mL}} \right| \frac{1 \text{ hr}}{60 \text{ min}} \left| \frac{10 \times 15 \times 1}{6} \right| \frac{150}{6} = 25 \frac{\text{gtt}}{\text{min}}$$

3

$$\frac{20 \text{ mU}}{\text{min}} \left| \frac{500 \text{ mL}}{10 \text{ U}} \right| \frac{1 \text{ U}}{1000 \text{ mU}} \left| \frac{60 \text{ min}}{1 \text{ hr}} \right| \frac{2 \times 5 \times 1 \times 6}{1 \times 1 \times 1} \left| \frac{60}{1} = 60 \frac{\text{mL}}{\text{hr}} \right.$$

4

$$\frac{50 \text{ mg}}{} \left| \frac{\text{mL}}{100 \text{ mg}} \right| \frac{5}{10} = 0.5 \text{ mL}$$

5

$$\frac{400 \text{ mg}}{} \left| \frac{\text{tablet}}{200 \text{ mg}} \right| \frac{4}{2} = 2 \text{ tablets}$$

Case Study 22   Bipolar Disorder

Orders requiring calculations: IV 0.9% NS at 75 mL/hr; lithium 300 mg, lithium 300 mg; clonazepam 0.5 mg; clonazepam 1 mg; doxepin 50 mg

1

$$\frac{75 \text{ mL}}{\text{hr}} \left| \frac{20 \text{ gtt}}{\text{mL}} \right| \frac{1 \text{ hr}}{60 \text{ min}} \left| \frac{75 \times 2 \times 1}{6} \right| \frac{150}{6} = 25 \frac{\text{gtt}}{\text{min}}$$

2

$$\frac{300 \text{ mg}}{} \left| \frac{\text{capsule}}{150 \text{ mg}} \right| \frac{30}{15} = 2 \text{ capsules}$$

3

$$\frac{0.5 \text{ mg}}{} \left| \frac{\text{tablet}}{0.5 \text{ mg}} \right| \frac{0.5}{0.5} = 1 \text{ tablet}$$

4

$$\frac{1 \text{ mg}}{} \left| \frac{\text{tablet}}{0.5 \text{ mg}} \right| \frac{1}{0.5} = 2 \text{ tablets}$$

5

$$\frac{50 \text{ mg}}{} \left| \frac{\text{tablet}}{25 \text{ mg}} \right| \frac{50}{25} = 2 \text{ tablets}$$

Case Study 23   Anorexia Nervosa

Orders requiring calculations: IV 1000 mL/8 hr; olanzapine (Zyprexa) 10 mg; fluoxetine (Prozac) 60 mg/day; amitriptyline 25 mg; cyproheptadine 32 mg/day

1

$$\frac{1000 \text{ mL}}{8 \text{ hr}} = 125 \frac{\text{mL}}{\text{hr}}$$

2

$$\frac{10 \text{ mg}}{} \left| \frac{\text{tablets}}{5 \text{ mg}} \right| \frac{10}{5} = 2 \text{ tablets}$$

3

$$\frac{60 \text{ mg}}{} \left| \frac{5 \text{ mL}}{20 \text{ mg}} \right| \frac{6 \times 5}{2} \left| \frac{30}{2} \right. = 15 \text{ mL}$$

4

$$\frac{25 \text{ mg}}{} \left| \frac{5 \text{ mL}}{10 \text{ mg}} \right| \frac{25 \times 5}{10} \left| \frac{125}{10} \right. = 12.5 \text{ mL}$$

5

$$\frac{32 \text{ mg}}{\text{day}} \left| \frac{\text{day}}{4 \text{ doses}} \right. = \frac{8 \text{ mg}}{\text{dose}}$$

$$\frac{8 \text{ mg}}{} \left| \frac{5 \text{ mL}}{2 \text{ mg}} \right| \frac{8 \times 5}{2} \left| \frac{40}{2} \right. = 20 \text{ mL}$$

Case Study 24   Clinical Depression

Orders requiring calculations: IV 100 mL/hr; glycopyrrolate (Robinul) 4.4 mcg/kg; Zoloft 50 mg PO every AM; Sinequan 25 mg PO tid; Parnate 30 mg/day PO in 2 divided doses

1

$$\frac{100 \text{ mL}}{\text{hr}} \left| \frac{10 \text{ gtt}}{\text{mL}} \right| \frac{1 \text{ hr}}{60 \text{ min}} \left| \frac{10 \times 10}{6} \right| \frac{100}{6} = 16.6 \text{ or } 17 \frac{\text{gtt}}{\text{min}}$$

2

$$\frac{4.4 \text{ mcg}}{\text{kg}} \left| \frac{\text{mL}}{200 \text{ mcg}} \right| \frac{1 \text{ kg}}{2.2 \text{ lb}} \left| \frac{175 \text{ lb}}{} \right| \frac{4.4 \times 1 \times 175}{200 \times 2.2} \left| \frac{770}{440} \right. = 1.75 \text{ or } 1.8 \text{ mL}$$

3

$$\frac{50 \text{ mg}}{} \left| \frac{\text{tablet}}{50 \text{ mg}} \right| \frac{5}{5} = 1 \text{ tablet}$$

4

$$\frac{25 \text{ mg}}{} \left| \frac{\text{capsule}}{25 \text{ mg}} \right| \frac{25}{25} = 1 \text{ capsule}$$

5

$$\frac{30 \text{ mg}}{\text{day}} \left| \frac{\text{day}}{2 \text{ doses}} \right| \frac{30}{2} = 15 \frac{\text{mg}}{\text{dose}}$$

$$\frac{15 \text{ mg}}{} \left| \frac{\text{tablet}}{10 \text{ mg}} \right| \frac{15}{10} = 1.5 \text{ tablets}$$

Case Study 25   Alzheimer's Disease

Orders requiring calculations: IV 1000 mL/8 hr; donepezil (Aricept) 5 mg; thioridazine (Mellaril) 25 mg; imipramine (Tofranil) 50 mg; temazepam (Restoril) 7.5 mg

1

$$\frac{1000 \text{ mL}}{8 \text{ hr}} \left| \frac{10 \text{ gtt}}{\text{mL}} \right| \frac{1 \text{ hr}}{60 \text{ min}} \left| \frac{100 \times 10 \times 1}{8 \times 6} \right| \frac{1000}{48} = 20.83 \text{ or } 21 \frac{\text{gtt}}{\text{min}}$$

2

$$\frac{5 \text{ mg}}{} \left| \frac{\text{tablet}}{5 \text{ mg}} \right| \frac{5}{5} = 1 \text{ tablet}$$

3

$$\frac{25 \text{ mg}}{} \left| \frac{\text{tablet}}{25 \text{ mg}} \right| \frac{25}{25} = 1 \text{ tablet}$$

4

$$\frac{50 \text{ mg}}{} \left| \frac{\text{tablet}}{25 \text{ mg}} \right| \frac{50}{25} = 2 \text{ tablets}$$

5

$$\frac{7.5 \text{ mg}}{} \left| \frac{\text{tablet}}{15 \text{ mg}} \right| \frac{7.5}{15} = 0.5 \text{ tablet}$$

Case Study 26   Otitis Media

Orders requiring calculations: amoxicillin 45 kg/day; acetaminophen 120 mg; ibuprofen 5 mg/kg; Zyrtec 2.5 mg; Pedialyte 75 mL/kg

1

$$\frac{45 \text{ mg}}{\text{kg/day}} \left| \frac{5 \text{ mL}}{125 \text{ mg}} \right| \frac{\text{day}}{2 \text{ doses}} \left| \frac{1 \text{ kg}}{2.2 \text{ lb}} \right| \frac{23 \text{ lb}}{} \left| \frac{45 \times 5 \times 1 \times 23}{125 \times 2 \times 2.2} \right| \frac{5175}{550} = 9.4 \frac{\text{mL}}{\text{dose}}$$

2

$$\frac{120 \text{ mg}}{} \left| \frac{\text{mL}}{100 \text{ mg}} \right| \frac{12}{10} = 1.2 \text{ mL}$$

3

$$\frac{5 \text{ mg}}{\text{kg}} \left| \frac{5 \text{ mL}}{100 \text{ mg}} \right| \frac{1 \text{ kg}}{2.2 \text{ lb}} \left| \frac{23 \text{ lb}}{} \right| \frac{5 \times 5 \times 1 \times 23}{100 \times 2.2} \left| \frac{575}{220} \right. = 2.6 \text{ mL}$$

4

$$\frac{2.5 \text{ mg}}{} \left| \frac{\text{mL}}{1 \text{ mg}} \right| \frac{2.5}{1} = 2.5 \text{ mL}$$

5

$$\frac{75 \text{ mL}}{\text{kg/8 hr}} \left| \frac{1 \text{ kg}}{2.2 \text{ lb}} \right| \frac{23 \text{ lb}}{} \left| \frac{75 \times 1 \times 23}{8 \times 2.2} \right| \frac{1725}{17.6} = 98 \frac{\text{mL}}{\text{hr}}$$

Case Study 27   Seizures

Orders requiring calculations: IV D5W/0.45% NS; Dilantin 2 mg/kg/min; diazepam 0.3/kg; acetaminophen 320 mg; ibuprofen 7.5 mg/kg

1

$$\frac{500 \text{ mL}}{8 \text{ hr}} \bigg| \frac{500}{8} = \frac{62.5 \text{ or } 63 \text{ mL}}{\text{hr}}$$

2

$$\frac{2 \text{ mg}}{\text{kg/15 min}} \bigg| \frac{50 \text{ mL}}{100 \text{ mg}} \bigg| \frac{1 \text{ kg}}{2.2 \text{ lb}} \bigg| \frac{60 \text{ lb}}{1 \text{ hr}} \bigg| \frac{60 \text{ min}}{15 \times 1 \times 2.2} \bigg| \frac{2 \times 50 \times 6 \times 6}{33} \bigg| \frac{3600}{33} = \frac{109 \text{ mL}}{\text{hr}}$$

3

$$\frac{0.3 \text{ mg}}{\text{kg}} \bigg| \frac{\text{mL}}{5 \text{ mg}} \bigg| \frac{1 \text{ kg}}{2.2 \text{ lb}} \bigg| \frac{60 \text{ lb}}{5 \times 2.2} \bigg| \frac{0.3 \times 1 \times 60}{11} \bigg| \frac{18}{11} = 1.63 \text{ or } 1.6 \text{ mL}$$

4

$$\frac{320 \text{ mg}}{100 \text{ mg}} \bigg| \frac{\text{mL}}{10} \bigg| \frac{32}{10} = 3.2 \text{ or } 3 \text{ mL}$$

5

$$\frac{7.5 \text{ mg}}{\text{kg}} \bigg| \frac{5 \text{ mL}}{100 \text{ mg}} \bigg| \frac{1 \text{ kg}}{2.2 \text{ lb}} \bigg| \frac{60 \text{ lb}}{10 \times 2.2} \bigg| \frac{7.5 \times 5 \times 1 \times 6}{22} \bigg| \frac{225}{22} = 10.2 \text{ or } 10 \text{ mL}$$

Case Study 28   Fever of Unknown Origin

Orders requiring calculations: acetaminophen 400 mg; ibuprofen 7.5 mg/kg; IV D5W/0.45% NS mL/hr and gtt/min; Unasyn 1500 mg

1

$$\frac{400 \text{ mg}}{500 \text{ mg}} \bigg| \frac{15 \text{ mL}}{5} \bigg| \frac{4 \times 15}{5} \bigg| \frac{60}{5} = 12 \text{ mL}$$

2

$$\frac{7.5 \text{ mg}}{\text{kg}} \bigg| \frac{5 \text{ mL}}{100 \text{ mg}} \bigg| \frac{1 \text{ kg}}{2.2 \text{ lb}} \bigg| \frac{80 \text{ lb}}{10 \times 2.2} \bigg| \frac{7.5 \times 5 \times 1 \times 8}{22} \bigg| \frac{300}{22} = 13.6 \text{ or } 14 \text{ mL}$$

3

$$\frac{500 \text{ mL}}{4 \text{ hr}} \bigg| \frac{500}{4} = \frac{125 \text{ mL}}{\text{hr}}$$

4

$$\frac{500 \text{ mL}}{4 \text{ hr}} \bigg| \frac{1 \text{ hr}}{60 \text{ min}} \bigg| \frac{60 \text{ gtt}}{\text{mL}} \bigg| \frac{500 \times 1}{4} \bigg| \frac{500}{4} = \frac{125 \text{ gtt}}{\text{min}}$$

5

$$\frac{1500 \text{ mg}}{30 \text{ min}} \bigg| \frac{50 \text{ mL}}{1.5 \text{ g}} \bigg| \frac{1 \text{ g}}{1000 \text{ mg}} \bigg| \frac{60 \text{ min}}{1 \text{ hr}} \bigg| \frac{15 \times 5 \times 6}{3 \times 1.5 \times 1} \bigg| \frac{450}{4.5} = \frac{100 \text{ mL}}{\text{hr}}$$

Case Study 29   TURP with CBI

Orders requiring calculations: IV D5W/0.45% NS in mL/hr and gtt/min; Cipro 400 mg; Colace 100 mg; dimenhydrinate 25 mg

1

$$\frac{1000 \text{ mL}}{8 \text{ hr}} \bigg| \frac{1000}{8} = \frac{125 \text{ mL}}{\text{hr}}$$

2

$$\frac{1000 \text{ mL}}{8 \text{ hr}} \bigg| \frac{20 \text{ gtt}}{\text{mL}} \bigg| \frac{1 \text{ hr}}{60 \text{ min}} \bigg| \frac{1000 \times 2 \times 1}{8 \times 6} \bigg| \frac{2000}{48} = 41.6 \text{ or } 42 \frac{\text{gtt}}{\text{min}}$$

3

$$\frac{400 \text{ mg}}{60 \text{ min}} \bigg| \frac{200 \text{ mL}}{400 \text{ mg}} \bigg| \frac{60 \text{ min}}{1 \text{ hr}} \bigg| \frac{200}{1} = \frac{200 \text{ mL}}{\text{hr}}$$

4

$$\frac{100 \text{ mg}}{100 \text{ mg}} \bigg| \frac{\text{capsule}}{100} \bigg| \frac{100}{100} = 1 \text{ capsule}$$

5

$$\frac{25 \text{ mg}}{50 \text{ mg}} \bigg| \frac{\text{mL}}{50} \bigg| \frac{25}{50} = 0.5 \text{ mL}$$

Case Study 30   Hypercholesterolemia

Orders requiring calculations: Chantix 0.5 mg for days 1–7; Lipitor 20 mg; cholestyramine resin 4 g; niacin 1.5 g/day

1

$$\frac{0.5 \text{ mg}}{0.5 \text{ mg}} \bigg| \frac{\text{tablet}}{0.5} \bigg| \frac{0.5}{0.5} = 1 \text{ tablet}$$

2

$$\frac{1 \text{ mg}}{0.5 \text{ mg}} \bigg| \frac{\text{tablet}}{0.5} \bigg| \frac{1}{0.5} = 2 \text{ tablets}$$

3

$$\frac{20 \text{ mg}}{10 \text{ mg}} \bigg| \frac{\text{tablets}}{1} \bigg| \frac{2}{1} = 2 \text{ tablets}$$

4

$$\frac{4 \text{ g}}{\text{dose}} \bigg| \frac{2 \text{ doses}}{\text{day}} \bigg| \frac{4 \times 2}{1} \bigg| \frac{8}{1} = \frac{8 \text{ g}}{\text{day}}$$

5

$$\frac{1.5 \text{ g}}{\text{day}} \bigg| \frac{\text{tablet}}{500 \text{ mg}} \bigg| \frac{1000 \text{ mg}}{1 \text{ g}} \bigg| \frac{1.5 \times 10}{5 \times 1} \bigg| \frac{15}{5} = \frac{3 \text{ tablets}}{\text{day}}$$

Case Study 31   Hypertension

Orders requiring calculations: mL/meal of fluids; nifedipine 60 mg; Colace 100 mg; hydrochlorothiazide 25 mg; weight gain

1

$$\frac{2\ \cancel{L}}{\cancel{day}}\ \left|\ \frac{\cancel{day}}{3\ \boxed{meals}}\ \right|\ \frac{1000\ \boxed{mL}}{1\ \cancel{L}}\ \left|\ \frac{2\times 1000}{3\times 1}\ \right|\ \frac{2000}{3}\ =\ 666.6\ or\ 667\ \frac{mL}{meal}$$

2

$$\frac{60\ \cancel{mg}}{}\ \left|\ \frac{\boxed{tablet}}{30\ \cancel{mg}}\ \right|\ \frac{6}{3}\ =\ 2\ tablets$$

3

$$\frac{100\ \cancel{mg}}{}\ \left|\ \frac{\boxed{capsule}}{100\ \cancel{mg}}\ \right|\ \frac{100}{100}\ =\ 1\ capsule$$

4

$$\frac{25\ \cancel{mg}}{}\ \left|\ \frac{\boxed{tablet}}{50\ \cancel{mg}}\ \right|\ \frac{25}{50}\ =\ 0.5\ tablet$$

5

$$\frac{5\ \cancel{kg}}{}\ \left|\ \frac{2.2\ \boxed{lb}}{1\ \cancel{kg}}\ \right|\ \frac{5\times 2.2}{1}\ \left|\ \frac{11}{1}\ \right|\ =\ 11\ lb$$

Case Study 32   Diabetic Ketoacidosis

Orders requiring calculations: IV 0.9% NS 20 mL/kg/hr; regular insulin 0.15 unit/kg; regular insulin 0.1 unit/kg/hr; IV D5W/0.45% NS; ampicillin sodium 500 mg

1

$$\frac{1000\ \boxed{mL}}{8\ \boxed{hr}}\ \left|\ \frac{1000}{8}\ \right|\ =\ 125\ \frac{mL}{hr}$$

2

$$\frac{0.15\ \cancel{units}}{kg}\ \left|\ \frac{250\ \boxed{mL}}{250\ \cancel{units}}\ \right|\ \frac{1\ \cancel{kg}}{2.2\ \cancel{lb}}\ \left|\ \frac{125\ \cancel{lb}}{}\ \right|\ \frac{0.15\times 1\times 125}{2.2}\ \left|\ \frac{18.75}{2.2}\ \right|\ =\ 8.52\ or\ 8.5\ mL$$

3

$$\frac{0.1\ \cancel{unit}}{kg\ \boxed{hr}}\ \left|\ \frac{250\ \boxed{mL}}{250\ \cancel{units}}\ \right|\ \frac{1\ \cancel{kg}}{2.2\ \cancel{lb}}\ \left|\ \frac{125\ \cancel{lb}}{}\ \right|\ \frac{0.1\times 1\times 125}{2.2}\ \left|\ \frac{12.5}{2.2}\ \right|\ =\ 5.68\ or\ 5.7\ \frac{mL}{hr}$$

4

$$\frac{10\ \boxed{mL}}{kg\ \boxed{hr}}\ \left|\ \frac{1\ \cancel{kg}}{2.2\ \cancel{lb}}\ \right|\ \frac{125\ \cancel{lb}}{}\ \left|\ \frac{10\times 1\times 125}{2.2}\ \right|\ \frac{1250}{2.2}\ =\ 568.1\ or\ 568\ \frac{mL}{hr}$$

5

$$\frac{500\ \cancel{mg}}{30\ \cancel{min}}\ \left|\ \frac{100\ \boxed{mL}}{1\ \cancel{g}}\ \right|\ \frac{1\ \cancel{g}}{1000\ \cancel{mg}}\ \left|\ \frac{60\ \cancel{min}}{1\ \boxed{hr}}\ \right|\ \frac{5\times 10\times 6}{3\times 1\times 1}\ \left|\ \frac{300}{3}\ \right|\ =\ 100\ \frac{mL}{hr}$$

Case Study 33   End-Stage Renal Failure

Orders requiring calculations: furosemide 120 mg; Zaroxolyn 10 mg; Vasotec 2.5 mg; Epogen 100 units/kg; calcium carbonate 10 g/day

1

$$\frac{120\ \cancel{mg}}{}\ \left|\ \frac{\boxed{tablet}}{80\ \cancel{mg}}\ \right|\ \frac{12}{8}\ =\ 1.5\ tablets$$

2

$$\frac{10\ \cancel{mg}}{}\ \left|\ \frac{\boxed{tablet}}{5\ \cancel{mg}}\ \right|\ \frac{10}{5}\ =\ 2\ tablets$$

3

$$\frac{2.5\ \cancel{mg}}{}\ \left|\ \frac{\boxed{tablet}}{2.5\ \cancel{mg}}\ \right|\ \frac{2.5}{2.5}\ =\ 1\ tablet$$

4

$$\frac{100\ \cancel{units}}{kg}\ \left|\ \frac{\boxed{mL}}{4000\ \cancel{units}}\ \right|\ \frac{1\ \cancel{kg}}{2.2\ \cancel{lb}}\ \left|\ \frac{140\ \cancel{lb}}{}\ \right|\ \frac{1\times 1\times 14}{4\times 2.2}\ \left|\ \frac{14}{8.8}\ \right|\ =\ 1.59\ or\ 1.6\ mL$$

5

$$\frac{10\ \cancel{g}}{day}\ \left|\ \frac{\boxed{tablet}}{1500\ \cancel{mg}}\ \right|\ \frac{1000\ \cancel{mg}}{1\ \cancel{g}}\ \left|\ \frac{\cancel{day}}{3\ \boxed{meals}}\ \right|\ \frac{10\times 10}{15\times 1\times 3}\ \left|\ \frac{100}{45}\ \right|\ =\ 2.2\ or\ 2\ \frac{tablets}{meals}$$

Case Study 34   Fluid Volume Deficit

Orders requiring calculations: IV 0.9% NS/2.5% dextrose 50 mL/kg; acetaminophen 400 mg; ibuprofen 7.5 mg/kg; mL/hr of PO fluids; mL/hr of Pedialyte

1

$$\frac{50\ \boxed{mL}}{kg/4\ \boxed{hr}}\ \left|\ \frac{1\ \cancel{kg}}{2.2\ \cancel{lb}}\ \right|\ \frac{35\ \cancel{lb}}{}\ \left|\ \frac{50\times 1\times 35}{4\times 2.2}\ \right|\ \frac{1750}{8.8}\ =\ 198.8\ or\ 199\ \frac{mL}{hr}$$

2

$$\frac{400\ \cancel{mg}}{}\ \left|\ \frac{\boxed{mL}}{100\ \cancel{mg}}\ \right|\ \frac{4}{1}\ =\ 4\ mL$$

3

$$\frac{7.5\ \cancel{mg}}{kg}\ \left|\ \frac{5\ \boxed{mL}}{100\ \cancel{mg}}\ \right|\ \frac{1\ \cancel{kg}}{2.2\ \cancel{lb}}\ \left|\ \frac{35\ \cancel{lb}}{}\ \right|\ \frac{7.5\times 5\times 1\times 35}{100\times 2.2}\ \left|\ \frac{1312.5}{220}\ \right|\ =\ 5.9\ or\ 6\ mL$$

4

$$\frac{1.5\ \cancel{oz}}{lb/24\ \boxed{hr}}\ \left|\ \frac{30\ \boxed{mL}}{1\ \cancel{oz}}\ \right|\ \frac{35\ \cancel{lb}}{}\ \left|\ \frac{1.5\times 30\times 35}{24\times 1}\ \right|\ \frac{1575}{24}\ =\ 65.6\ or\ 66\ \frac{mL}{hr}$$

5

$$\frac{53\ \cancel{oz}}{24\ \boxed{hr}}\ \left|\ \frac{30\ \boxed{mL}}{1\ \cancel{oz}}\ \right|\ \frac{53\times 30}{24\times 1}\ \left|\ \frac{1590}{24}\ \right|\ =\ 66.25\ or\ 66\ \frac{mL}{hr}$$

Case Study 35 — Increased Intracranial Pressure

Orders requiring calculations: IV 0.9% NS; Dilantin 10 mg/kg; mannitol 0.25 g/kg; dexamethasone 10 mg; furosemide 0.5 mg/kg

1

$$\frac{1000\ \text{mL}}{10\ \text{hr}} \cdot \frac{1000}{10} = \frac{100\ \text{mL}}{\text{hr}}$$

2

$$\frac{10\ \text{mg}}{\text{kg}} \cdot \frac{20\ \text{mL}}{1000\ \text{mg}} \cdot 75\ \text{kg} \cdot \frac{1 \times 2 \times 75}{10} \cdot \frac{150}{10} = 15\ \text{mL}$$

3

$$\frac{0.25\ \text{g}}{\text{kg/hr}} \cdot \frac{500\ \text{mL}}{100\ \text{g}} \cdot 75\ \text{kg} \cdot \frac{0.25 \times 5 \times 75}{1} \cdot \frac{93.7}{1} = 93.7\ \text{or}\ 94\ \frac{\text{mL}}{\text{hr}}$$

4

$$\frac{10\ \text{mg}}{120\ \text{mg}} \cdot \frac{5\ \text{mL}}{12} \cdot \frac{1 \times 5}{12} \cdot \frac{5}{12} = 0.41\ \text{or}\ 0.4\ \text{mL}$$

5

$$\frac{0.5\ \text{mg}}{\text{kg}} \cdot \frac{\text{mL}}{10\ \text{mg}} \cdot 75\ \text{kg} \cdot \frac{0.5 \times 75}{10} \cdot \frac{37.5}{10} = 3.75\ \text{or}\ 3.7\ \text{mL}$$

Case Study 36 — Breast Cancer

Orders requiring calculations: IV D5W/1/2 NS at 100 mL/hr; filgrastim (Neupogen) 5 mcg/kg/day; metoclopramide (Reglan) 2 mg/kg; 1 unit of PRBC; and diphenhydramine (Benadryl) 25 mg

1

$$\frac{100\ \text{mL}}{\text{hr}} \cdot \frac{15\ \text{gtt}}{\text{mL}} \cdot \frac{1\ \text{hr}}{60\ \text{min}} \cdot \frac{10 \times 15 \times 1}{6} \cdot \frac{150}{6} = 25\ \frac{\text{gtt}}{\text{min}}$$

2

$$\frac{5\ \text{mcg}}{\text{kg/day}} \cdot \frac{\text{mL}}{300\ \text{mcg}} \cdot \frac{1\ \text{kg}}{2.2\ \text{lb}} \cdot 150\ \text{lb} \cdot \frac{5 \times 1 \times 15}{30 \times 2.2} \cdot \frac{75}{66} = 1.1\ \text{or}\ 1\ \frac{\text{mL}}{\text{day}}$$

3

$$\frac{2\ \text{mg}}{\text{kg}} \cdot \frac{1\ \text{kg}}{2.2\ \text{lb}} \cdot 150\ \text{lb} \cdot \frac{2 \times 1 \times 150}{2.2} \cdot \frac{300}{2.2} = 136.3\ \text{or}\ 136\ \text{mg}$$

4

$$\frac{450\ \text{mL}}{3\ \text{hr}} \cdot \frac{450}{3} = \frac{150\ \text{mL}}{\text{hr}}$$

5

$$\frac{25\ \text{mg}}{50\ \text{mg}} \cdot \frac{\text{mL}}{50} \cdot \frac{25}{50} = 0.5\ \text{mL}$$

Case Study 37 — Severe Abdominal Pain

Orders requiring calculations: weight; IV D5W/0.45% NS @ 1000 mL/8 hr; Cleocin 300 mg; Claforan 50 mg/kg; morphine sulfate 3 mg

1

$$\frac{88\ \text{lb}}{2.2\ \text{lb}} \cdot \frac{1\ \text{kg}}{2.2} \cdot \frac{88 \times 1}{2.2} \cdot \frac{88}{2.2} = 40\ \text{kg}$$

2

$$\frac{1000\ \text{mL}}{8\ \text{hr}} \cdot \frac{1000}{8} = 125\ \frac{\text{mL}}{\text{hr}}$$

3

$$\frac{300\ \text{mg}}{20\ \text{min}} \cdot \frac{50\ \text{mL}}{300\ \text{mg}} \cdot \frac{60\ \text{min}}{1\ \text{hr}} \cdot \frac{50 \times 6}{2 \times 1} \cdot \frac{300}{2} = \frac{150\ \text{mL}}{\text{hr}}$$

4

$$\frac{50\ \text{mg}}{\text{kg}} \cdot \frac{10\ \text{mL}}{2\ \text{g}} \cdot \frac{1\ \text{g}}{1000\ \text{mg}} \cdot 40\ \text{kg} \cdot \frac{5 \times 1 \times 1 \times 4}{2 \times 1} \cdot \frac{20}{2} = 10\ \text{mL}$$

$$\frac{60\ \text{mL}}{30\ \text{min}} \cdot \frac{60\ \text{min}}{1\ \text{hr}} \cdot \frac{60 \times 6}{3 \times 1} \cdot \frac{360}{3} = \frac{120\ \text{mL}}{\text{hr}}$$

5

$$\frac{3\ \text{mg}}{4\ \text{mg}} \cdot \frac{\text{mL}}{4} \cdot \frac{3}{4} = 0.75\ \text{or}\ 0.8\ \text{mL}$$

Case Study 38 — Acute Asthma Attack

Orders requiring calculations: IV D5W/1/2 NS at 1000 mL/10 hr; weight 176 lb; Solu-Medrol 80 mg; azithromycin (Zithromax) 500 mg; cimetidine (Tagamet) 300 mg

1

$$\frac{1000\ \text{mL}}{10\ \text{hr}} \cdot \frac{1000}{10} = \frac{100\ \text{mL}}{\text{hr}}$$

2

$$\frac{176\ \text{lb}}{2.2\ \text{lb}} \cdot \frac{1\ \text{kg}}{2.2} \cdot \frac{176 \times 1}{2.2} \cdot \frac{176}{2.2} = 80\ \text{kg}$$

3

$$\frac{80\ \text{mg}}{125\ \text{mg}} \cdot \frac{2\ \text{mL}}{125} \cdot \frac{80 \times 2}{125} \cdot \frac{160}{125} = 1.28\ \text{or}\ 1.3\ \text{mL}$$

4

$$\frac{500\ \text{mg}}{250\ \text{mg}} \cdot \frac{\text{capsular}}{25} \cdot \frac{50}{25} = 2\ \text{capsulars}$$

5

$$\frac{50\ \cancel{\text{mL}}}{20\ \cancel{\text{min}}}\ \bigg|\ \frac{60\ \cancel{\text{min}}}{1\ \text{\textcircled{hr}}}\ \bigg|\ \frac{50\times6}{2\times1}\ \bigg|\ \frac{300}{2} = 150\ \frac{\text{mL}}{\text{hr}}$$

Case Study 39 — Right Total Hip Replacement

Orders requiring calculations: IV D5W/NS at 1000 mL/10 hr; atenolol 50 mg; lisinopril 5 mg; enoxaparin (Lovenox) 40 mg; dimenhydrinate 50 mg; and morphine 10 mg

1

$$\frac{50\ \cancel{\text{mg}}}{25\ \cancel{\text{mg}}}\ \bigg|\ \frac{\text{\textcircled{tablet}}\ 50}{25} = 2\ \text{tablets}$$

2

$$\frac{5\ \cancel{\text{mg}}}{2.5\ \cancel{\text{mg}}}\ \bigg|\ \frac{\text{\textcircled{tablet}}\ 5}{2.5} = 2\ \text{tablets}$$

3

$$\frac{40\ \cancel{\text{mg}}}{80\ \cancel{\text{mg}}}\ \bigg|\ \frac{0.8\ \text{\textcircled{mL}}}{8}\ \bigg|\ \frac{4\times0.8}{8}\ \bigg|\ \frac{3.2}{8} = 0.4\ \text{mL}$$

4

$$\frac{50\ \cancel{\text{mg}}}{50\ \cancel{\text{mg}}}\ \bigg|\ \frac{\text{\textcircled{mL}}\ 5}{5} = 1\ \text{mL}$$

5

$$\frac{10\ \cancel{\text{mg}}}{8\ \cancel{\text{mg}}}\ \bigg|\ \frac{\text{\textcircled{mL}}\ 10}{8} = 1.25\ \text{or}\ 1.3\ \text{mL}$$

Case Study 40 — Colon Resection

Orders requiring calculations: IV NS with KCl 20 mEq/L at 1000 mL/12 hr; cefoxitin 1 g; Ranitidine 50 mg; tamsulosin (Flomax) 0.8 mg; and Os-Cal 1.25 g

1

$$\frac{1000\ \text{\textcircled{mL}}}{12\ \text{\textcircled{hr}}}\ \bigg|\ \frac{1000}{12} = 83.3\ \text{or}\ 83\ \frac{\text{mL}}{\text{hr}}$$

2

$$\frac{50\ \text{\textcircled{mL}}}{30\ \cancel{\text{min}}}\ \bigg|\ \frac{60\ \cancel{\text{min}}}{1\ \text{\textcircled{hr}}}\ \bigg|\ \frac{50\times6}{3\times1}\ \bigg|\ \frac{300}{3} = 100\ \frac{\text{mL}}{\text{hr}}$$

3

$$\frac{100\ \text{\textcircled{mL}}}{20\ \cancel{\text{min}}}\ \bigg|\ \frac{60\ \cancel{\text{min}}}{1\ \text{\textcircled{hr}}}\ \bigg|\ \frac{100\times6}{2\times1}\ \bigg|\ \frac{600}{2} = 300\ \frac{\text{mL}}{\text{hr}}$$

4

$$\frac{0.8\ \cancel{\text{mg}}}{0.4\ \cancel{\text{mg}}}\ \bigg|\ \frac{\text{\textcircled{capsule}}\ 0.8}{0.4} = 2\ \text{capsules}$$

5

$$\frac{1.25\ \cancel{\text{g}}}{1250\ \cancel{\text{mg}}}\ \bigg|\ \frac{\text{\textcircled{capsule}}\ 1000\ \cancel{\text{mg}}}{1\ \cancel{\text{g}}}\ \bigg|\ \frac{1.25\times100}{125\times1}\ \bigg|\ \frac{125}{125} = 1\ \text{capsule}$$

Case Study 41 — Left Total Knee Replacement

Orders requiring calculations: IV D5/LR with 20 mEq KCl; cefazolin 1g IV; cefazolin 500 mg; enoxaparin (Lovenox) 30 mg; and ferrous sulfate 0.3 g

1

$$\frac{1000\ \text{\textcircled{mL}}}{8\ \text{\textcircled{hr}}}\ \bigg|\ \frac{1000}{8} = 125\ \frac{\text{mL}}{\text{hr}}$$

2

$$\frac{100\ \text{\textcircled{mL}}}{30\ \cancel{\text{min}}}\ \bigg|\ \frac{60\ \cancel{\text{min}}}{1\ \text{\textcircled{hr}}}\ \bigg|\ \frac{100\times6}{3\times1}\ \bigg|\ \frac{600}{3} = 200\ \frac{\text{mL}}{\text{hr}}$$

3

$$\frac{50\ \text{\textcircled{mL}}}{30\ \cancel{\text{min}}}\ \bigg|\ \frac{60\ \cancel{\text{min}}}{1\ \text{\textcircled{hr}}}\ \bigg|\ \frac{50\times6}{3\times1}\ \bigg|\ \frac{300}{3} = 100\ \frac{\text{mL}}{\text{hr}}$$

4

$$\frac{30\ \cancel{\text{mg}}}{40\ \cancel{\text{mg}}}\ \bigg|\ \frac{0.4\ \text{\textcircled{mL}}}{4}\ \bigg|\ \frac{3\times0.4}{4}\ \bigg|\ \frac{1.2}{4} = 0.3\ \text{mL}$$

5

$$\frac{0.3\ \cancel{\text{g}}}{300\ \cancel{\text{mg}}}\ \bigg|\ \frac{\text{\textcircled{tablet}}\ 1000\ \cancel{\text{mg}}}{1\ \cancel{\text{g}}}\ \bigg|\ \frac{0.3\times10}{3\times1}\ \bigg|\ \frac{3}{3} = 1\ \text{tablet}$$

Case Study 42 — Chest Pain

Orders requiring calculations: IV nitroglycerin 10 mcg/min; ASA 160 mg; and morphine 2.5 mg

1

$$\frac{10\ \cancel{\text{mcg}}}{\text{min}}\ \bigg|\ \frac{250\ \text{\textcircled{mL}}}{50\ \cancel{\text{mg}}}\ \bigg|\ \frac{1\ \cancel{\text{mg}}}{1000\ \cancel{\text{mcg}}}\ \bigg|\ \frac{60\ \cancel{\text{min}}}{1\ \text{\textcircled{hr}}}\ \bigg|\ \frac{1\times25\times1\times6}{5\times10\times1}\ \bigg|\ \frac{150}{50} = 3\ \frac{\text{mL}}{\text{hr}}$$

2

$$\frac{15\ \cancel{\text{mL}}}{\text{hr}}\ \bigg|\ \frac{50\ \cancel{\text{mg}}}{250\ \cancel{\text{mL}}}\ \bigg|\ \frac{1000\ \text{\textcircled{mcg}}}{1\ \cancel{\text{mg}}}\ \bigg|\ \frac{1\ \cancel{\text{hr}}}{60\ \text{\textcircled{min}}}\ \bigg|\ \frac{15\times5\times100\times1}{25\times1\times6}\ \bigg|\ \frac{7500}{150} = 50\ \frac{\text{mcg}}{\text{min}}$$

3

$$\frac{160 \text{ mg}}{} \; \Big| \; \frac{\text{tablet}}{80 \text{ mg}} \; \Big| \; \frac{16}{8} = 2 \text{ tablets}$$

4

$$\frac{2.5 \text{ mg}}{} \; \Big| \; \frac{\text{mL}}{5 \text{ mg}} \; \Big| \; \frac{2.5}{5} = 0.5 \text{ mL}$$

5

$$\frac{7.5 \text{ mg}}{} \; \Big| \; \frac{\text{mL}}{5 \text{ mg}} \; \Big| \; \frac{7.5}{5} = 1.5 \text{ mL}$$

Case Study 43 — **Pneumococcal Meningitis**

Orders requiring calculations: Weight lb to kg; IV bolus; acetaminophen 15 mg/kg/dose; ceftriaxone 50 mg/kg/dose; and vancomycin 60 mg/kg/day

1

$$\frac{44 \text{ lb}}{} \; \Big| \; \frac{1 \text{ kg}}{2.2 \text{ lb}} \; \Big| \; \frac{44}{2.2} = 20 \text{ kg}$$

2

$$\frac{10 \text{ mL}}{\text{kg}} \; \Big| \; \frac{20 \text{ kg}}{} \; \Big| \; \frac{10 \times 20}{} = 200 \text{ mL}$$

3

$$\frac{15 \text{ mg}}{\text{kg/dose}} \; \Big| \; \frac{20 \text{ kg}}{} \; \Big| \; \frac{2.5 \text{ mL}}{80 \text{ mg}} \; \Big| \; \frac{15 \times 2 \times 2.5}{} \; \Big| \; \frac{75}{8} = 9.3 \text{ or } 9 \; \frac{\text{mL}}{\text{dose}}$$

4

$$\frac{50 \text{ mg}}{\text{kg/dose}} \; \Big| \; \frac{20 \text{ kg}}{} \; \Big| \; \frac{50 \times 20}{} \; \Big| \; \frac{1000}{} = 1000 \; \frac{\text{mg}}{\text{dose}}$$

$$\frac{1000 \text{ mg}}{30 \text{ min}} \; \Big| \; \frac{50 \text{ mL}}{1 \text{ g}} \; \Big| \; \frac{1 \text{ g}}{1000 \text{ mg}} \; \Big| \; \frac{60 \text{ min}}{1 \text{ hr}} \; \Big| \; \frac{5 \times 60}{3 \times 1} \; \Big| \; \frac{300}{3} = 100 \; \frac{\text{mL}}{\text{hr}}$$

5

$$\frac{60 \text{ mg}}{\text{kg/day}} \; \Big| \; \frac{20 \text{ kg}}{} \; \Big| \; \frac{\text{day}}{4 \text{ doses}} \; \Big| \; \frac{60 \times 20}{4} \; \Big| \; \frac{1200}{4} = 300 \; \frac{\text{mg}}{\text{dose}}$$

$$\frac{300 \text{ mg}}{30 \text{ min}} \; \Big| \; \frac{100 \text{ mL}}{500 \text{ mg}} \; \Big| \; \frac{60 \text{ min}}{1 \text{ hr}} \; \Big| \; \frac{30 \times 10 \times 6}{3 \times 5 \times 1} \; \Big| \; \frac{1800}{15} = 120 \; \frac{\text{mL}}{\text{hr}}$$

Case Study 44 — **Diabetic Ketoacidosis**

Orders requiring calculations: Weight lb to kg; IV bolus; IV NS with KCl 20 mEq/L; regular insulin 0.1 unit/kg/hr; and ondansetron IV push 0.1 mg/kg

1

$$\frac{54 \text{ lb}}{} \; \Big| \; \frac{1 \text{ kg}}{2.2 \text{ lb}} \; \Big| \; \frac{54}{2.2} = 24.5 \text{ kg}$$

2

$$\frac{10 \text{ mL}}{\text{kg}} \; \Big| \; \frac{24.5 \text{ kg}}{} \; \Big| \; \frac{10 \times 24.5}{} \; \Big| \; \frac{245}{} = 245 \text{ mL}$$

3

$$\frac{3.5 \text{ mL}}{\text{kg/hr}} \; \Big| \; \frac{24.5 \text{ kg}}{} \; \Big| \; \frac{3.5 \times 24.5}{} \; \Big| \; \frac{85.7}{} = 85.7 \text{ or } 86 \; \frac{\text{mL}}{\text{hr}}$$

4

$$\frac{0.1 \text{ unit}}{\text{kg/hr}} \; \Big| \; \frac{24.5 \text{ kg}}{} \; \Big| \; \frac{250 \text{ mL}}{25 \text{ units}} \; \Big| \; \frac{0.1 \times 24.5 \times 250}{25} \; \Big| \; \frac{612.5}{25} = 24.5 \; \frac{\text{mL}}{\text{hr}}$$

5

$$\frac{0.1 \text{ mg}}{\text{kg}} \; \Big| \; \frac{24.5 \text{ kg}}{} \; \Big| \; \frac{\text{mL}}{2 \text{ mg}} \; \Big| \; \frac{0.1 \times 24.5}{2} \; \Big| \; \frac{2.45}{2} = 1.2 \text{ or } 1 \text{ mL}$$

Case Study 45 — **C-Section Delivery**

Orders requiring calculations: zidovudine 2 mg/kg/dose IV; zidovudine 1 mg/kg/hr continuous IV infusion; cefazolin 1 g IVPB; and metoclopramide (Reglan) 10 mg IV push

1

$$\frac{164 \text{ lb}}{} \; \Big| \; \frac{1 \text{ kg}}{2.2 \text{ lb}} \; \Big| \; \frac{164 \times 1}{2.2} \; \Big| \; \frac{164}{2.2} = 74.5 \text{ kg}$$

2

$$\frac{2 \text{ mg}}{\text{kg}} \; \Big| \; \frac{74.5 \text{ kg}}{} \; \Big| \; \frac{50 \text{ mL}}{200 \text{ mg}} \; \Big| \; \frac{2 \times 74.5 \times 5}{20} \; \Big| \; \frac{745}{20} = 37.2 \text{ or } 37 \text{ mL}$$

3

$$\frac{1 \text{ mg}}{\text{kg/hr}} \; \Big| \; \frac{100 \text{ mL}}{400 \text{ mg}} \; \Big| \; \frac{74.5 \text{ kg}}{} \; \Big| \; \frac{1 \times 1 \times 74.5}{4} \; \Big| \; \frac{74.5}{4} = 18.6 \text{ or } 19 \; \frac{\text{mL}}{\text{hr}}$$

4

$$\frac{1 \text{ g}}{30 \text{ min}} \; \Big| \; \frac{60 \text{ min}}{1 \text{ hr}} \; \Big| \; \frac{100 \text{ mL}}{1000 \text{ mg}} \; \Big| \; \frac{1000 \text{ mg}}{1 \text{ g}} \; \Big| \; \frac{6 \times 100}{3 \times 1} \; \Big| \; \frac{600}{3} = 200 \; \frac{\text{mL}}{\text{hr}}$$

5

$$\frac{10 \text{ mg}}{} \; \Big| \; \frac{\text{mL}}{5 \text{ mg}} \; \Big| \; \frac{10}{5} = 2 \text{ mL}$$

Case Study 46   Iron Deficiency Anemia

Orders requiring calculations: ferrous sulfate 325 mg daily PO; ascorbic acid 1500 mg PO every day in three divided doses; folic acid (Folate) 400 mcg PO once daily; vitamin B_6 25 mg PO three times daily; doxylamine 12.5 mg PO three times daily

1

$$\frac{325\ \text{mg}}{\text{dose}} \cdot \frac{\text{tablet}}{325\ \text{mg}} \cdot \frac{325}{325} = 1\ \frac{\text{tablet}}{\text{dose}}$$

2

$$\frac{1500\ \text{mg}}{\text{day}} \cdot \frac{\text{tablet}}{500\ \text{mg}} \cdot \frac{\text{day}}{3\ \text{doses}} \cdot \frac{15}{5 \times 3} \cdot \frac{15}{15} = 1\ \frac{\text{tablet}}{\text{dose}}$$

3

$$\frac{400\ \text{mcg}}{\text{dose}} \cdot \frac{\text{tablet}}{0.4\ \text{mg}} \cdot \frac{1\ \text{mg}}{1000\ \text{mcg}} \cdot \frac{4 \times 1}{0.4 \times 10} \cdot \frac{4}{4} = 1\ \frac{\text{tablet}}{\text{dose}}$$

4

$$\frac{25\ \text{mg}}{\text{dose}} \cdot \frac{\text{tablet}}{50\ \text{mg}} \cdot \frac{25}{50} = 0.5\ \frac{\text{tablet}}{\text{dose}}$$

5

$$\frac{12.5\ \text{mg}}{\text{dose}} \cdot \frac{\text{tablet}}{25\ \text{mg}} \cdot \frac{12.5}{25} = 0.5\ \frac{\text{tablet}}{\text{dose}}$$

Case Study 47   Lyme Disease

Orders requiring calculations: IV 0.9% NS infusing at 100 mL/hr; ceftriaxone (Rocephin) 50 mg/kg/day (up to 2 g) in two divided doses every 12 hours IV; amoxicillin 25 mg/kg/day in two divided doses every 12 hours PO

1

$$\frac{100\ \text{mL}}{\text{hr}} \cdot \frac{1\ \text{hr}}{60\ \text{min}} \cdot \frac{20\ \text{gtt}}{\text{mL}} \cdot \frac{100 \times 1 \times 2}{6} \cdot \frac{200}{6} = 33.3\ \text{or}\ 33\ \frac{\text{gtt}}{\text{min}}$$

2

$$\frac{50\ \text{mg}}{\text{kg/day}} \cdot \frac{40\ \text{kg}}{} \cdot \frac{\text{day}}{2\ \text{doses}} \cdot \frac{50 \times 40}{2} \cdot \frac{2000}{2} = 1000\ \frac{\text{mg}}{\text{dose}}$$

3

$$\frac{100\ \text{mL}}{30\ \text{min}} \cdot \frac{60\ \text{min}}{1\ \text{hr}} \cdot \frac{100 \times 6}{3 \times 1} \cdot \frac{600}{3} = 200\ \frac{\text{mL}}{\text{hr}}$$

4

$$\frac{25\ \text{mg}}{\text{kg/day}} \cdot \frac{40\ \text{kg}}{} \cdot \frac{25 \times 40}{} \cdot \frac{1000}{} = 1000\ \frac{\text{mg}}{\text{day}}$$

5

$$\frac{1000\ \text{mg}}{\text{day}} \cdot \frac{\text{day}}{2\ \text{doses}} \cdot \frac{5\ \text{mL}}{250\ \text{mg}} \cdot \frac{100 \times 5}{2 \times 25} \cdot \frac{500}{50} = 10\ \frac{\text{mL}}{\text{dose}}$$

Case Study 48   Infectious Mononucleosis

Orders requiring calculations: acyclovir (Zovirax) 400 mg PO tid for 10 days; prednisone 40 mg PO every 12 hours for a short-course 5-day burst; ibuprofen >102.5°F 400 mg PO every 6 hours prn not to exceed 3.2 g/day to alternate with acetaminophen 1000 mg PO every 8 hours prn not to exceed 4 g/day

1

$$\frac{400\ \text{mg}}{\text{dose}} \cdot \frac{\text{capsule}}{200\ \text{mg}} \cdot \frac{4}{2} = 2\ \frac{\text{capsules}}{\text{dose}}$$

2

$$\frac{40\ \text{mg}}{\text{dose}} \cdot \frac{\text{tablet}}{20\ \text{mg}} \cdot \frac{2\ \text{doses}}{\text{day}} \cdot \frac{4 \times 2}{2} \cdot \frac{8}{2} = 4\ \frac{\text{tablets}}{\text{day}}$$

3

$$\frac{400\ \text{mg}}{\text{dose}} \cdot \frac{\text{tablets}}{200\ \text{mg}} \cdot \frac{4\ \text{doses}}{\text{day}} \cdot \frac{4 \times 4}{2} \cdot \frac{16}{2} = 8\ \frac{\text{tablets}}{\text{day}}$$

4

$$\frac{1000\ \text{mg}}{\text{dose}} \cdot \frac{\text{tablets}}{500\ \text{mg}} \cdot \frac{3\ \text{doses}}{\text{day}} \cdot \frac{10 \times 3}{5} \cdot \frac{30}{5} = 6\ \frac{\text{tablets}}{\text{day}}$$

5

$$\frac{8\ \text{tablets}}{\text{day}} \cdot \frac{200\ \text{mg}}{\text{tablets}} \cdot \frac{8 \times 200}{} \cdot \frac{1600}{} = 1600\ \frac{\text{mg}}{\text{day}}\quad \text{*Yes, not to exceed 3.2 g/day}$$

$$\frac{6\ \text{tablets}}{\text{day}} \cdot \frac{500\ \text{mg}}{\text{tablets}} \cdot \frac{6 \times 500}{} \cdot \frac{3000}{} = 3000\ \frac{\text{mg}}{\text{day}}\quad \text{*Yes, not to exceed 4 g/day}$$

Case Study 49   H1N1 Influenza (Swine Flu)

Orders requiring calculations: IV D5W/0.9 NS 1000 mL/8 hr; oseltamivir (Tamiflu) 75 mg PO every 12 hours × 5 days; acetaminophen 650 mg PO every 8 hours prn not to exceed 4 g/day; ibuprofen 400 mg PO for fever >102.5°F 400 mg PO every 6 hours prn not to exceed 3.2 g/day; promethazine with codeine 10 mg PO every 4 hours prn not to exceed 30 mL/24 hr

1

$$\frac{1000\ \text{mL}}{8\ \text{hr}} \cdot \frac{1000}{8} = 125\ \frac{\text{mL}}{\text{hr}}$$

2

$$\frac{75 \;\text{(mg)}}{\cancel{\text{dose}}} \;\Bigg|\; \frac{2 \;\cancel{\text{doses}}}{\cancel{\text{day}}} \;\Bigg|\; \frac{5 \;\cancel{\text{days}}}{} \;\Bigg|\; \frac{75 \times 2 \times 5}{} \;\Bigg|\; \frac{750}{} = 750 \;\text{mg}$$

3

$$\frac{650 \;\cancel{\text{mg}}}{\text{(dose)}} \;\Bigg|\; \frac{\text{(tablets)}}{325 \;\cancel{\text{mg}}} \;\Bigg|\; \frac{650}{325} = 2 \;\frac{\text{tablets}}{\text{dose}}$$

4

$$\frac{400 \;\cancel{\text{mg}}}{\text{(dose)}} \;\Bigg|\; \frac{\text{(tablets)}}{200 \;\cancel{\text{mg}}} \;\Bigg|\; \frac{4}{2} = 2 \;\frac{\text{tablets}}{\text{dose}}$$

5

$$\frac{10 \;\cancel{\text{mg}}}{\text{(dose)}} \;\Bigg|\; \frac{5 \;\text{(mL)}}{10 \;\cancel{\text{mg}}} \;\Bigg|\; \frac{5}{} = 5 \;\frac{\text{mL}}{\text{dose}}$$

2

$$\frac{300 \;\text{(mg)}}{\cancel{\text{kg/day}}} \;\Bigg|\; \frac{20 \;\cancel{\text{kg}}}{} \;\Bigg|\; \frac{\cancel{\text{day}}}{4 \;\text{(doses)}} \;\Bigg|\; \frac{300 \times 20}{4} \;\Bigg|\; \frac{6000}{4} = 1500 \;\frac{\text{mg}}{\text{dose}}$$

3

$$\frac{1500 \;\cancel{\text{mg}}}{\text{(dose)}} \;\Bigg|\; \frac{1 \;\cancel{\text{g}}}{1000 \;\cancel{\text{mg}}} \;\Bigg|\; \frac{50 \;\text{(mL)}}{1.5 \;\text{g}} \;\Bigg|\; \frac{15 \times 5}{1.5} \;\Bigg|\; \frac{75}{1.5} = 50 \;\frac{\text{mL}}{\text{dose}}$$

4

$$\frac{50 \;\text{(mL)}}{30 \;\cancel{\text{min}}} \;\Bigg|\; \frac{60 \;\cancel{\text{min}}}{1 \;\text{(hr)}} \;\Bigg|\; \frac{50 \times 6}{3 \times 1} \;\Bigg|\; \frac{300}{3} = 100 \;\frac{\text{mL}}{\text{hr}}$$

5

$$\frac{80 \;\cancel{\text{mg}}}{\text{(dose)}} \;\Bigg|\; \frac{5 \;\text{(mL)}}{160 \;\cancel{\text{mg}}} \;\Bigg|\; \frac{8 \times 5}{16} \;\Bigg|\; \frac{40}{16} = 2.5 \;\frac{\text{mL}}{\text{dose}}$$

Case Study 50   **Bronchiolitis**

Orders requiring calculations: IV therapy 500 mL 0.9% NS over 8 hours; Unasyn 300 mg per kg of body weight per day administered via intravenous infusion in equally divided doses every 6 hours; acetaminophen 80 mg per dose PO every 6 hours (160 mg/5 mL infant suspension drops)

1

$$\frac{500 \;\text{(mL)}}{8 \;\text{(hr)}} \;\Bigg|\; \frac{500}{8} = 62.5 \;\text{or}\; 63 \;\frac{\text{mL}}{\text{hr}}$$

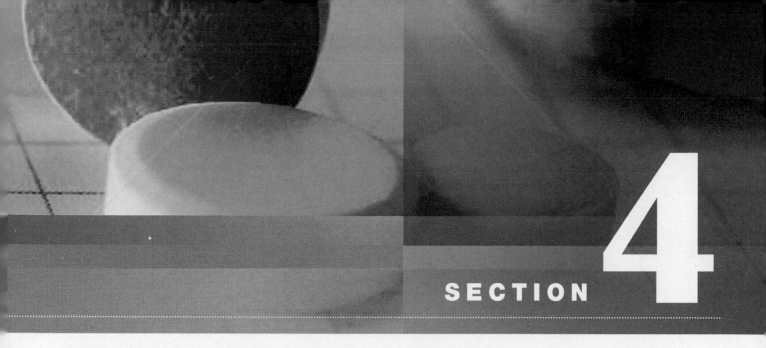

Comprehensive Post-Tests

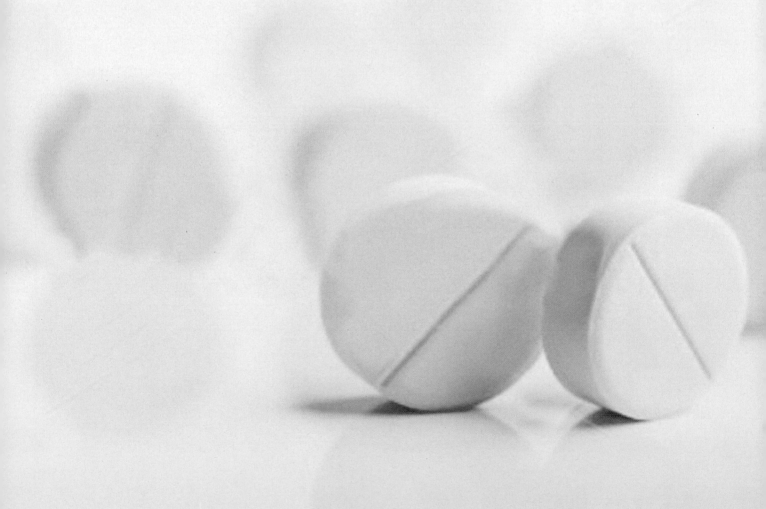

Comprehensive Post-Test 1

Name _____ Date _____

1. Order: Lopressor 12.5 mg PO daily for severe heart failure

   Supply: Lopressor 25 mg/tablets

   ✳ **How many tablets will you give?** _____

2. Order: Synthroid 0.2 mg PO daily for hypothyroidism

   Supply: Synthroid 200 mcg/tablets

   ✳ **How many tablets will you give?** _____

3. Order: Micro K 30 mEq PO daily for hypokalemia

   Supply: Micro K 10 mEq/capsules

   ✳ **How many capsules will you give?** _____

4. Order: Phenergan 12.5 mg IV every 4 hours for nausea

   Supply: Phenergan 25 mg/mL

   ✳ **How many milliliters will you give?** _____

5. Order: 1000 mL of D5W/0.45 NS to infuse over 12 hours

   Drop factor: 15 gtt/mL

   ✳ **Calculate the number of drops per minute.** _____

6. Order: heparin 2500 units/hr IV for thrombophlebitis

   Supply: heparin 25,000 units/500 mL

   ✳ **Calculate milliliters per hour to set the IV pump.** _____

7. Order: Infuse heparin at 45 mL/hr IV for thrombophlebitis

   Supply: heparin 25,000 units/500 mL

   ✳ **How many units per hour is the patient receiving?** _____

8. Order: Infuse 250 mL bolus of 0.9% NS at 33 gtt/min

   Supply: 250 mL 0.9% NS with 20 gtt/mL tubing

   ✳ **How many hours will it take to infuse the IV bolus?** _____

9. Order: Pentamidine: 4 mg/kg IV daily for 14 days for patient weighing 130 lb for severe *Pneumocystis carinii* pneumonia

   Supply: Pentamidine 300 mg/250 mL D5W to infuse over 60 min

   ✳ **Calculate the milliliters per hour to set the IV pump.** _____

(Comprehensive Post-Test 1 continues on page 278)

10. Order: naloxone (Narcan) 0.01 mg/kg IV for narcotic overdose for child weighing 35 kg

    Supply: naloxone (Narcan) 0.4 mg/mL

    ✳ **How many milliliters will you give?** _____

11. Order: Epogen 150 units/kg SQ three times weekly due to anemia secondary to chemotherapy for a patient weighing 80 kg

    Supply: Epogen 20,000 units/mL

    ✳ **How many milliliters will you give?** _____

12. Order: acyclovir 5 mg/kg IV every 8 hours for 7 days for cutaneous herpes simplex for a patient weighing 70 kg

    Supply: acyclovir 1-g vial

    Nursing drug reference: Reconstitute each 1-g vial with 10 mL of sterile water and further dilute in 100 mL 0.9% NS and infuse over 1 hour

    ✳ **How many milliliters will you draw from the vial after reconstitution?** _____

    ✳ **Calculate the milliliters per hour to set the IV pump.** _____

    ✳ **Calculate the drops per minute with a drop factor of 20 gtt/mL.** _____

13. Order: vancomycin 1 g IV every 12 hours for severe staphylococcal infection

    Supply: vancomycin 5-g vial

    Nursing drug reference: Reconstitute each 5-g vial with 10 mL of sterile water and further dilute in 250 mL of D5W and infuse over 60 minutes

    ✳ **How many milliliters will you draw from the vial after reconstitution?** _____

    ✳ **Calculate the milliliters per hour to set the IV pump.** _____

    ✳ **Calculate the drops per minute with a drop factor of 10 gtt/mL.** _____

14. Order: regular insulin 8 units/hour for hyperglycemia

    Supply: regular insulin 100 units/250 mL 0.9% NS

    ✳ **Calculate milliliters per hour to set the IV pump.** _____

15. Order: nitroprusside 0.8 mcg/kg/min for hypertensive crisis

    Supply: nitroprusside 50 mg/500 mL D5W

    The patient weighs: 143 lb

    ✳ **Calculate milliliters per hour to set the IV pump.** _____

16. Order: Mycostatin oral suspension 500,000 units swish/swallow for oral candidiasis

    Supply: Mycostatin 100,000 units/mL

    ✳ **How many teaspoons will you give?** _____

17. Order: Dilaudid 140 mL/hr

    Supply: Dilaudid 30 mg/1000 mL D5/NS

    ✳ **Calculate milligrams per hour the patient is receiving.** _____

18. Order: aminophylline 44 mg/hr for status asthmaticus

    Supply: aminophylline 1 g/250 mL D5W

    ✳ **Calculate milliliters per hour to set the IV pump.** _____

19. Order: 1000 mL NS to infuse at 60 gtt/min

    Drop factor: 15 gtt/mL

    ✳ **Calculate how many hours it will take for the IV to infuse.** _____

20. Order: dopamine (Intropin) 5 mcg/kg/min IV for cardiogenic shock secondary to myocardial infarction

    Supply: dopamine 200 mg/250 mL D5W

    Patient weight: 90 kg

    ✳ **Calculate the milliliters per hour to set the IV pump.** _____

Comprehensive Post-Test 2

Name _____ Date _____

1. Order: phenobarbital 60 mg PO daily for seizures

   Supply on hand: phenobarbital 30 mg/tablet

   ✳ **How many tablets will you give?** _____

2. Order: chloral hydrate 250 mg PO 30 minutes before HS as sedative

   Supply on hand: chloral hydrate 250 mg/5 mL

   ✳ **How many milliliters will you give?** _____

3. Order: digitoxin 0.3 mg PO daily for maintenance dose after digitalization

   Supply on hand: digitoxin 100-mcg tablets

   ✳ **How many tablets will you give?** _____

4. Order: potassium chloride 20 mEq PO tid for hypokalemia

   Supply: potassium chloride 40 mEq/15 mL

   ✳ **How many teaspoons will you give?** _____

5. Order: 500 mL D5W to infuse over 12 hours

   Drop factor: 60 gtt/mL

   ✳ **Calculate the number of drops per minute.** _____

6. Order: heparin 1500 units/hr for thrombophlebitis

   Supply: heparin 25,000 units/500 mL

   ✳ **Calculate milliliters per hour to set the IV pump.** _____

7. Order: Infuse heparin at 20 mL/hr for thrombophlebitis

   Supply: heparin 25,000 units in 250 mL

   ✳ **How many units per hour is the patient receiving?** _____

8. Order: Infuse bolus of 0.9% NS at 100 gtt/min

   Supply: 250 mL 0.9% NS with 60 gtt/mL tubing

   ✳ **How many hours will it take to infuse the IV bolus?** _____

9. Order: fluconazole 200 mg IVPB over 60 minutes for systemic candidal infections

   Supply: fluconazole 200 mg/100 mL with 20 gtt/mL tubing

   ✳ **Calculate the number of drops per minute.** _____

10. Order: furosemide 2 mg/kg PO daily for congestive heart failure

    Supply: furosemide 10 mg/mL oral solution

    ❋ **How many milliliters will you give a child weighing 10 lb?** _____

11. Order: Neupogen 6 mcg/kg SQ twice daily for chronic neutropenia

    Supply: Neupogen 300 mcg/mL

    ❋ **How many milliliters will you give a patient weighing 175 lb?** _____

12. Order: ampicillin 500 mg IV every 6 hours for urinary tract infection

    Supply: ampicillin 1-g vial

    Nursing drug reference: Reconstitute each 1-g vial with 10 mL of sterile water and further dilute in 50 mL of 0.9% NS and infuse over 15 minutes.

    ❋ **How many milliliters will you draw from the vial after reconstitution?** _____

    ❋ **Calculate the milliliters per hour to set the IV pump.** _____

    ❋ **Calculate the drops per minute with a drop factor of 10 gtt/mL.** _____

13. Order: acyclovir 10 mg/kg IV every 8 hours for varicella zoster in immuno-suppressed patient weighing 140 lb

    Supply: acyclovir 1-g vial

    Nursing drug reference: Reconstitute each 1-g vial with 10 mL of sterile water and further dilute in 100 mL of 0.9% NS and infuse over 1 hour.

    ❋ **How many milliliters will you draw from the vial after reconstitution?** _____

    ❋ **Calculate the milliliters per hour to set the IV pump.** _____

    ❋ **Calculate the drops per minute with a drop factor of 10 gtt/mL.** _____

14. Order: epinephrine 1 mcg/min IV for bradycardia

    Supply: epinephrine 1 mg/250 mL 0.9% NS

    ❋ **Calculate the milliliters per hour to set the IV pump.** _____

(Comprehensive Post-Test 2 continues on page 282)

15. Order: Isuprel 5 mcg/min IV for heart block

    Supply: Isuprel 2 mg in 500 mL D5W

    ❋ **Calculate the milliliters per hour to set the IV pump.** _____

16. Order: dobutamine 2.5 mcg/kg/min IV for management of heart failure for a patient weighing 130 lb

    Supply: dobutamine 250 mg in 1000 mL of 0.9% NS

    ❋ **Calculate the milliliters per hour to set the IV pump.** _____

17. Order: dopamine 10 mcg/kg/min IV for management of hypotension secondary to decreased cardiac output for a patient weighing 120 lb

    Supply: dopamine 400 mg in 500 mL D5W

    ❋ **Calculate the milliliters per hour to set the IV pump.** _____

18. Order: aminophylline is infusing at 24 mL/hr for respiratory distress for a patient weighing 80 kg

    Supply: aminophylline is 250 mg in 250 mL in D5W

    ❋ **How many milligrams per kilogram per hour is the patient receiving?** _____

19. Order: amrinone infusing at 47 mL/hr for a patient weighing 100 kg for short-term treatment of congestive heart failure

    Supply: amrinone 100 mg/100 mL 0.45% NS

    ❋ **How many micrograms per kilogram per minute is the patient receiving?** _____

20. Order: aminophylline loading dose of 5.6 mg/kg to infuse over 30 minutes for a patient weighing 50 kg followed by 0.6 mg/kg/hr maintenance dose for COPD

    Supply: aminophylline 500 mg in 500 mL of D5W

    ❋ **How many milliliters per hour will you set the IV pump for the loading dose?** _____

    ❋ **How many milliliters per hour will you set the IV pump for the maintenance dose?** _____

Educational Theory of Dimensional Analysis

Dimensional analysis is a problem-solving method based on the principles of cognitive theory. Bruner (1960) theorized that learning is dependent on how information is structured, organized, and conceptualized. He proposed a cognitive learning model that emphasized the acquisition, organization (structure), understanding, and transfer of knowledge—focusing on "how" to learn, rather than "what" to learn. Learning involves associations established according to the principles of continuity and repetition.

Dimensional analysis (also called factor-label method, conversion-factor method, units analysis, and quantity calculus) provides a systematic way to set up problems and helps to organize and evaluate data. Hein (1983) emphasized that dimensional analysis gives a clear understanding of the principles of the problem-solving method that correlates with the ability to verbalize what steps are taken leading to critical thinking. He described dimensional analysis as a useful method for solving a variety of chemistry, physics, mathematics, and daily life problems. He identified that dimensional analysis is often the problem-solving method of choice because it provides a straightforward way to set up problems, gives a clear understanding of the principles of the problem, helps the learner to organize and evaluate data, and assists in identifying errors if the setup of the problem is incorrect.

Goodstein (1983) described dimensional analysis as a problem-solving method that is very simple to understand, reduces errors, and requires less conceptual reasoning power to understand than does the ratio–proportion method. She expressed that "even though the ratio–proportion method was at one time the primary problem-solving method, it has been largely replaced by a dimensional analysis approach in most introductory chemistry textbooks...this method condenses multi-step problems into one orderly extended solution."

Peters (1986) identified dimensional analysis as a method used for solving not only chemistry problems but also a variety of other mathematical problems that require conversions. He defined dimensional analysis as a method that can be used whenever two quantities are directly proportional to each other and one quantity must be converted to the other using a conversion factor or conversion relationship.

Literature that has examined the quality of higher education and professional education in the United States (National Institute of Education, 1984) recommends that educators increase the emphasis of the intellectual skills of problem solving and critical thinking. Also recommended is an increased emphasis on the mastery of concepts rather than specific facts. Other literature on curriculum revolution in nursing (Bevis, 1988; Lindeman, 1989; Tanner, 1988) recommends that learning not be characterized merely as a change in behavior or the acquisition of facts, but in seeing and *understanding* the significance of the whole. Because it focuses on "how" to learn, rather than "what" to learn, dimensional analysis supports conceptual mastery and higher-level thinking skills that have become the core of the curriculum change that is sweeping through all levels of education and, most importantly, nursing education.

Bibliography

Bevis, E. (1988). New directions for a new age. In National League for Nursing, *Curriculum revolution: Mandate for change* (pp. 27–52). New York: National League for Nursing (Pub. No. 15–2224).

Bruner, J. (1960). *The process of education.* New York: Random House.

Craig, G. (1995). The effects of dimensional analysis on the medication dosage calculation abilities of nursing students. *Nurse Educator, 20*(3), 14–18.

Craig, G. P. (1997). The effectiveness of dimensional analysis as a problem-solving method for medication calculations from the nursing student perspective. Unpublished doctoral dissertation, Drake University, Des Moines, IA.

Goodstein, M. (1983). Reflections upon mathematics in the introductory chemistry course. *Journal of Chemical Education, 60*(8), 665–667.

Hein, M. (1983). *Foundations of chemistry* (4th ed.). Encino, CA: Dickenson Publishing Company.

Lindeman, C. (1989). Curriculum revolution: Reconceptualizing clinical nursing education. *Nursing and Health Care, 10*(1), 23–28.

National Institute of Education. (1984). *Involvement in learning: Realizing the potential of American higher education.* Washington, DC: National Institute of Education.

Peters, E. (1986). *Introduction to chemical principles* (4th ed.). Saratoga, CA: Saunders College Publishing.

Tanner, C. (1988). Curriculum revolution: The practice mandate. *Nursing and Health Care, 9*(8), 426–430.

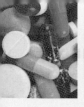
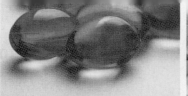
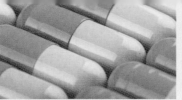
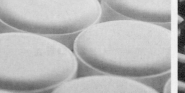
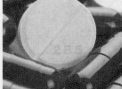

Index

Note: Page numbers followed by f, t, and b indicate figures, tables, and boxes respectively.

A

abacavir (Ziagen), dosage calculation for
  one-factor, 188
  two-factor, 199
abortion, spontaneous, case study of, 234–235
acetaminophen, *see* Tylenol (acetaminophen)
acquired immunodeficiency syndrome (AIDS), case study
  of, 222
acyclovir
  dosage calculation for, two-factor, 134
  IV therapy considerations, 129
adalat (nifedipine), dosage calculation for, one-factor, 177
administration routes, 65
  enteral, 81–88
  intravenous (*see* intravenous therapy)
  parenteral, 86–92
advil (ibuprofen), dosage calculation for, 71
AIDS (acquired immunodeficiency syndrome), case study of, 222
Alzheimer's disease, case study of, 238–239
amikacin (Amikin), dosage calculation for, three-factor, 204
aminophylline, dosage calculation for, 206
  IV therapy, 123–125
  three-factor, 161, 169
amiodarone (Cordarone IV), dosage calculation for, 208
amoxicillin, dosage calculation for, 208
ampicillin. *See* Unasyn (ampicillin)
amrinone, dosage calculation for, three-factor, 160
ancef, dosage calculation for
  three-factor, 156
  two-factor, 120
anemia, sickle cell, case study of, 222–223
anorexia nervosa, case study of, 237
anticoagulants, administration of, 87
apothecaries' measurement system, 33–34
  abbreviations, 32b–34b
  defined, 33
  other system equivalents for, 38t, 39, 43
  volume in, 33, 34b, 34f, 38t
  weight in, 33, 34b, 34f, 38t
Arabic number system, 5, 6t
  converting between Roman and, 3, 6–8, 18, 21
  defined, 5
ascorbic acid, dosage calculation for, 205
aspirin, dosage calculation for, 69–70
atenolol (Tenormin), dosage calculation for, 207
atropine sulfate, dosage calculation for, 189–190
  two-factor, 115, 189
  using drug label, 90
azactam, dosage calculation for, two-factor, 142
azithromycin (Zithromax), dosage calculation for, 208

B

batch number, of a drug, 75
Benadryl (diphenhydramine), dosage calculation for,
  three-factor, 200
bipolar disorder, case study of, 236–237
bone marrow transplantation, case study of, 224
bronchopulmonary dysplasia, case study of, 233
bronchiolitis, case study of, 258

C

caplets, administration of, 81, 81f
capsules, administration of, 81, 81f

Celsius temperature, 36
  conversion to Fahrenheit, 36b, 36f, 39
ceptaz (ceftazidime), dosage calculation for, two-factor, 198
cerebral palsy, case study of, 234
chronic obstructive pulmonary disease (COPD), case study of, 220
Cimetidine, 82
Cipro (Ciprofloxacin)
  dosage calculation for, using drug label, 77
  drug label, components of, 76
cirrhosis, case study of, 226–227
claforan, dosage calculation for
  three-factor, 168
  two-factor, 119
cleocin, dosage calculation for
  one-factor, 186
  three-factor, 156, 200
clindamycin, dosage calculation for, three-factor, 168
clinical depression, case study of, 238
colestid (colestipol hydrochloride), dosage calculation for, two-factor, 193
compazine (prochlorperazine), dosage calculation for
  one-factor, 180, 183
  using drug label, 83, 87
congestive heart failure (CHF), case study of, 219–220
conversion factors, in dimensional analysis, 48, 68
COPD (chronic obstructive pulmonary disease), case study of, 220
cortef (hydrocortisone cypionate), dosage calculation for, two-factor, 193
coumadin, administration of, 87
cup, medication, 34b, 34f, 38t, 81f
cystic fibrosis, case study of, 229, 230

D

decimals, 12–14
  converting between fractions and, 3, 16–17, 20
  dividing, 3, 15, 19, 21
  multiplying, 3, 13, 19, 21
  rounding, 13, 75
deep vein thrombosis, case study of, 223–224
demerol, dosage calculation for, 205
denominator
  in dimensional analysis, 47
  in fractions, 9
depo-Provera, dosage calculation for, one-factor, 188
depression, case study of, 238
diabetic ketoacidosis, case study of, 244
digits, 5
digoxin, dosage calculation for, 205
  three-factor, 167
  two-factor, 189
dilantin
  dosage calculation for, three-factor, 156
  IV therapy considerations, 129
dilaudid, dosage calculation for, 85, 206
  two-factor, 190
diluent, defined, 116
dimensional analysis
  defined, 47, 73, 155
  denominator in, 47
  educational theory of, 283
  elements of, 47
  numerator in, 47
  one-factor, 68–74
    defined, 68
    problem solving using, 68–74, 77–106

dimensional analysis (*continued*)
    random method, 68, 73
    sequential method, 68
  random method, 68, 73
  sequential method, 68–70
  solving problems with, 48–56
    gallons to milliliters example, 50
    liter to ounces example, 48–49
    steps in, 48, 68
  three-factor, 149–159
    defined, 150, 155
    problem solving using, 149
  two-factor, 112
    defined, 112
    involving drop factors, 125–129
    involving intermittent infusion, 129–132
    involving IV therapy, 121–124
    involving reconstitution, 116–121
    involving weight, 112–114
    problem solving using, 133–137
dividing line, of fraction, 9
division
  of decimals, 3, 14–15, 19, 21
  of fractions, 3, 10–12, 19, 21
dobutamine, dosage calculation for, three-factor, 152–154
documentation, in medication administration, 65
dopamine, dosage calculation for, 207
  three-factor, 157–158, 160, 200–204
dosage, in medication administration, 65
dram (dr), 33b, 33f, 38t
drop factors
  defined, 125
  medication problems involving, 125–128
  tubing considerations in, 125, 125t
drop (gtt), 34b, 34f, 38t
drug, *see also under* medication *entries*
  in medication administration, 64–65
drug label
  components of, 75–77
  solving problems using, 77–81, 96–100
    enteral, 81–85
    parenteral, 86–92
D5W solution, dosage calculation for, 205–206
  three-factor, 202
  two-factor, 190
dysplasia, bronchopulmonary, case study of, 233

E

emphysema, case study of, 220–221
end-stage renal failure, case study of, 244–245
enteral medications, 81–86
epivir (lamivudine), dosage calculation for, two-factor, 195
epoetin (Procrit), dosage calculation for, three-factor, 204
epogen, dosage calculation for
  three-factor, 166
  two-factor, 140
erythromycin dosage calculation for
  IV therapy, 130
  IV therapy considerations, 129
  two-factor, 121
eskalith (lithium carbonate), dosage calculation for, one-factor, 188
esmolol hydrochloride, dosage calculation for, three-factor, 204
expiration date, of a drug, 75–77

F

Fahrenheit temperature, 36
  conversion to Celsius, 36b, 36f, 40, 43
fever of unknown origin (FUO), case study of, 241
filgrastim, dosage calculation for, three-factor, 166
fluid dram (fl dr), 33b, 33f
fluid ounce (fl oz), 33b, 33f
fluid volume deficit, case study of, 245–246
fortaz, dosage calculation for, two-factor, 121, 133, 191
fractions, 9–12
  components of, 9
  converting between decimals and, 3, 16–17, 20

defined, 9
  dividing, 3, 11–12, 19, 21
  multiplying, 3, 9–11, 18, 21
fragmin, dosage calculation for, one-factor, 185
furosemide, dosage calculation for
  one-factor, 178
  three-factor, 155, 161, 199
  two-factor, 114, 139

G

gallon (gal)
  conversions, 33b, 33f, 38t
  dimensional analysis conversion, 50
gantrisin, dosage calculation for, two-factor, 199
generic name, of a drug
  defined, 74
  identification of, 64, 76–77
gentamicin, dosage calculation for
  three-factor, 172, 205, 203
  two-factor, 112–116
given quantity
  in dimensional analysis, 47, 68
  in three-factor problem solving, 149
  in two-factor problem solving, 112
glyset (miglitol), dosage calculation for, one-factor, 187
grain (gr), 33b, 33f, 38t
gram (g), 31, 32b, 32f, 38t
gravity flow, IV therapy, 125–129

H

halcion (triazolam), 77
  dosage calculation for
    one-factor, 177
    using drug label, 79
hemabate, dosage calculation for, one-factor, 184
heparin
  administration of, 87
  dosage calculation for, 206
    IV therapy, 122, 124
    parenteral, 90–91, 97
    two-factor, 133, 135
H1N1 Influenza (Swine Flu), case study of, 257
household measurement system, 33, 34b, 34f
  abbreviations, 32b, 34b
  importance of, 31
  other system equivalents for, 38t
hydrea, dosage calculation for, three-factor, 201
hydromorphone, dosage calculation for
  one-factor, 182
  using drug label, 90, 104
hyperbilirubinemia, case study of, 234
hypercholesterolemia, case study of, 242–243
hyperemesis gravidarum, case study of, 227
hypertension, case study of, 242–243
hypoglycemia, signs and symptoms of, 86

I

increased intracranial pressure, case study of, 246
infectious mononucleosis, case study of, 256–257
infusion pump, 129. *See also* intermittent infusion
insulin
  administration of, 86
  dosage calculation for, 91, 97, 205
  types of, 86
  using drug label, 89
insulin syringe, 86, 86f
intake and output, monitoring of, 35, 35f, 40, 41
intermittent infusion, medication problems involving, 129–132
intracranial pressure, increased, case study of, 246
intravenous pumps, 121. *See also* intravenous therapy
intravenous therapy
  drop factors, 125–129
  gravity flow, 125
  intermittent infusion, 129–132
  types of tubing for, 125, 125t
iron deficiency anemia, case study of, 254–255